D1564718

Diet, Life Expectancy, and Chronic Disease

Diet,
Life Expectancy,
and Chronic Disease

Studies of Seventh-day Adventists
and Other Vegetarians

GARY E. FRASER

OXFORD
UNIVERSITY PRESS
2003

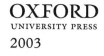

OXFORD
UNIVERSITY PRESS

Oxford   New York
Auckland   Bangkok   Buenos Aires   Cape Town   Chennai
Dar es Salaam   Delhi   Hong Kong   Istanbul   Karachi   Kolkata
Kuala Lumpur   Madrid   Melbourne   Mexico City   Mumbai
Nairobi   São Paulo   Shanghai   Taipei   Tokyo   Toronto

Published by Oxford University Press, Inc.
198 Madison Avenue, New York, New York, 10016
http://www.oup-usa.org

Oxford is a registered trademark of Oxford University Press

Library of Congress Cataloging-in-Publication Data
Fraser, Gary E.
Diet, life expectancy, and chronic disease:
studies of Seventh-day Adventists and other vegetarians /
Gary E. Fraser.
p. cm.
Includes bibliographical references and index.
ISBN 0-19-511324-1
1. Vegetarianism—Health aspects.
2. Vegetarianism—Religious aspects—Seventh-day Adventists.
3. Seventh-day Adventists—Health and hygiene.
4. Seventh-day Adventists—Diseases.
5. Diet in disease.
I. Title.   RM236.F736 2003   613.2'62—dc21   2002037905

9 8 7 6 5 4 3 2 1

Printed in the United States of America
on acid-free paper

To Sharon

Preface

For nearly 140 years, Seventh-day Adventists have been encouraged to avoid meat and emphasize fruits, vegetables, and nuts in their diets. One rationale for this has been that such a diet promotes better health. There have been vegetarians, some very prominent, for thousands of years. Until the nineteenth century, however, improved health was an uncommon motivation. More typically, the driving force was animal rights or the perceived virtue of an ascetic lifestyle in certain other religious groups.

John Wesley, Sylvester Graham, William Alcott, and Russell Trall (Barkas, 1975; Numbers, 1992; Whorton, 1994) are among the American reformers who 150 to 200 years ago became convinced that a vegetarian way of life promoted health. Adventists joined this mix in 1863, and a health message continues today to be an important part of their tradition. However, most people now demand scientific evidence, rather than faith alone, as a criterion for action.

The famous Framingham Study was launched in 1948, and within 10 years an extensive study of the health of California Adventists also got under way with the aid of federal funding. By subjecting their health experiences to scientific scrutiny, Adventists in theory faced the possibility that research evidence would not support their claims. This has not been the case, although research results may suggest minor changes in the Adventist positions.

Almost by definition, a religious group gives credence to subjectivity and to claims that can be neither proved nor disproved. In studies of Adventists over the years, this interface with the supposedly objective methods of epidemiologic research has created an interesting tension. Fortunately, as a group, Adventists have placed great emphasis on education and traditional health care. They own and run many highly regarded medical centers throughout the United States and also overseas. Thus, for many

Adventists, the rigorous investigation of one tenet of their faith that could be subjected to scientific methods was intriguing—indeed, attractive.

Our studies in California have always been guided during data collection by an external committee of some of the country's leading non-Adventist epidemiologists. Published reports, as usual, are rigorously peer-reviewed before publication. Despite this, it must be acknowledged that all evidence, even the seemingly objective, is interpreted through the filter of the investigators', and now the readers', past experiences and prejudices. These are the "spectacles behind the eyes" referred to by Russell Hanson (1969) and by the eminent physicist–cleric John Polkinghorne (1993). This problem with interpretation of evidence is not at all unique to studies of Adventists. It affects most researchers as they evaluate their own cherished data and hypotheses.

Until quite recently, vegetarians were commonly regarded as a little eccentric, and in some cases this was probably justified. Health professionals were not confident that such a diet was beneficial. Indeed, serious reservations about nutritional adequacy were commonly expressed.

As far as I know, the evidence that links vegetarianism directly to health and life expectancy has not been comprehensively reviewed before. This is also true of health research among Adventists, where more than 320 publications in the peer-reviewed literature are spread over 40 years through dozens of different journals. This book is in part a response to the requests of health professionals and lay-persons to summarize this information in a more compact and accessible form.

Another motivation has been to give readers some insight into nutritional epidemiology. Many people, even health professionals, are confused by the frequently conflicting reports of the effects of diet on health status that appear in newspapers and on television screens. I have tried to provide explanations for the conflicts by describing the difficulties in this line of research and giving some guidelines for interpreting the evidence. Undoubtedly, some people will be surprised at how few conclusions we can draw with confidence. But enough is clear about the benefits of vegetarian diets, or diets that tilt in this direction, to recommend them with confidence.

The intended readership for this book is primarily health professionals, including physicians, nurses, health educators, nutritionists, and epidemiologists, who may find it a useful reference. Nonprofessionals may also find the book of interest, however, as I have made an effort to keep the language relatively nontechnical or, where technical terms are unavoidable, to explain them in a glossary. The glossary is extensive, and readers who encounter unfamiliar terms are encouraged to use it. The summaries at the end of each chapter, and also the contents of the final chapter, will help all readers understand my interpretation of the evidence.

This book should be of interest to members of the Seventh-day Adventist Church. Many, particularly in California but also elsewhere, have spent a good deal of time filling out long dietary questionnaires without ever having had a comprehensive report on the results of their efforts. I hope that this work will fill a void for them and also will serve as a "thank you" for the time and efforts of all who participated. The evidence it presents about a long-held position of the Adventist church on dietary practice will comfort some and may encourage other, less-committed, vegetarians to reconsider.

The chapters are ordered to first report health and lifestyle comparisons between Adventists and non-Adventists living in the same areas (1–4). As it turned out that Adventists in general do better, the next chapters (5–8) address the question of which facets of the diet might at least partly explain these differences. Of course, Adventists differ from non-Adventists in ways aside from what they eat. So Chapter 9 deals (as well as we can) with the possible influence of psychosocial factors and differences in religious commitment on physical health.

Chapters 10 and 11 report the evidence about health effects from studies of non-Adventist vegetarians and other health-conscious individuals. Chapter 12 considers risk factor values in vegetarians as compared to others, and here, too, much of the information comes from non-Adventist vegetarians. Chapter 13 continues the same theme, but the focus is on the risk factor values and the health experiences of a particular type of vegetarians, the vegans, who do not eat any animal products.

Chapters 14 and 15 appear rather different from the others. Although the emphasis on a vegetarian diet is clear, these chapters have a much more practical, behavioral approach, rather than the epidemiologic approach of the rest of the book. Some readers may have an interest in changing to a vegetarian diet, and I hope these chapters will be helpful.

Loma Linda, California   G.E.F.

Acknowledgments

First, my wife, Sharon, claims that she has missed me on the many evenings and occasional Sundays spent in preparing this book. I am extremely grateful for her willingness to overlook these indiscretions. My time in this work has been partially funded, and in particular I must recognize Loma Linda University (Dr. Lyn Behrens) and the North American Division and General Conference of Seventh-day Adventists (Drs. DeWitt Williams and Alan Handysides) for their support. The National Institutes of Health and the U.S. Public Health Service have provided many large grants to support the collection and analysis of data in California Adventists over a period of 40 years. Special thanks to DeWitt Williams who carefully reviewed most of the manuscript, pointing out many minor omissions and inconsistencies. My thanks also to colleagues who authored or coauthorized three of the chapters, specifically Drs. Graham Stacey, Jerry Lee, Helen Hopp-Marshak, Kiti Freier, and Ella Haddad.

My assistants Hanni Bennett and, more recently, Jean Bindels have cheerfully endured countless revisions of this manuscript on the word processor. David Shavlik has provided expert data management and data analysis with relatively few complaints. Before him, Dr. Larry Beeson was the data manager of these studies for many years. The other epidemiologists who have contributed important data and interpretation have often been my predecessors and colleagues here at Loma Linda University. In California these especially include the following past faculty of Loma Linda University: Drs. Frank Lemon, Richard Walden, Roland Phillips, Jan Kuzma, David Snowdon, and Paul Mills. Other valued colleagues and contributors to this literature from the United Kingdom are Dr. Tim Key, Mr. Paul Appleby (Oxford University), and Dr. Margaret Thorogood (London School of Hygiene and Tropical Medicine).

Contents

If the money we use to purchase and eat the muscles of cows, pigs, chickens, turkeys, and fish were put into vegetables, fruits, and lipid-lowering drugs, our health would skyrocket. . . . There is still a holocaust going on—just ask the cows (100,000/day killed in the USA) or pigs (250,000/day) or chickens (15,000,000/day). The healthier are our nonhuman animals, the healthier are the human ones. We kill them, and then, they kill us!*

William C. Roberts, MD
Editor, *American Journal of Cardiology*

*Reprinted from *Am J Cardiol* 83:817, 1999. Shifting from decreasing risk to actually preventing and arresting atherosclerosis; with permission from Excerpta Medica Inc.

Diet, Life Expectancy, and Chronic Disease

1

Why We Study the Health of Adventists

WHO ARE SEVENTH-DAY ADVENTISTS?

Who are Seventh-day Adventists, anyway? How can their lifestyle help others become more healthy?

Seventh-day Adventists are a conservative religious group that includes more than 13 million members worldwide. They were first organized as a denomination in 1863 in the eastern United States. Their roots can be found largely in Methodism. While they share many of the doctrines of mainline Protestant churches, Adventists differ from most in their relatively strict observance of Saturday, rather than Sunday, as their day of rest. They also differ from some Protestants groups by:

- Looking forward to a soon-to-occur, literal second coming of Jesus Christ
- Believing that the dead remain in a state of unconsciousness until this event
- Traditionally emphasizing the value of biblical prophecy
- Being creationists

A key figure during the early years of the Adventist church was Ellen G. White. She was a forceful and talented speaker and, along with her husband James, a wise administrator. On numerous occasions she claimed to have received heaven-sent messages, several of which were related to lifestyle and health. These episodes would often occur during times of prayer, and they affected her profoundly, casting her into a trancelike state, sometimes for lengthy periods. She became a prolific writer (Goen, 1971), documenting her visionary experiences and also writing commentaries on most parts of the Bible.

In the same year that their church was organized (1863), the small Adventist group also began to emphasize the role of lifestyle in promoting health, happiness, and enhanced spirituality. Thus, Adventists have strongly recommended their distinctive lifestyle for 140 years, although only the use of alcohol and tobacco, and the consumption of biblically unclean foods such as pork, are actually prohibited. In addition, the church recommends that Adventists avoid the consumption of other meats and poultry, fish, coffee, tea, other caffeine-containing beverages, rich and highly refined foods, and hot condiments and spices. The church also recommends that Adventists exercise regularly. In light of these recommendations, at least half of American Adventists today either are lacto-ovo vegetarians or eat meat less than once a week, but they follow other specific recommendations to varying degrees.

Ellen White inspired the adoption of these lifestyle recommendations. Indeed, beginning in the mid-1860s, she wrote extensively (White, 1905; White, 1938; White, 1951) in her efforts to encourage changes that she claimed would lead to better health. Her ideas were not in themselves unique, but they formed an original mix. Three of her many written statements are cited in the footnote to this chapter.[1]

Other health reformers of the mid-nineteenth century and of earlier periods were also active in advocating similar changes. These included clerics such as John Wesley (founder of the Methodist church), who wrote extensively on health; the Bible Church pastor William Metcalfe, who introduced vegetarianism into the United States in an organized fashion; the Presbyterian minister Sylvester Graham (of Graham Cracker fame); and the Millerite preacher–physician Larkin B. Coles. Many religious people became concerned about the abuse of alcohol—leading to the establishment of a strong interdenominational temperance movement. The early Adventists were no exception to this movement—Ellen White and other Adventists were very active temperance reform advocates.

The Adventists' interest in health quickly led to the establishing of health-care institutions for both their own use, and to the spreading of the health message to others. This message included the arguments that appropriate lifestyle changes could prevent disease, improve the existing poor health conditions, and enhance the religious experience. Battle Creek, Michigan, became the site of the Western Health Reform Institute, the first such health institution. By 1878 the institute was succeeded by the much larger Battle Creek Medical and Surgical Sanitarium, which was directed by the dynamic young Dr. John Harvey Kellogg. Although the Battle Creek Sanitarium quickly became a world-famous institution, John Kellogg parted ways with the Adventist church around 1905 because of his disagreements with the church leaders about theology, administrative style, and, later, some of the medical methods that he advocated.

Before he left the Adventist church, Kellogg and his brother Will had already invented flake cereals and peanut butter. This soon led to the founding of the Kellogg food company, now a household name (Schwarz,

1970). Although it is not now an Adventist business, it certainly began as such, and the same motives noted above have led to the organization of several other well-known health food companies that are, or until recently have been, owned by Adventists. These companies include Loma Linda Foods, La Loma Foods, Worthington Foods in the United States; Granose Foods in the United Kingdom; and, perhaps most prominent, the Sanitarium Health Food Company in Australasia, where Weetbix, Marmite, and peanut butter are national staples. Besides producing breakfast foods, many of these companies have also specialized in plant-based protein foods and drinks, using soy, wheat gluten, and peanut proteins.

Dr. Harry Miller, an Adventist surgeon who went to China as a missionary in the early years of the twentieth century, noted the frequent use of soybeans, especially among adults, in the Far East. He also observed that severe malnutrition was common in infants, perhaps due partly to the lack of cow's milk as a protein source. By the mid-1930s, he succeeded in developing ways to make soy milk both more palatable and less likely to cause an intestinal upset due to colonic fermentation of undigested carbohydrates from the soybeans. He demonstrated soy milk's effectiveness as an infant food (Miller and Wen, 1936) and then promoted its use worldwide (Shurtleff, 1981). Thus, he became a strong advocate for the health benefits of soy 70 years ago, prefiguring the current interest of the scientific community in this food.

The Adventist church has developed a system of health-care institutions around the world. The best known of these centers is probably Loma Linda University Medical Center in California, established in 1905 by Ellen White after the Battle Creek Sanitarium was lost when John Harvey Kellogg left the church. Adventists have also been in the forefront of promoting personal health in the community and are well known for running vegetarian cooking schools and operating health-screening vans. They were among the first to develop group-based, quit-smoking programs, particularly the well-known "Five-Day Plan," which was developed by the Adventist physician J. Wayne McFarland and the clergyman-counselor Elman J. Folkenberg (Office of Cancer Communications, National Cancer Institute, 1977).

That most Adventists do follow many of the church's recommendations regarding lifestyle, and have done so for generations, is a testimony to the powerful impact of incorporating the subject of health into a system of religious beliefs. Adventists have never believed that good health practices are a measure of religious virtue, but they do see the choice of good health habits as a valuable spiritual discipline.

Others have speculated about the possible beneficial effects of religion on the changing of social norms and the promoting of adherence to healthy behaviors. Vaux (1976), for example, described the concept of "purity in life," which enters into Judeo-Christian belief systems. If the body and its health are considered sacred, then maintenance of health becomes a "core belief." This will powerfully influence motivation and action. While there are few religious groups that formally incorporate health issues into their belief structure, Adventists do so, and it is a natural fit for Christianity, Judaism, or Islam. Vaux also described a second concept, "peace in existence," arguing that "beliefs that elicit contentment and purposiveness in the life" "directly affect health attitudes and behaviors" (p. 528). It is possible that a sense of well-being and of purpose elicits a desire to "guard one's health" and may lead to "a desire for more life, rising with a new thrill each day" (p. 530).

Finally, the knowledge and social support that are derived from belonging to a group that subscribes often to similar nontraditional values and health behaviors can be a powerful aid. It is true of Adventists that most of their friends are church members, a situation well suited to social learning, as propounded by Bandura (1977).

ADVANTAGES THAT THIS GROUP PRESENTS
FOR EPIDEMIOLOGIC RESEARCH

Why are researchers interested in studying the health of Seventh-day Adventists as a group? Are they healthier than others? Have they found some special fountain of youth that so many are searching for?

Several features of this special population make them an attractive group for epidemiologic research. Such research can be plagued by both measurement problems and poor compliance when subjects are required to complete lengthy questionnaires or attend clinics. In order to test complicated dietary hypotheses, where particular foods or nutrients involve moderate-sized relative risks (say, 1.5–2.0), it is best to have several hundred new cases of disease available for the analysis. Otherwise, statistical power for detecting the effects of the risk factors is quite limited. Hence, in prospective research, the defined study population must contain a large number of subjects, typically tens of thousands, as particular chronic diseases are quite uncommon.

Obtaining baseline health-habit data from thousands of subjects is an expensive exercise, even when using a mailed questionnaire, particularly if it is necessary to send reminder letters to a large percentage of the population, or perhaps send questionnaires to twice the number who will finally respond. Adventists are by definition interested in health and have generally shown their willingness to complete lengthy questionnaires.

The accuracy of responses provided by individuals in the study is critical to both statistical power and the avoidance of bias. Random errors in questionnaire responses will most commonly bias relative risks toward the appearance of no effect and thereby diminish the chances of detecting any actual effects. Therefore, the accuracy of data improves the efficiency of such studies. Adventists are generally well educated and, because of their special interest in diet and their own dietary habits, are able to report relatively accurately about what they eat.

Many have the idea that members of such a group are relatively alike in their habits, and in some respects this is the case. For instance, the church requires abstinence from tobacco and alcohol. There is almost uniform adherence to the former, and although some alcohol is consumed, this was found to be so in fewer than 10 percent of those involved in our studies—and even these generally drink only small quantities of alcohol. Only 1.8% admitted any use of tobacco, and 4% cited the consumption of pork. Consequently, it is certainly true that the unique health experience enjoyed by Adventists as a group is partially related to the relative absence of tobacco and alcohol among them. This means that it is not possible to investigate the independent contributions of these two factors by studies within the population because virtually all abstain. There is indeed no useful comparison group! However, when testing theories relating to diet, exercise, and psychosocial and other variables, the relatively uniform absence of use of tobacco and alcohol means that investigators do not need to be concerned that subgroup differences in the use of alcohol or tobacco may distort estimates of effect.

Perhaps most important in making Adventists a fertile ground for study is the great variety found in their practice of certain key behaviors. When it comes to questions of diet, exercise, and psychosocial factors, uniformity in the group is certainly not found. Regarding diet, in particular, Adventists are quite dissimilar. The church only recommends abstinence from flesh foods and allows the eating of eggs and dairy products with no restrictions. Consequently, only about 3% of the Adventists in our studies are vegans; about 27% are lacto-ovo vegetarians; about 20% eat meat less than once each week; and the remainder, on average, eat meat more than four times each week.

Vegetables, nuts, and fruits are, on average, eaten in greater quantities than the usual amounts, but sizable subgroups still eat very small amounts of these foods. Therefore, within the group there is also a wider-than-usual range of exposures to these foods. This is an important aid to the efficiency and statistical power of research studies, particularly where measurement errors are a problem (White et al., 1994). If a food does have an effect, the opportunity then exists to demonstrate this: subgroups that eat very large amounts of the food can be compared with others who eat it rarely or not at all. For example, our findings on nut consumption and heart disease (see Chapter 5) would hardly have been possible had it not been for the extraordinary finding that 24% of Adventists eat nuts five or more times each week, but the 34% who eat nuts less than once each week were also necessary as a sizable comparison group.

TWO TYPES OF PROSPECTIVE STUDIES USED IN THIS RESEARCH

Two different kinds of studies, both prospective in nature, have often been used to investigate the health of Adventists. These studies allow different ideas to be examined and should be interpreted with a clear understanding of their strengths and limitations.

The first type of study gathers data that allow a comparison of rates of disease among Adventists, as a group, with those from the general population in the same location. This type of study has an advantage in that the factor of interest, that is being an Adventist, is easily and accurately defined and measured. If disease rates, for instance, are lower among the Adventists than among the non-Adventists, one can reasonably conclude that there is something about the Adventist lifestyle—whether it be the absence of smoking, vegetarianism, other dietary differences, or psychosocial or religious factors—that prevents disease. Some have even suggested that genetic differences may be involved, though there is no evidence to support this idea or much reason to suspect it.

The weakness of this kind of data lies in the temptation to overinterpret the evidence obtained. These studies do not allow for the isolation of specific, potential causal factors, and indeed it is usually difficult to even know all of the factors that may provide differences between Adventists and others. Most of the older, and often smaller, studies were of this sort. They were valuable because they clearly indicated that there was something interesting here. However, more careful and detailed work is necessary to allow more specific conclusions.

Adventism is a way of life, almost a subculture. If Adventists live longer, or experience less frequent chronic disease, a natural question is, Which of the Adventists' lifestyle characteristics are responsible for this? It would be unreasonable to suggest that all aspects of the Adventist lifestyle are helpful, or at least equally helpful. To answer this question, it is useful to compare the health experience of Adventists who have different health habits. There are less likely to be important unmeasured and unthought-of differences among different Adventists than there would be in a comparison with an external population. Hence, confounding or confusion among different variables is reduced in this second type of study.

The second type of study is a comparison that is done within the Adventist group rather than with an external population. This immediately implies the need to measure specific lifestyle attributes of individuals. The need to measure, for example, dietary intake (foods and nutrients), exercise, obesity, and medical history is both a strength and a weakness of this type of study. It is a strength because we can potentially define some of the detailed characteristics of Adventist individuals that may explain the differences observed in the first type of study.

However, this specificity of measurement in the second type of study is also a weakness, because unlike the ability to accurately measure the label "Adventism," the ability to accurately measure such complicated behaviors as diet and physical activity is limited. Then the whole problem of the effects of measurement errors on the analysis needs discussion. This is a very important question in the context of these studies, and in the author's view, the fact that most of the published literature on diet and disease has ignored this difficulty has led to much confusion among lay and professional persons alike regarding the relationship between diet and health. A more detailed discussion of the possible effects of measurement errors is found in Chapter 5 and elsewhere (Thomas et al., 1993).

Another problem with the second type of study is that by comparing Adventists with other Adventists, we will inevitably restrict the available range of values of some variables. These are variables that measure habits that Adventists subscribe to in a more uniform way. For instance, we find that a very small proportion of Adventists smoke, drink alcohol, or eat red meat several times each day. Thus, we cannot accurately evaluate the effects of these levels of such habits. Yet, individuals who smoke, drink alcohol, or eat meat very frequently are not rare in the general population and will in part be responsible for the differences that we observe between Adventists and non-Adventists in the first type of study.

In summary, the first type of study leads to a general conclusion that something about these people is causing a difference in health experience. The Adventist Mortality Study (AMS) (see the Appendix) is an example of such a design—analyses compared rates of disease among California Adventists with those of non-Adventists in the concurrent American Cancer Society (ACS) Study. The second type of study attempts to isolate individual factors and examine their effects in increasing or decreasing risk. An example is the analysis based on Adventist Health Study (AHS) data. However, measurement errors are a potential problem in this type of analysis and will often (but not always) lead to an underestimate of effects.

HEALTH PRACTICES OF ADVENTISTS: THE DATA

It is one thing to recommend a particular way of life but another to get people to follow the recommendation. Physicians are well acquainted with the difficulties they have in successfully encouraging patients to exercise regularly or eat more healthfully. Before examining the health of Adventists, we must understand the nature of their health habits as actually practiced. That the church makes a recommendation may or may not result in close adherence to it. Hence, it is useful to examine the results of surveys that have sought to gather objective information.

The supposed objectivity of such survey information does indeed deserve further consideration. Most of the detailed studies of Adventists have been conducted at Loma Linda University, an Adventist institution. Hence, it is possible that Adventists may feel some pressure to appear to conform with church standards when responding to surveys. It is almost impossible to rule out some minor effects of this sort, but important biases are unlikely.

First, regarding most foods, the church only makes recommendations. It is widely understood among members that adherence is voluntary and that there are variations in commitment to these matters. Hence, with the exception of items such as the use of alcohol, pork, and tobacco, there are no external consequences of poor compliance.

Second, in the surveys at Loma Linda, we have clearly notified subjects of our commitment to confidentiality, and we have had no lapses in the security of our data. Individuals' names are never entered into computer files that are connected to their lifestyle data, and only one or two senior investigators have the knowledge that would link a name to an identifying number on the computer file.

Third, the frequency of missing data in the Adventist Health Study data set is no greater for sensitive questions than for other items having no sensitivity to religion. In addition, there is no greater degree of nonresponsiveness in regard to these sensitive items among Adventists as compared to non-Adventist members of Adventist households. In keeping with this, a small proportion of Adventists admitted the use of alcohol (8.9%), tobacco (1.8%), and pork (4%).

In this chapter, we describe the way in which California Adventists actually live by noting the proportions of them that fall into particular categories of behavior. The focus here is on diet, exercise, and psychosocial factors. The effects that these variables may have on important intermediary risk indicators, such as levels of blood pressure and blood lipids, and also the direct effect on the risk of disease, will be described in later chapters.

Since the interest in studies of Adventists relates in large part to their diet, we must understand how Adventists with different dietary patterns differ in other ways. Vegetarian status is an indicator of many other differences, and unless one carefully analyzes and interprets the data, it will not be clear whether it is the vegetarian status or the other associated variables that truly affect risk of cancer, heart disease, or early death. Therefore, we must also compare vegetarian and nonvegetarian Adventists in regard to their consumption of nonmeat foods, physical activity, obesity, education, age, and gender.

The Heart Attack Risk Factor Study

To illustrate the habits of Adventists who have been involved in our research, this book draws on two sets of data: the Heart Attack Risk Factor (HARF) Study (Fraser et al., 1987), and the Adventist Health Study (Beeson et al., 1989). The Adventist Health Study is a prospective investigation of 34,000 California Adventists, and its design is described in detail in the Appendix.

The objective of the HARF Study was to compare health behaviors and coronary risk factors between a representative group of Adventist men and their non-Adventist neighbors. In 1982, we randomly selected 13 of the 127 Adventist congregations in Orange and Los Angeles counties. From these selected churches, all non-Hispanic white males aged 35 to 55 years were invited to participate, and 90% (160 men) did so by completing a questionnaire and providing a blood specimen. A middle-aged non-Adventist male neighbor (living at least six doors away from the Adventist) was matched by age to each Adventist participant.

The value of this study design is, first, that most of the eligible Adventists were included—thus giving little opportunity for the bias often found in descriptive studies with a large percentage of volunteers. Second, the comparison with neighborhood men was not affected by differences in socioeconomic status, as the neighborhood matching very adequately ensured comparability according to education and income.

The Diet of Adventists

Dietary habits can be described in two main ways: either in terms of the foods that we choose to eat, or by the total nutrients and chemicals that the foods contain. Of course, particular nutrients may be common to many foods. Information from the use of both methods is presented next. It should always be remembered that since the chemical constituents of foods

Table 1–1. Mean (Standard Deviation in Parentheses) Daily Intake of Common Foods in Middle-aged Adventist Men and Their Neighbors (157 Pairs): The Heart Attack Risk Factor Study

Food	Unit	Adventists	Neighbors	p Value
Cream	Tablespoon	0.18 (0.69)	0.31 (1.08)	<.10
Coffee	Cup	1.20 (1.77)	3.30 (2.98)	<.0005
Alcohol	Drink	0.008 (0.29)	1.93 (2.88)	<.001
Green salads	3/4 cup	0.89 (0.86)	0.62 (0.58)	<.001
Citrus fruits	Medium	0.45 (0.53)	0.27 (0.44)	<.03
Bananas	Medium	0.43 (0.51)	0.21 (0.30)	<.0001
Melons	Medium	0.13 (0.29)	0.13 (0.35)	NS
Other fresh fruits	Medium	0.67 (0.83)	0.36 (0.70)	<.005
Canned fruits	1/2 cup	0.23 (0.34)	0.09 (0.23)	<.002
Raisins/dates	2 tablespoons	0.28 (0.48)	0.11 (0.41)	<.001
Other dried fruit	2 tablespoons	0.07 (0.24)	0.02 (0.07)	<.02
Total fruit	Medium	2.68 (1.98)	1.47 (1.57)	<.0001
Tomatoes	Medium	0.37 (0.40)	0.22 (0.25)	<.0001
White bread	1 slice	0.44 (1.01)	0.99 (1.47)	<.0005
Whole wheat bread	1 slice	1.61 (1.67)	0.99 (1.24)	<.0005
Butter	1 pat	0.37 (0.91)	0.78 (1.21)	<.005
Margarine	1 pat	1.26 (1.38)	0.88 (1.10)	<.005
Eggs	1 egg	0.50 (0.57)	0.59 (0.56)	NS
Beef	3 oz	0.40 (0.51)	0.75 (0.70)	<.0005
Pork	3 oz	0.002 (0.014)	0.14 (0.22)	<.0005
Chicken	3 oz	0.22 (0.38)	0.34 (0.37)	<.005
Fish	3 oz	0.12 (0.17)	0.21 (0.34)	<.005
Meat analogues	3 oz	0.28 (0.43)	0.03 (0.15)	<.0005

NS, nonsignificant.

are only partially understood, foods may show effects on health that are not predicted by their known constituents. The difficulties of making accurate dietary measurements are well described (Willett, 1998a), but the data shown in Tables 1–1 to 1–6 minimize the random errors from individual dietary recalls by using average levels to represent large groups of subjects.

By studying the daily intake of a variety of foods by the Adventist men and neighbors (see Table 1–1) enrolled in the Heart Attack Risk Factor Study, we immediately find differences between the two groups. Data showed that Adventists consumed less meat, alcohol, cream, coffee, butter, and white bread, and more fruit, green salads, whole wheat bread, margarine, and meat analogues. When converted to nutrients (see Table 1–2), differences are more modest, though still evident. The Adventist diet is marked by an intake of about 300 fewer calories and about 16% fewer fat calories. In this study this is due largely to the consumption of less saturated and monounsaturated fat, resulting in a higher polyunsaturated/saturated fat (P/S) ratio. Dietary cholesterol was also lower by 25%, which,

Table 1-2. Daily Mean (Standard Deviation in Parentheses) Macronutrient Intake Comparing Adventists with Their Neighbors (157 Pairs): The Heart Attack Risk Factor Study

Nutrient (unit)	Adventists	Neighbors	p Value
Calories	2255 (781.0)	2547 (1128.6)	<.01
Carbohydrate (g)	267 (105.8)	243 (111.2)	NS
Fat (g)	101 (45.8)	119 (59.8)	<.005
Protein (g)	80 (30.4)	87 (43.2)	<.06
Crude fiber (g)	6.9 (3.3)	4.4 (2.3)	<.001
Saturated fat (g)	23.5 (11.5)	29.0 (14.8)	<.001
Linoleic acid (g)	24.4 (13.4)	24.0 (14.9)	NS
Oleic acid (g)	33.8 (15.9)	42.5 (21.9)	<.001
Cholesterol (mg)	312 (188.7)	419 (242.9)	<.001
P/S ratio[a]	1.09 (0.42)	0.88 (0.37)	<.001
Keys' dietary score	192.8 (8.97)	198.4 (8.86)	<.001

NS, nonsignificant.

[a]Ratio of polyunsaturated to saturated fats, often used as a summary measure of the type of fat in the diet.

Source: Fraser GE et al., IHD risk factors in middle-aged Seventh-day Adventist men and their neighbors, *Am J Epidemiol* 126:638–646, 1987, by permission of Oxford University Press.

along with the higher P/S ratio, led to a significantly lower Keys score (Jacobs et al., 1979)—which predicts the effects of diet on blood cholesterol levels. Crude fiber intake was 57% greater in Adventist men.

Thus church recommendations and traditions, although only partially followed, have resulted in markedly different food choices but a more modest difference in the intake of nutrients when Adventists are compared with non-Adventists. Generally, the dietary choices of Adventists reflect more healthful habits.

Another look at the dietary habits among a larger population of Adventists, this time both men and women, was provided by the Adventist Health Study. Dietary information was gathered via a food frequency questionnaire distributed to 34,192 non-Hispanic white subjects, and also from 147 subjects in a Special Nutrition Substudy (see the Appendix). In the Special Nutrition Substudy, we developed indices of nutrient intake by comparing food frequency data with the more accurate average of five 24-hour recalls provided by these individuals. The indices were then used to convert the food frequency information to estimates of nutrient intake for the whole cohort. As there is no non-Adventist comparison group in this study, these data are used to depict differences among the dietary habits of Adventists. Particularly interesting is a comparison of other characteristics of those Adventists who reported different frequencies of meat consumption. These different frequency categories are labeled vegetarian, almost vegetarian (or semivegetarian), and nonvegetarian, and are defined as follows:

Vegetarian: no meat, fish, or poultry consumption

Almost vegetarian or semivegetarian: frequency of meat, fish, and poultry intake combined is less than weekly

Nonvegetarian: consumption of some meat at least once each week

Among non-Hispanic white Adventists, 29% were vegetarian, 21.3% were semivegetarian, and 49.2% were nonvegetarian. Although the categories are defined by meat consumption, there are probably many other differences between these groups, and it may be these, rather than the meat intake, that determine a different disease experience. First, there is the question of whether such powerful health predictors as Adventists' age, sex, and education define their meat consumption. Second, we evaluate whether other dietary characteristics differ among those who fall into different vegetarian categories.

Whether vegetarian Adventists are likely to be older or younger than others is addressed in Table 1–3. When interpreting Tables 1–3 and 1–4, it is useful to know that a value of 1.0 is given when the proportion of Adventists in that age group (or in the educational groups shown in Table 1–4) is neither higher nor lower than the overall average in that category of meat consumption. In fact, it can be seen that younger subjects are nonvegetarians about 18% to 20% more often than expected, whereas Adventists aged 80 years and older are about 36% more likely to be vegetarians than expected.

Whether vegetarian Adventists are on average more or less educated than other Adventists is shown in Table 1–4. Those who did not graduate from high school are 16% less likely to be vegetarians than the average, whereas college graduates are more than 31% more likely to be vegetarians than expected.

Similar analyses show that women are modestly more likely to be vegetarians than men, as men are overrepresented by 10% in the nonvegetarian category ($p < .0001$) when data are adjusted for age (detailed data are not shown). Exercise habits were also associated with the vegetarian dietary pattern ($p < .0001$), but only to a small degree. When data are ad-

Table 1–3. Association of Vegetarian Status with Age[a]: The Adventist Health Study

Age (years)	Vegetarian	Almost Vegetarian	Nonvegetarian
25–44	.90	.94	1.18
45–64	.88	.95	1.20
65–79	.93	1.10	.98
80+	1.36	1.02	.72

[a]Adjusted for gender; $p < .0001$.

Table 1–4. Association of Vegetarian Status with Education:[a] The Adventist Health Study

Education	Vegetarian	Almost Vegetarian	Nonvegetarian
Less than high school	.84	1.01	1.19
High school graduate or some college	.91	.98	1.12
College graduate or postgraduate degree	1.31	1.01	.75

[a]Adjusted for age and gender, $p < .0001$.

justed for age and gender, those who exercised vigorously at least three times weekly were more likely to be vegetarians than expected, by about 7%.

The age differences in the proportions who are vegetarians and those who are not may represent a generational effect, or it could be that as Adventists age, they become more concerned about health and more conservative in their choices. Our data cannot distinguish between these two possibilities. Better-educated persons in other populations also tend to choose vegetarianism (Fraser et al., 2000), and this may reflect their better understanding of the health and ecologic consequences of their choices, or even a greater willingness to explore new foods.

It is likely that vegetarians eat differently than nonvegetarians in ways that are separate from their lack of meat consumption. As might be expected (see Table 1–5), the nonvegetarians in our study ate considerably more meat than the "almost vegetarians," and most of this meat was beef. This is surprising since red meats are generally considered less healthy than fish or chicken, and it may indicate that among nonvegetarian Adventist subjects health is not the main motivation for their choices. Vegetarian Adventists also eat more fruit and vegetables such as tomatoes, legumes, and nuts, but they eat eggs and doughnuts and drink coffee less frequently. Vegetarians are more likely to use margarine than butter on bread, are more likely to choose whole-grain bread than white bread, and are much less likely to consume any alcohol. They also ate commercial, plant-based protein foods (meat analogues) more frequently, no doubt in part as alternatives for meat.

Differences in food intake according to vegetarian status also cause some differences in nutrient intake among the three groups (see Table 1–6). Many of these differences are small, but the values for vegetarians usually show a pattern thought to be more healthful. The P/S ratio is substantially lower in nonvegetarians, and the dietary cholesterol is greater, although cholesterol intakes in all Adventist groups are relatively low. The trends expected in the intake of vegetable or animal sources of both fat and protein are indeed seen. Dietary calcium is modestly greater in the vegetarians, which is interesting as concerns are often expressed regarding the ad-

Table 1-5. Comparison of Intake of Common Foods between Vegetarian and Nonvegetarian Adventists[a]: The Adventist Health Study

	Vegetarian	Almost Vegetarian — White Subjects	Nonvegetarian	White Subjects	All Black Subjects[b]
Percentage of the population	32.0	22.8	45.2	100	100
SERVINGS PER WEEK					
Fruits					
Canned	3.17	2.78	2.30	2.69	1.85
Dried	3.13	2.56	1.81	2.40	2.19
Citrus	2.92	2.65	2.50	2.67	3.33
Winter	5.64	5.07	4.55	5.02	4.47
Other	4.26	3.97	3.57	3.88	3.98
All fruit	19.12	17.03	14.73	16.66	15.82
Tomatoes	3.77	3.65	3.54	3.64	3.15
Legumes	2.30	1.87	1.23	1.72	1.67
Nuts	3.89	3.26	2.19	2.98	2.49
Green salads	4.72	4.67	4.72	4.71	4.07
Soft margarine on bread	6.19	6.22	5.96	6.09	4.49
Eggs	1.25	1.64	2.17	1.75	1.77
Doughnuts	0.38	0.51	0.89	0.64	0.74
Coffee	0.34	1.39	5.10	2.73	0.74
Beef	0	0.20	3.05	1.42	1.94
Poultry	0	0.09	0.72	0.35	0.71
Fish	0	0.10	0.61	0.30	0.46
Meat analogues	3.48	3.05	1.35	2.42	3.08
PERCENTAGES					
Prefers whole grain bread	96.7	94.5	82.5	89.7	87.4
Some beer or wine	0.5	1.5	11.3	5.6	5.6
Some hard liquor	0.3	0.5	5.8	3.0	4.5

[a]Adjusted for age and gender, non-Adventists excluded.

[b]Not divided into vegetarian categories due to smaller numbers and a much lower response rate that may make these data less representative of all black Adventists.

Table 1–6. Comparison of Average Daily Nutrient Intake between Vegetarian and Nonvegetarian Non-Hispanic White Adventists:[a] The Adventist Health Study

	Vegetarian	Almost Vegetarian	Nonvegetarian
Energy (kcal)	2064	2053	2031
Total fat (g)	83.5	83.7	85.2
Polyunsaturated fat (g)	21.4	20.8	19.3
Monounsaturated fat (g)	28.2	28.3	29.7
Saturated fat (g)	23.3	24.0	28.8
P/S ratio	0.92	0.87	0.67
Keys' score (mg/DL)	188.5	190.2	198.5
Vegetable fat (g)	57.5	55.5	48.0
Animal fat (g)	22.8	24.4	32.0
Cholesterol (mg)	193.6	211.6	271.9
Protein (g)	69.3	69.9	71.7
Vegetable protein (g)	38.9	36.8	32.6
Animal protein (g)	30.3	31.4	36.4
Fiber (g)	8.57	8.02	7.07
Calcium (mg)	1010	1019	992
Magnesium (mg)	384	374	350
Vitamin E[b] (mg)	9.28	8.89	7.66

[a]Adjusted for age and gender.

[b]From foods alone, supplements excluded.

equacy of calcium intake by vegetarians. Intake of vitamin E, an antioxidant vitamin that may afford some protection against cardiovascular disease, is also higher in the vegetarians.

There is very little published information about the dietary or exercise habits of black Americans and their effects on the group's mortality. The Adventist Health Study included 1739 black subjects who gave dietary information (Fraser et al., 1997b). It is interesting to compare the dietary habits of black and white Adventists (see Table 1–5). In many respects, these two ethnic groups of Adventists have quite similar dietary patterns. In fact, the black Adventists typically eat fruit, vegetables, and nuts a little less frequently than the whites and drink much less coffee. However, they eat meats about 50% more frequently and, somewhat unexpectedly (given their higher meat intake), also eat meat analogues more frequently than do white Adventists.

Measuring Physical Activity

As is true for diet, it is very difficult to measure physical activity with precision, given that individuals are almost always involved in some degree of movement, and the range of different types of activity is very large and hard to quantify in surveys. Consequently, one should at least use the same questions to evaluate exercise habits when making comparisons between different people. This was possible in the HARF Study (Fraser et al., 1987), and Adventist men reported a greater number of "sweaty exercise" sessions each week (about 50% more) than their non-Adventist neighbors of similar ages. They also had a significantly lower resting heart rate, which may indicate a greater degree of physical fitness consequent on the exercise. Another evaluation of exercise habits—this one done among 1028 black Adventists living in southern states (Murphy et al., 1997)—found that 46% participated in physical exercise three or more times per week; 26%, one time to two times per week; and 26%, less than once per week.

Selected Psychosocial Characteristics

Studies of psychosocial variables among populations that include both Adventists and non-Adventists are very few in number and limited in scope. Various psychosocial variables are suspected of affecting risk of chronic disease (Brezinka and Kittel, 1986; Eysenck, 1992), and prominent among them are those indicating higher or lower levels of social support.

Social support, resulting from supportive interactions with others, has been thought of as an antidote to stress. It is often measured in terms of whether or not a subject is married and whether the person maintains an active church affiliation or active membership in clubs or social societies. A distinction can be made between the size of a social network and the subjects' perception of the level of support actually obtained.

Some interesting differences between Adventists and their neighbors were shown by the HARF Study (Fraser et al., 1997a). The questionnaire included a section on social support networks and revealed certain perceptions about the emotional consequences of these networks. Adventists were more likely to be currently married (see Table 1–7), but the average number of children did not differ between the two groups.

Although the Adventists had a greater number of trusted relatives and perhaps close friends (see Table 1–8), the frequency of contacts with chil-

Table 1–7. Marital Status (Percentages) for Adventist Males and Their Neighbors (157 Pairs), Aged 35–55 Years: The Heart Attack Risk Factor Study

Marital Status	Adventists	Neighbors	p Value
Ever married	98.1	96.3	NS
Present status			$p < .05$
Married	91.2	80	
Separated	1.3	4.4	
Divorced	5.6	10.6	
Widowed	0	1.3	
Never married	1.9	3.7	

NS, nonsignificant.

Source: Fraser GE et al., Selected social support variables in middle-aged Seventh-day Adventist men and their neighbors, *J Religion Health* 36:231–239, 1997, by permission.

Table 1-8. Average Number of Children, Trusted Friends, and Relatives per Person, and Satisfaction with Contacts, Adventist Males and Their Neighbors (157 Pairs): The Heart Attack Risk Factor Study

	Adventists	Neighbors	p Value
No. of children	2.6	2.4	NS
Contact with children			<.10
Very satisfied	91	89	
Somewhat satisfied	55	49	
Not very satisfied	8	15	
Not at all satisfied	3	4	
No. of trusted relatives	4.0	3.1	<.005
Contact with trusted relatives			NS
Very satisfied	69	70	
Somewhat satisfied	66	65	
Not very satisfied	20	19	
Not at all satisfied	2	3	
No. of close friends	4.7	4.1	<.10
Contact with close friends			NS
Very satisfied	80	77	
Somewhat satisfied	62	65	
Not very satisfied	11	11	
Not at all satisfied	3	4	

NS, nonsignificant.

Source: Fraser GE et al., Selected social support variables in middle-aged Seventh-day Adventist men and their neighbors, *J Religion Health* 36:231–239, 1997, by permission.

dren, trusted relatives, and close friends did not differ (data are not shown), and there was no apparent difference revealed in the degree of satisfaction with the frequency of these contacts.

No clear differences between Adventists and their neighbors were revealed in the frequency of feeling lonely, but a substantially greater proportion of Adventists felt that "people really cared for them" (see Table 1-9). It is not surprising that Adventists also attend church much more

Table 1-9. Frequency of Feeling Cared For and Feeling Lonely: Adventist Males and Their Neighbors (156 Pairs): The Heart Attack Risk Factor Study

	How Often Do You Feel that Other People Really Care for You? ($p < .001$)		How Often Do You Feel Lonely? (NS)	
	Adventists	Neighbors	Adventists	Neighbors
Frequently	117	81	4	12
Occasionally	32	60	47	54
Rarely	7	12	70	61
Never	0	3	35	29

NS, nonsignificant.

Source: Fraser GE et al., Selected social support variables in middle-aged Seventh-day Adventist men and their neighbors, *J Religion Health* 36:231–239, 1997, by permission.

frequently, with 84% attending each week as compared to only 30% of their neighbors. However, no significant difference was revealed in membership in other social groups/organizations.

SUMMARY

1. Seventh-day Adventists have a long and distinguished international history of promoting better health habits among their members and also in the wider community.
2. California Adventists have a lifestyle that is distinct from other Californians. A majority of the Adventists adhere to behaviors that may sometimes fall short of the church's recommendations but that still represent a substantial departure from those of other Californians. Many Adventists are vegetarians who eat more fruit and vegetables than others but fewer nonmeat animal products.
3. Several studies have compared the disease experience of Adventists with that of non-Adventists in the same communities. (See the Appendix for study designs.)
4. More detailed information is provided by studies, done within the Adventist group, that compare members who subscribe to different habits. However, this strength is offset by the problem of measurement errors that occur when we attempt to measure the details of complex behaviors such as dietary intake and physical activity and their effects on health.
5. Adventist middle-aged men exercise more frequently than their neighbors, on average. In addition, they have a somewhat larger network of social support by being more involved in an organization with a significant social function (their church), are more likely to benefit from the support of a spouse, have more trusted relatives, and are more likely to feel cared for by others.
6. As compared to nonvegetarian Adventists, the vegetarians are on average older and better educated. In addition to the absence of meat consumption, they have other dietary characteristics closer to those recommended by the American Heart Association (Nutrition Committee, AHA, 2000), by the World Cancer Research Fund, and by the American Institute for Cancer Research (Potter, 1997). Consequently, analyses related to vegetarian status will need careful interpretation or adjustment for the effects of other factors. Otherwise, it will not be clear whether the causal factor in disease experience is the absence of meat or other factors that also characterize the vegetarian Adventists.

NOTES

1. "Foods should be prepared with simplicity, yet with a nicety which will invite the appetite. You should keep grease out of your food. It defiles any preparation of food you may make. Eat largely of fruits and vegetables" (White, 1868/1948), p. 63.

"Cancers, tumors, and all inflammatory diseases are largely caused by meat-eating. . . . The mortality caused by meat-eating is not discerned; if it were, we would hear no more arguments and excuses in favor of the indulgence of the appetite for dead flesh" (White, 1896), p. 278.

"Grains, fruits, nuts, and vegetables constitute the diet chosen for us by our Creator. These foods, prepared in as simple and natural a manner as possible, are the most healthful and nourishing. They impart a strength, a power of endurance, and a vigor of intellect, that are not afforded by a more complex and stimulating diet" (White, 1905), p. 81.

2

Coronary Heart Disease Rates among Adventists and Others

Deaths from coronary heart disease have decreased by half or more in the United States over the last 30 years (Gillum, 1993; Havlik and Feinleib, 1979). Despite this, it is still a major killer in the United States and most Western countries, as well as being leading cause of morbidity. Among the manifestations of this disease are myocardial infarction (heart attack), sudden death, congestive heart failure, serious arrhythmia, and angina pectoris.

Coronary heart disease (CHD) is a consequence of the atherosclerotic process as it affects the coronary arteries and thus diminishes the blood and oxygen supply to the heart muscle. Atherosclerosis is an accumulation of cholesterol, cholesterol esters, collagen, and inflammatory cells beneath the lining of arteries (Ross, 1993). We now understand that this process depends on higher values of LDL cholesterol and a relatively oxidizing environment (Witztum, 1994). The oxidized LDL cholesterol filters into the artery wall and tends to remain there, forming a plaque that may protrude into the open space (lumen) of the artery.

The cholesterol deposits provoke an inflammatory response that may weaken the integrity of this fatty mass, allowing it to rupture into the bloodstream. Then a clot, or thrombus, often forms at this site and completely closes the artery, resulting in the death of a portion of the heart muscle supplied by that artery—a myocardial infarction. The disorganization of electrical activity in the heart produced either by the scar from a heart attack or by the decreased supply of oxygen to the surviving heart muscle may provoke serious arrhythmia or even sudden death.

Lifestyle choices, particularly dietary habits and cigarette smoking, can alter this cascade of events at several points by changing the levels of blood cholesterol (Criqui et al., 1980; Jacobs et al., 1979); the oxidation state of the blood (Gilligan et al., 1994; Morrow et al., 1995); and the likelihood of forming a blood clot (Marckmann et al., 1994; Miller, 1992; Meade et al., 1987; Nilsson et al., 1990). In addition, atherosclerotic arteries are often in a state of spasm as compared to normal arteries, further narrowing the lumen. This spasm occurs because muscle cells in the walls of affected arteries are less sensitive to the relaxing effects of endogenous nitric oxide and thus become more constricted than they normally are. Fortunately, reducing LDL cholesterol can markedly improve this condition (Schmieder and Schobel, 1995), as can quitting cigarette smoking (Heitzer et al., 1996) and possibly increased physical activity as well (Clarkson et al., 1999).

Many Adventists have dietary habits and an intake of fat and fiber at levels recommended by the American Heart Association (Nutrition Committee, AHA, 2000) to prevent coronary artery disease. They do not smoke cigarettes, and they engage in more than an average amount of physical activity. Hence, it may be expected that rates of fatal and nonfatal heart attacks would be somewhat lower than those in the non-Adventist population. Indeed, this is the case for both men and women, as we will see below.

CARDIOVASCULAR MORTALITY RATES IN NON-AMERICAN ADVENTISTS AND NON-ADVENTISTS

As described in the Appendix, a number of studies done in other countries have used national registries to compare the mortality rates of Adventists and non-Adventists in the same communities. These comparisons are often expressed by using a statistic known as the standardized mortality ratio (SMR). To find a standardized mortality ratio, the expected number of CHD deaths is calculated as if the national rates had applied to the Adventist population. The SMR is the ratio of the number of deaths actually observed in the Adventists to the number of deaths expected.

Adventist men, particularly those below 75 years of age, appear to be substantially protected against cardiovascular mortality as their SMRs are usually significantly less than 1.0 (see Table 2–1). This is the case for both coronary and cerebrovascular events (strokes). The situation for women is less clear, with Japanese data suggesting protection, but being based on relatively small numbers, and Norwegian data also suggesting a modest degree of protection but with relatively wide confidence intervals. We can be 95% certain that the true value of the SMR lies within the 95% confidence interval, this allowing for chance fluctuations that affect any observed data. There are no separate data for cerebrovascular deaths among Norwegian or Dutch women.

In Norway there were clear trends in cardiovascular disease rates according to whether subjects joined the Adventist church at an age under

Table 2–1. Comparison of Cardiovascular Mortality in Adventists and Non-Adventists: Non-American Results

Country	Disease Endpoint	Standardized Mortality Ratio (95% Confidence Interval)		
		Both Sexes	Men	Women
Netherlands	Ischemic heart disease	0.43 (0.35–0.52)		
	Cerebrovascular disease	0.54 (0.43–0.67)		
Norway	Cardiovascular diseases		0.80[a]	0.93[a]
	≤75 years		0.65 (0.55–0.77)	0.90 (0.78–1.03)
	>75 years		0.89 (0.80–1.00)	0.93 (0.87–1.01)
	Coronary heart disease		0.73[a]	NA
	≤75 years		0.55 (0.43–0.69)	NA
	>75 years		0.91 (0.76–1.09)	NA
	Cerebrovascular disease		0.88[a]	NA
	≤75 years		0.89 (0.60–1.27)	NA
	>75 years		0.88 (0.71–1.08)	NA
Japan	Ischemic heart disease		1.00[a,b]	0.67*[a]
	Cerebrovascular disease[a]		0.38**[a]	0.43**[a]

*$p < .05$ (29 events), **$p < .01$; NA, not available.

[a]Confidence interval not given and unable to be calculated from published data.

[b]Based on 18 events.

Sources of data: Kuratsune et al, 1986; Berkel and deWaard, 1983; Fonnebo, 1992.

19 years, an age from 19 to 34 years, or an age over 35 (Fønnebø, 1992). For men, the SMRs for these three situations are, respectively, 44, 76, and 87 ($p < .05$, trend); and for women, 52, 79, and 102 ($p < .001$, trend)—where a value of 100 represents the risk in a population of non-Adventists that have a similar age structure. These interesting trends suggest the possibility that there may be some unique effects of lifestyle at different stages of the life cycle. The effects seem to be greater at younger ages. But it is important to realize that the results are equally consistent with a "duration of exposure" effect, as those joining at an earlier age will, on average, have been exposed to the Adventist lifestyle for a longer period.

In summary, this international evidence indicates that Adventists have lower cardiovascular mortality rates than non-Adventists in the same communities. These differences appear to be stronger in men, and, for coronary disease, especially in younger men.

CORONARY HEART DISEASE IN CALIFORNIA ADVENTISTS AND NON-ADVENTISTS

Mortality from coronary heart disease among younger Adventist men was less than one-third that of their non-Adventist counterparts (see Fig. 2–1; Phillips et al., 1980a). This reduced risk is less evident in older Adventist subjects, but the lower rates are seen consistently throughout adult life. Expressed as differences in CHD mortality rates, these are lower by approximately 170 events/100,000 per year in younger Adventist men, with

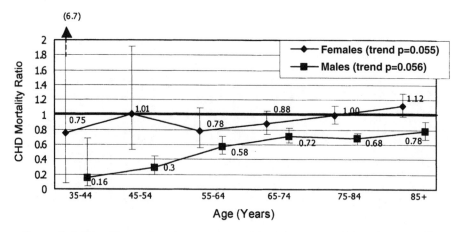

Figure 2–1 Mortality ratios that compare Adventist to non-Adventist mortality rates, by age and sex. 1960–1976 (Adventists) and 1960–1971 (non-Adventists). *Source:* Adventist Mortality and American Cancer Society Studies (see Appendix).

this difference widening to mortality rates lower by 1000 events/100,000 per year in older Adventists. Thus the smaller proportionate reduction in CHD mortality in older Adventist men nevertheless translates to a greater difference in risk as a consequence of the much higher overall rates of CHD mortality seen at older ages.

By contrast, the CHD mortality rates for Adventist women are less clearly different from those of the non-Adventist ACS Study participants, although those for younger Adventist women do tend to be lower. Comparing Adventists with non-Adventists, the CHD mortality rate ratios (95% confidence intervals) are 0.66 (0.62–0.71) for men, and 0.98 (0.90–1.06) for women if the data are averaged over all age groups by using the Mantel–Haenszel procedure.

It appears that in men, and less clearly in women, there is a modification of the Adventist/non-Adventist comparison according to age. In women below the age of 75 years, there is a 10% to 20% advantage for the Adventists, but as the great majority of coronary events in Adventist women occur at ages above 75 years, the lack of effects occurring at these ages predominates in the summary Mantel–Haenszel rate ratio statistic reported in the preceding paragraph. These results are consistent with those seen in Norway (Table 2–1).

A further comparison has been made between fatal CHD events and definite cases of myocardial infarction in California studies of the more recent Adventist Health Study (AHS) cohort and the non-Hispanic white subjects in the Stanford Five-City cohort of non-Adventists (Fortmann et al., 1995). This comparison covers the years 1978–1982 in the Adventist study and 1979–1985 in the Stanford study of non-Adventists, the latter being the years when Stanford data were available. The comparison was confined to subjects aged 45–74 years, as the Stanford study did not have data on older people. We could again compare results for similar calendar years, and there were the added advantages, when compared to the ACS/AMS comparison mentioned earlier, that the same detailed diagnostic criteria (Gillum et al., 1984) were used in both studies, and that the data included both nonfatal and fatal events.

Cardiac event rate ratios were calculated for each of the seven calendar years of the comparison period, with these ratios being standardized according to the age structure of the 1970 U.S. population. No obvious time trends in these ratios were noted. This suggests that the volunteer status of the Adventists had little effect, since, if it were important, it is expected that rates in Adventists would rise during a follow-up year as the effects of the volunteerism dissipated. Nevertheless, we excluded the first year of the follow-up, 1977, from these analyses to guard against any such effect. A healthy volunteer effect is much less likely if at the time of vol-

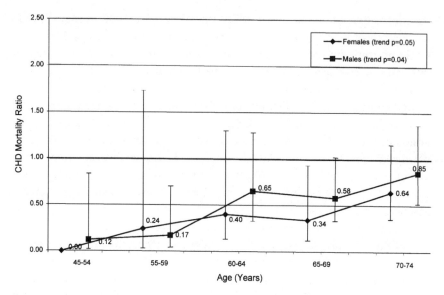

Figure 2-2 Mortality ratios that compare Adventist to non-Adventist First Event definite fatal CHD rates, by age and sex. Adventist and Stanford Study non-Hispanic white subjects. (Average across calendar years applying inverse standard error weights to year-specific standard event rate ratios.) *Source* (of Stanford data): Fortmann SP, personal communication.

unteering a person has no knowledge of an impending disease event as then it could not influence the decision to participate in the study. This should be the situation when dealing with an incident or a new event, as is true in these analyses.

For both total CHD and myocardial infarction, there is a steep rise in the rate ratio with age, showing that the reduction in heart disease among Adventists is greatest at younger ages (see Figs. 2–2 and 2–3). This is similar to results from the ACS/AMS comparison (see Fig. 2–1). It is generally considered that first, or incident, events, as here, give a clearer comparison, because people who had already known disease at the study baseline may have changed their lifestyle as a consequence of the disease, thus distorting causal associations.

The strong dependence on the age factor could be accounted for if younger Adventists were more careful about their lifestyles than were older Adventists. However, the opposite appears to be true, as vegetarianism (a reasonable surrogate for a number of health habits of Adventists) is more common among older Adventists (see Chapter 1). Thus, it appears that the physiologic impact of lifestyle is less dramatic in the very old, a situation also suggested by the results of other studies (Benfante et al., 1989; Psaty et al., 1990; Stevens et al., 1998).

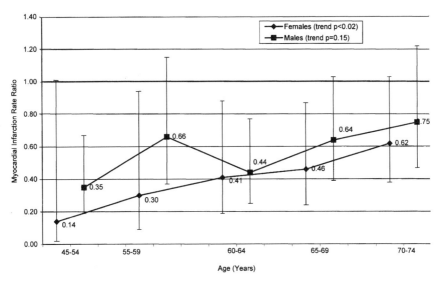

Figure 2–3 Rate ratios that compare Adventist to non-Adventist first event definite myocardial infarction rates, by age and sex. Adventist and Stanford Study non-Hispanic white subjects. (Average across calendar years, applying inverse standard error weights to year-specific standard event rate ratios.) *Source* (of Stanford data): Fortmann SP, personal communication.

Finally, when we summarize across age groups (45–74 years) and calendar years for all fatal CHD events, the standardized ratios (Adventists/Five-City studies) and their 95% confidence intervals for the different CHD endpoints are shown in Table 2–2. Similar figures also give the rates of CHD events in vegetarian Adventists as compared to those of non-Adventists. The summary rate ratios for this age range are substantially lower for the Adventists, and still lower for the vegetarian Adventists.

It is noteworthy that there is little to separate the relative advantage of Adventist men from that of Adventist women in these latter comparisons— which contrasts with the ACS/AMS comparison. The Adventist women have a clear advantage in the Stanford study comparison, an advantage which is less evident in the data from 10 to 15 years earlier. One explanation may be that the more recent comparison covers only the younger portion of the age range described in the ACS/AMS comparison, and it seems that it is at these younger ages where the lower Adventist rates are particularly striking.

Aside from dietary factors, an obvious contributor to the risk differences between Adventists and non-Adventists is the use of tobacco among non-Adventists and its virtual absence in the Adventist group. This would

Table 2-2. Summary Rate Ratios for Coronary Heart Disease (CHD) Endpoints Comparing Vegetarians and All Adventists in the Adventist Health Study to Stanford Five-City Non-Hispanic White Subjects and Summarizing over Both Calendar Years and Ages 45–74 Years

Endpoint	Adventist Group	Standardized Rate Ratios (95% Confidence Intervals)	
		Men	Women
All definite fatal CHD	All Adventists	0.73 (0.58–0.90)	0.57 (0.41–0.79)
	Vegetarians	0.53 (0.34–0.84)	0.22 (0.09–0.53)
First event definite fatal CHD	All Adventists	0.51 (0.37–0.69)	0.48 (0.31–0.74)
	Vegetarians	0.38 (0.20–0.71)	0.18 (0.06–0.55)
All definite myocardial infarction	All Adventists	0.53 (0.43–0.64)	0.38 (0.29–0.51)
	Vegetarians	0.27 (0.16–0.43)	0.37 (0.21–0.65)
First event definite myocardial infarction	All Adventists	0.53 (0.42–0.68)	0.42 (0.30–0.59)
	Vegetarians	0.26 (0.14–0.47)	0.53 (0.30–0.93)

be particularly expected to affect the comparison for males, given the higher smoking rates in non-Adventist men than in non-Adventist women.

A comparison between Adventist and non-Adventist nonsmokers was possible in the earlier AMS and ACS studies. The CHD mortality rate ratio summarized across all ages, is a little higher at 0.76 ($p < .01$) for men, and, as expected, is virtually unchanged for women at 1.01. Because all subjects in this comparison were nonsmokers, much of the risk reduction for Adventist men must have been due to factors other than the absence of cigarette smoking. This may also be true for the modestly lower risk revealed for younger and middle-aged Adventist women of the AMS study.

Differences in educational status may also confuse this comparison. Both the AMS and ACS study groups were better educated than the average Californian, and the ACS comparison group was slightly better educated, on average, than the Adventists—which would usually promote a lower, rather than higher, risk status among the non-Adventists (Kaplan et al., 1993). Thus the comparison is probably slightly biased toward the null (or no-difference) result by modest differences in educational attainment.

DECLINE IN CHD MORTALITY AMONG CALIFORNIA ADVENTISTS

From the mid-1960s, there has been a continual decline in CHD mortality trends in the United States that now exceeds 50% (Gillum, 1993; Havlik and Feinleib, 1979), and similar changes have been seen in many other Western countries. Mortality statistics have been standardized by age and sex in these published trend analyses, thereby excluding any artifact due to changes in the demographic structure of the population. There has been a great deal of discussion (Hunink et al., 1997; McGovern et al., 1996) as to the cause of this decline in CHD mortality trends that has typically affected all age, sex, and racial groups. The causes are thought to involve not only a mix of more effective primary prevention efforts, resulting in decreased cigarette smoking, better control of hypertension, and better eating habits, but also improved secondary prevention from more effective medical care in recent years.

Would the Adventists—a low-risk group that, on average, had already implemented many of the major preventive measures even by the 1960s (and in fact long before then)—participate in this continuing decline in CHD mortality? One could postulate that there would be only small reductions in the rates of new heart disease among Adventists over the years for which we have data, perhaps due to modest improvement in blood pressure control as a result of the new medications that have become available. By contrast, Adventists with existing CHD would have benefited as much

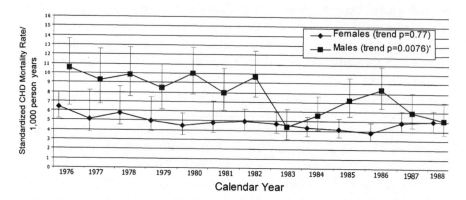

Figure 2-4 Time trends for age-standardized CHD mortality rates for male and female Adventists over the years 1976–1988: all definite CHD mortality. (Mortality rates standardized to the age structure of the 1976 AHS population. ICD9 coding of the death certificate.)

as others from advances in medications for heart disease, the use of coronary care units, and interventional procedures such as bypass surgery and, more recently, balloon angioplasty. Thus, one might predict a blunted decline in CHD mortality among the Adventists, with any reduced risk being explained mostly by secondary prevention and improved treatment for those who have already developed coronary disease.

Trends for all fatal, definite CHD events among Adventists (see Fig. 2–4) do show a significant reduction in mortality (approximately 40%) between 1978 and 1988, but for men only. In fact, this occurred largely among men with established CHD at the study baseline (see Fig. 2–5). A similar analysis (not shown) in subjects where there was no known CHD at the beginning of the study—that is, incident or new events—found little evidence of time trends for men ($p = .40$) or for women ($p = .95$).

Thus, these results are consistent with the above hypotheses. There has been no perceptible decline for either men or women when considering only incident CHD deaths—that is, deaths in subjects with no previous history of heart disease. Such events would show little impact from advances in medical care, as most occur in the community outside hospitals (Fraser, 1978; Kannel and Thomas, 1982), and any decline here would implicate primary prevention, which has probably shown little change among Adventists.

The decreasing mortality in men with previously established disease presumably indicates improved medical care and, conceivably, more attention to risk factors once the diagnosis of CHD was made.

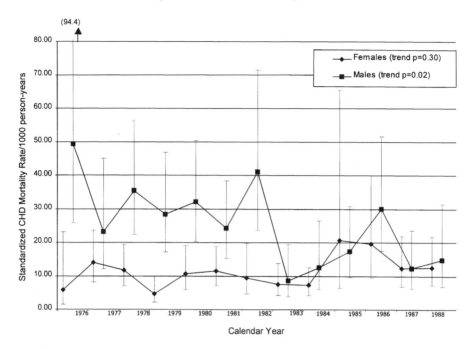

Figure 2–5 Time trends for age-standardized CHD mortality rates for male and female Adventists over the years 1976–1988: Nonincident definite CHD mortality. (Mortality rates standardized to the age structure of the 1976 AHS population. ICD9 coding of the death certificate.)

There is little evidence of trend in total CHD mortality rates or in CHD rates among Adventist women with disease at the baseline, which may suggest that medical advances have been less important for women. This is in keeping with other evidence (Bell et al., 1993; Cowley et al., 1987; Davis, 1987; Greenberg and Mueller, 1993; O'Connor et al., 1993).

SUMMARY

1. Based on the known and suspected effects of diet, exercise, and cigarette smoking on risk of CHD, it was expected that California Adventists would experience lower rates of coronary disease than other Californians. This expectation is indeed borne out by the data, but with the additional insight that the effect is much stronger in younger individuals and in vegetarians.
2. The lower risks for Adventists are broadly similar for both CHD mortality and morbidity among men and younger women. Despite the lower proportionate protection for older Adventist men, the absolute risk dif-

ferences are actually greater here, due to the much higher rates of disease in this age group.

3. Norwegian data suggest that for both sexes, a younger age when joining the Adventist church, or equivalently a longer exposure to the Adventist lifestyle, is more strongly associated with lower cardiovascular mortality.

4. Although part of the explanation for the lower rates among Adventists lies in the absence of cigarette smoking, this probably explains only a modest portion of the reduced risk for Adventist men and probably even less for the women, given the lower rates of smoking among non-Adventist women.

5. The decline in CHD mortality rates that has been such a striking feature across the U.S. population during the last 30 years is seen only among Adventist men, and then only among those with existing CHD at the beginning of the study. This is consistent with the idea that this population has experienced little decline in CHD mortality that could be ascribed to changes in health habits, as their habits have, on average, conformed to current recommendations for decades. However, improvements in medical management have probably reduced mortality among Adventist men with existing disease.

6. The evidence presented above could be interpreted as a large-scale demonstration that the lifestyle often recommended to prevent coronary disease has indeed been effective within this segment of the American population.

3

Cancer Rates among Adventists and Others

Cancer is fundamentally a disorder of the control mechanisms for cell multiplication and location. Normal cells have built-in mechanisms that limit their rate of multiplication, so that new cells appear only where others have died—at least after childhood growth has ceased. Organs maintain their shape and functional integrity by these means. Control mechanisms ensure that most normal cells of fixed organs do not move about and never enter the blood or lymphatic circulation and then settle and multiply in some distant organ (a metastasis).

Yet this is what happens in many cancers, which, after metastasis, are usually incurable with current therapies. Even those cancers that have not metastasized if untreated may grow rapidly to form tumors in their organ of origin. These may interfere with the organ's function or may damage other surrounding structures.

The flaws that underlie a cell's escape from control are largely located in the DNA of the cell nucleus. In other words, if certain critical genes become damaged or mutated, the cell will no longer behave normally (Ruoslahti, 1996; Weinberg, 1996). The body does have several back-up or emergency mechanisms, and evidence suggests that a cell must actually accumulate multiple mutations before cancer results.

DNA can be damaged by several different processes. A small proportion of cancers are hereditary. The damaged DNA in these cases is inherited from the person's parents. Other causes of damage are radiation, including natural radiation, and exposure to chemicals that bind and alter DNA. These include certain chemicals found in tobacco smoke and also free radicals. The latter are highly reactive molecules that are formed naturally by the body's metabolism but usually are quickly deactivated. Although most cancers are not caused by viruses, cancers of the uterine cervix and liver (and a few other rare tumors) clearly result in part from damage that certain viruses cause to the cell nucleus during their infection (Trichopoulos et al., 1996).

Aging alone may result in the accumulation of unrepaired genetic damage sufficient to cause cancer, simply because of lengthy exposure to environmental hazards. In fact, there are well-known mechanisms by which the cell detects and repairs damaged DNA, but the repair mechanisms become less efficient with age and allow a greater proportion of errors to remain. Another mechanism that normally prevents the accumulation of damaged DNA is apoptosis, or programmed cell death, whereby cells detect their own unrepairable errors and then "commit suicide." But the apoptotic control genes may themselves be damaged over time, and then cells with serious errors in their DNA survive rather than self-destruct (Weinberg, 1996).

In older cells, the biochemical mechanisms that "mop up" the harmful free radicals are less efficient, and this results in a more damaging cellular environment (Banks and Fossel, 1997). The liver produces a host of enzymes that will chemically bind and neutralize many cancer-producing chemicals. With age, however, these enzymes also become less efficient (Abrass, 1990). Finally, along with most other body systems, the immune system becomes less effective in the aged (Hirokawa, 1992). This is important as abnormal cells that can develop into the early stages of cancer are neither detected as usual by the immune system nor destroyed by lymphocytes or macrophages.

While cancer cells are produced (or initiated) with some regularity in all of us, the great majority are detected and are either destroyed or undergo apoptosis. Even if such a cell survives, however, unless it divides quite rapidly, it may never form a tumor of sufficient size to cause any symptoms during the remaining years of one's life. Thus, although initiation of cancer cells is essential, promotion of rapid growth will also determine how quickly the tumor grows and whether it ever causes clinical problems. Factors that can promote more rapid cell growth include hormones such as estrogen and insulin, and certain chemicals that alter gene expression so as to increase cell division. Greater intake of dietary fat and calories may also enhance tumor growth (Potter, 1997). Vitamin D, however, may have antipromotion activity.

Thus, it is clear that although genetic factors are very much involved, environmental exposures and personal choices will also influence risk (Schottenfeld and Fraumeni, 1996). Certain occupations involve the risk of exposure to cancer-producing chemicals or radiation. Obesity in postmenopausal women raises blood estrogen levels, and in both sexes it often induces higher insulin levels. The timing of pregnancies and the duration of the reproductive life in women will also influence hormone levels. Regular exercise and a less calorie-dense diet helps prevent obesity and may enhance immune function. If healthy choices can delay the biochemical changes of aging (and this is as yet unproven), then a delayed decline in the effectiveness of protective enzyme systems and of the immune system would decrease risk.

Dietary choices can reduce or enhance cancer risk in a number of different ways. Diets rich in fruit and vegetables can prevent obesity and can limit the excess calorie intake that may promote tumor growth. Dietary antioxidants deactivate free radicals, and other dietary factors stimulate the detoxifying liver enzymes; more details are given in Chapter 6.

Epidemiologists generally agree that common cancers are environmentally induced to an important extent (National Academy of Sciences, 1982). In particular, it has been estimated that dietary changes have the potential to reduce cancer deaths by 35% in the United States (Doll and Peto, 1981). Thus, it is possible that Adventists, who have a generally more conservative lifestyle, obtain more exercise than others, and, on average, eat more fruit and vegetables and less meat than others, might have a different experience with some, or perhaps all, cancers.

CANCER RATES BETWEEN ADVENTISTS AND NON-ADVENTISTS IN OTHER COUNTRIES

As with the coronary heart disease comparisons, the population-based studies in California, Norway, the Netherlands, Japan, and Denmark provide an opportunity to compare mortality or incidence rates for several different sites of cancer among Adventists with those rates among non-Adventists in the same locations. To identify cancer cases and deaths in Norway, the Netherlands, Denmark, and Japan, national registries were used for studying cases among both Adventists and non-Adventists. In the Netherlands, church records were also used to ascertain who among the Adventists being studied were still alive. If the latter created any bias, it would presumably elevate Adventist rates due to a more complete study follow-up. Further details of study designs and numbers of cancer events can be found in the Appendix (Table A–7).

The international evidence suggests that there are modest reductions in rates for all sites of cancer among younger Adventist men and perhaps younger Adventist women, with this being more evident for mortality than for incidence (see Table 3–1). This statement summarizes the results from

Table 3–1. Comparison of All-Site Standardized Cancer Mortality and Incidence Ratios for Adventists and Non-Adventists: Studies Outside the United States

Country	Men	Women
AGE-STANDARDIZED MORTALITY RATIOS (95% CONFIDENCE INTERVAL)		
Japan	0.30[*][a]	0.78[a]
Netherlands	0.50 (0.41–0.60)[b]	
Norway		
All ages	0.92[a]	0.99[a]
≤75 years	0.78 (0.61–0.99)	0.94 (0.79–1.11)
>75 years	1.04 (0.87–1.27)	1.04 (0.88–1.21)
STANDARDIZED INCIDENCE RATIOS (95% CONFIDENCE INTERVAL)		
Denmark	0.7 (0.5–0.9)	NA
Norway		
All ages	0.91 (0.81–1.03)	0.97 (0.89–1.06)
≤75 years	0.82[a]	0.93[a]
>75 years	1.03[a]	1.03[a]

[*]$p < .01$, but only 7 cancers observed (26 in Japanese women); NA, not available.

[a]Confidence intervals not given and cannot be calculated from published data.

[b]Men and women combined.

Sources: Kuratsune et al., 1986; Berkel and deWaard, 1983; Fønnebø and Helseth, 1991; Jensen, 1983.

Norway (Fønnebø and Helseth, 1991); Japan (Kuratsune et al., 1986); Denmark (Jensen, 1983); and the Netherlands (Berkel and deWaard, 1983).

Comparisons of site-specific cancers (see Table 3–2) from the Netherlands show mortality ratios that are much lower than the null value of 1.0 (a value of 1.0 would indicate that results for Adventists and non-Adventists do not differ). This is true for all four cancer sites that show adequate study numbers. Cancer incidence ratios from Norway and Denmark imply more modest reductions than those seen in Adventist mortality rates, but confidence intervals are wide. In summary, there is an indication of lower mortality and incidence rates for breast and digestive system cancers in Adventists, but little evidence of an advantage for genital cancers in either sex.

Any evidence of protection against cancer mortality in Norwegian Adventists is confined to subjects under 75 years of age, who had an SMR of 78 (95% confidence interval, 61–99) (Fønnebø, 1992; Fønnebø and Helseth, 1991). On dividing subjects into those who joined the church at ages less than 19 years, 19–34 years, and 35 years of age or older, an all-site cancer mortality advantage was seen only in the first two groups (Fønnebø, 1992). The SMRs for these different ages of joining the church are 88, 67, and 106, respectively, for men, and 75, 79, and 114 for women, suggesting protection for those who joined the church at earlier ages. As for coronary disease, this can be interpreted either as an "age at joining" effect or a "duration of exposure" effect (see Chapter 2).

Table 3–2. A Comparison of Site-Specific Standardized Cancer Mortality (SMR) and Incidence Ratios (SIR) for Adventists and Non-Adventists: Studies Outside the United States[a]

Cancer Site or Type	Country	SMR or SIR	95% Confidence Interval
CANCER MORTALITY (SMR)			
Breast	Netherlands	0.50	0.41–0.60
Lung	Netherlands	0.45	0.23–0.79
Colorectal	Netherlands	0.43	0.24–0.71
Stomach	Netherlands	0.59	0.34–0.96
CANCER INCIDENCE (SIR)			
Breast[b]	Norway	0.91	0.70–1.17
Respiratory[b]	Norway	0.59	0.36–0.91
Gastrointestinal[b]	Norway	0.85	0.69–1.03
Digestive organs	Denmark (men only)	0.80	0.5–1.1
Colorectal	Denmark (men only)	0.80	NA
Stomach	Denmark (men only)	1.1	0.5–2.0
Prostate[b]	Norway	0.98	0.64–1.45
Male genital	Denmark	0.9	0.4–1.7
Female genital[b]	Norway	1.14	0.89–1.44
Urinary	Norway	0.83	0.53–1.24
Hemopoietic	Norway	1.06	0.73–1.49

NA, not available.

[a]Results quoted only for sites where at least 10 deaths/cases were observed in the Adventists. This excludes Japanese data. Age and sex (as appropriate) standardization.

[b]Results for cancers occurring before age 75 years.

Sources: Berkel and deWaard, 1983; Fønnebø and Helseth, 1991; Jensen, 1983.

CALIFORNIA STUDIES

Cancer Mortality Comparisons between Adventists and Other Californians

Cancer mortality ratios nearly always favored the Adventists when Adventist Mortality Study findings were compared with those of the concurrent California ACS study of non-Adventists (see Table 3–3) (Phillips et al., 1980a). It is clear that some of this advantage is due to the absence of cigarette smoking. If we exclude both Adventists and non-Adventists who had ever smoked, we see a large shift toward the null value in the Adventist–non-Adventist mortality ratio for the total of all cancers (in men) and for cancers of the lung (in both sexes). This indicates that smoking is an important predictor of mortality from lung cancer, and from some other cancers, and so explains a part of the reduction for Adventists.

When smokers are excluded from the analysis, the Adventists still showed considerably lower mortality from lung, colorectal, and breast cancers, and from all cancers combined. The evidence supporting reduced

Table 3–3. Comparison of Cancer Mortality for California Adventists and Non-Adventists: The Adventist Mortality (1960–1976) and American Cancer Society (1960–1971) Studies[a]

Cancer Site or Type	Sex	Age-Adjusted Mortality Ratios	
		All Subjects	Never-Smoking Adventists and Non-Adventists
All cancer	M	0.60**	0.85
	F	0.76**	0.78**
Lung	M	0.18**	0.67
	F	0.31**	0.42**
Colorectal	M	0.62**	0.67
	F	0.58**	0.56**
Stomach	M	1.41	1.02
	F	0.89	0.80
Lymphoma and leukemia	M	0.86	0.93
	F	1.00	0.89
Prostate	M	0.92	0.93
Breast	F	0.85	0.81*

*$p < .05$—tests the null hypothesis that the mortality ratio = 1.0; **$p < .01$.

[a]Mantel-Haenszel stratified analyses.

Source: Adapted from Phillips et al., 1980a.

mortality was then clearer in women (estimated 22% reduction), although similar nonsignificant trends were seen in men for all cancers combined, and for lung and colorectal cancers. This reduced mortality can no longer be ascribed to the absence of smoking and most likely relates to differences in dietary and other lifestyle characteristics between Adventists and others.

Cancer Incidence Rates Comparing Adventists and Other Californians

The problem with the results described above is that for many sites, most new cancers were excluded from the analysis. This is because only those that ended in death were detected in these mortality studies. For common cancers such as those of the breast, colon, and prostate, most people survive. Hence the results cited above pertain to only a minority of events.

The more recent Adventist Health Study was designed to find all new cancers during the follow-up of both fatal and nonfatal cases. If a comparable database that included all new cancer cases among non-Adventists at around the same time period (1976–1982) could be found, a more informative comparison would be possible.[1] There were two tumor registries operating for populations in California at this time, both covering major urban areas: the Los Angeles County Tumor Registry (Mack, 1977) and the Oakland Bay Area Tumor Registry (*Surveillance, Epidemiology and End Results*, 1998). Although the geographic overlap with the Adventist cohort is imperfect, as Adventists lived all around the state of California, these are the best comparable incidence data for non-Adventists that are available.

The expected numbers of events for Adventists were calculated based on weightings of the two age-specific tumor registry rates that reflect the geographic distribution of the Adventists between northern and southern California. These are the numbers of events expected if non-Adventist rates had been applied in the Adventist population. They are compared with the numbers of cancers actually observed among the Adventists in order to form incidence ratios standardized by age groups (Table 3–4).

To ensure fair comparisons, both the International Classification of Disease (ICD) codes that determine a cancer site, and the ICD0 codes that determine the histologies or cell types of interest at that site, were decided before the analysis. Only epithelial cancers were included for a particular organ, as they represent the great majority of tumors at that location. Rare tumor types, such as carcinoid tumors or sarcomas, were thus excluded from site-specific analyses, but are included in the comparison for all sites. Skin cancers, aside from melanomas, were excluded from all comparisons.

Cancers that had reached a more advanced stage of progression when first diagnosed were often identified separately from those that were already considered invasive. The latter category excludes in situ and microinvasive tumors. This distinction may be important because, if the Adventists had, on average, better access to medical care, and were more health conscious, a relatively large number of their cancers might have been found at earlier stages. Then any advantage for Adventists would be more evident when invasive tumors were considered separately.

In comparison to Californians of similar ages in the Los Angeles and the Oakland Bay areas during the same calendar years (Table 3–4), both male and female California Adventists experienced significantly lower rates of new cancers at many, but not all, sites. Overall, the rate of invasive colon cancer was lower by 33%, that of stomach cancer by 59%, invasive bladder cancer by 61%, kidney cancer by 60%, lung cancer by 80%, and pancreatic cancer by 34%. For cancers of women's reproductive organs, the rate of invasive breast cancer was lower by 23%, that of invasive ovarian cancer by 30%, and invasive cervical cancer by 54%, but there was evidence of possibly higher rates in Adventist women for uterine cancer. Among Adventist men, there was no evidence of a lower incidence for either invasive or all prostate cancers. The rate of invasive melanoma was lower among Adventists by only 11%, a difference compatible with chance, and cancers of the nervous system, leukemias, and lymphomas were not

Table 3-4. Comparison of Cancer Incidence in California Adventists and That Calculated from General Population Tumor Registries in Los Angeles County and the Oakland Bay Area (1976–1982)

Cancer Site or Type	Histology	Males		Females		Total	
		Standardized Incidence Ratio	95% Confidence Interval	Standardized Incidence Ratio	95% Confidence Interval	Standardized Incidence Ratio	95% Confidence Interval
Colon	All	0.55	0.41–0.74	0.75	0.61–0.93	0.67	0.57–0.80
	Invasive	0.54	0.40–0.73	0.75	0.61–0.93	0.67	0.56–0.80
Stomach	Invasive	0.43	0.23–0.80	0.38	0.19–0.76	0.41	0.26–0.65
Bladder	All	0.42	0.28–0.63	0.55	0.34–0.90	0.46	0.34–0.63
	Invasive	0.38	0.25–0.59	0.40	0.22–0.72	0.39	0.27–0.55
Kidney	Invasive	0.32	0.13–0.76	0.52	0.23–1.16	0.40	0.22–0.73
Melanoma	Invasive	0.90	0.55–1.47	0.89	0.56–1.39	0.89	0.64–1.24
Lymphoma	Invasive	1.33	0.93–1.90	1.16	0.84–1.60	1.23	0.97–1.56
Leukemia	Invasive	1.04	0.67–1.59	0.92	0.60–1.42	0.98	0.73–1.32
Lung	Invasive	0.17	0.11–0.25	0.25	0.17–0.37	0.20	0.15–0.27
Pancreas	Invasive	0.53	0.29–0.96	0.75	0.49–1.14	0.66	0.34–0.74
Brain/nervous system	Invasive	1.32	0.75–2.33	1.10	0.62–1.94	1.20	0.80–1.79
Breast	All	NA	NA	0.78	0.68–0.89	NA	NA
	Invasive	NA	NA	0.77	0.67–0.89	NA	NA
Ovary	Invasive	NA	NA	0.70	0.48–1.03	NA	NA
Cervix	All	NA	NA	0.46	0.31–0.68	NA	NA
	Invasive	NA	NA	0.41	0.21–0.83	NA	NA
Uterus	Invasive	NA	NA	1.27	1.05–1.53	NA	NA
Prostate	All	1.09	0.93–1.28	NA	NA	NA	NA
	Invasive	1.03	0.88–1.21	NA	NA	NA	NA
All smoking-related sites	Invasive	0.24	0.19–0.31	0.40	0.32–0.49	0.31	0.26–0.36
All sites	Invasive	0.61	0.55–0.67	0.74	0.69–0.80	0.69	0.65–0.73

NA, not applicable.

NA is used for sex-specific cancers.

clearly different among Adventists. For all smoking-related sites, there is a 69% rate reduction for Adventists, as might be expected, and for all sites combined the reduction is 31%.

There were small differences in the Adventist/non-Adventist comparison when "all" as compared to only "invasive" cancers were distinguished for several of the cancer sites. In nearly every case the Adventists showed lower relative risks when attention was restricted to invasive tumors. This is consistent with the conjecture that Adventists may have a relatively larger number of cancers diagnosed at an early stage, perhaps due to a greater interest in preventive screening and better access to health care.

Thus the evidence shows that Adventists have lower rates of both cancer incidence and mortality for cancer at many anatomic sites. In Norway, this was more evident for cancer incidence in persons below 75 years of age (Table 3–1). When a similar age division was made in the California AHS, rates were typically still lower among Adventists over 74 years of age, but for most common cancers the standardized incidence ratios were usually closer to 1.0 than before. Three of the cancers that gave little indication of lower rates for all age groups among Adventists—uterine, prostate, and lymphomas (Table 3–4)—also showed a similar situation at these older ages. For all cancers combined, the standardized incidence ratio in subjects 75 years of age and older was 0.77 (95% confidence interval, 0.70–0.85), still a 23% reduction in risk.

Thus, the Norwegian results are somewhat confirmed, although in California rates for elderly Adventists are still significantly lower than those for elderly non-Adventists. This suggests that the protective factors associated with Adventism become relatively less effective as the population ages, but some effects continue. As discussed later for cardiovascular disease mortality and for mortality from all causes (see Chapter 7), it seems likely that this is due to the increasing importance of genetic and metabolic effects in the elderly that are less responsive to behavioral factors.

For several cancers, the much lower Adventist risk will at least be due partially to the absence of cigarette smoking. This is so for cancers of the lung, bladder, and perhaps stomach and cervix. However, for all of these, other factors are also important. Unfortunately, the tumor registries did not collect data on smoking habits, so it is not possible to compare rates for Adventists with those for nonsmoking non-Adventists in the more recent AHS comparison.

Studies comparing Adventists who have different habits (but all nonsmokers) strongly suggest that dietary factors are important determinants of many cancers (see Chapter 6), and this is confirmed by studies of other populations. Hence the lower rates for Adventists as compared to others are probably related in part to dietary differences. Other possible explanatory factors include more physical activity, relatively less obesity, and the virtual absence of alcohol use among Adventists.

There are a few anatomic sites for which the pattern of lower cancer rates for Adventists is *not* seen. The sites that most consistently show little or no Adventist advantage are the lymphatic system and the prostate in men and the uterus in women. Cancers for these sites are relatively common ones, and so confidence intervals are not excessively wide in the California Adventist data, indicating that chance is an unlikely cause of these null results. There was also little to suggest that Adventists had lower rates of these cancers in the earlier AMS/ACS data or in results from Norway (see Tables 3–2 and 3–3).

A diagnostic bias may confuse the comparison between Adventists and non-Adventists regarding rates of prostate cancer. Even invasive prostate cancers are often quite indolent and compatible with long and relatively asymptomatic survival. Thus both early-stage and invasive cancers may be found when screening asymptomatic subjects. As Adventists are probably more likely to have regular screenings, including digital rectal examinations and prostate specific antigen (PSA) testing, there may be a tendency for cancers to be found, and even treated, that would never have been found without the use of the screening procedure. Such a bias may also be possible for uterine cancer, but it is somewhat less plausible. An alternative is that Adventists may not have lower rates of prostate or uterine cancers, but this would be a little surprising, at least for prostate cancer, as there is stronger evidence here than for most cancer sites that diet can reduce risk (see Chapter 6).

It seems reasonable to conclude that the lifestyle differences between Adventists and others (including cigarette smoking) probably play an important part in the etiology of cancers of the colon, stomach, bladder, kidney, lung, pancreas, breast, ovary, and cervix. This analysis does not strongly support such a role for nervous system cancers, melanoma, lymphoma, leukemia, and cancer of the uterus. However, as already mentioned for prostate cancer, distortions and biases are possible, and such conclusions can only be tentative.

SUMMARY

1. When compared to others, Adventists have lower mortality rates for many cancers. This was so for studies in California, Europe, and Japan.
2. Cancer incidence rates are also lower among Adventists for many anatomic sites, often dramatically so. In older subjects, differences between Adventists and others are less extreme but, in the California data, continue to be seen for most cancers.

3. In Norway, reduced cancer rates were seen only for those that became Adventists before the age of 35, though more evidence is needed on this point.

4. The lower rates of most cancers in Adventists are probably due to a combination of factors, including the absence of cigarette smoking, differences in dietary habits, more physical activity, and less alcohol intake.

5. None of the studies find significantly lower rates of prostate cancer for Adventists. While there may be a diagnostic bias involved, it is possible that the Adventist lifestyle does not protect against this cancer, or it may be counterbalanced by other, unknown factors. Other cancer types in which protection is less evident are uterine and nervous system cancers, melanoma, lymphoma, and leukemia.

NOTES

1. I wish to recognize the effort and expertise of Dr. Wendy Cozen and Kathleen Danley, of the Los Angeles County Tumor Registry (University of Southern California), who both contributed in an important way to the analyses in this section.

4

The Longevity of Adventists as Compared with Others

For many of us, life expectancy is among the most important expressions of personal health. However, most would agree that this needs to be accompanied by a good quality of life, except perhaps for a short period before death. Vegetarians live longer than others, as we will see, and probably also have a better quality of life.

The definitive proof of improved quality of life must await future research, but an educated guess is possible. Some of the causes of mortality that are more frequent in nonvegetarians are the same disorders that result in prolonged periods of morbidity before death. Indeed, we have found that vegetarian Adventists use fewer medications and are less likely than nonvegetarians to have had an overnight hospital stay, surgery, or an X-ray during the previous year (Knutsen, 1994). Further evidence of an improved quality of life comes from a recent longitudinal analysis of 1741 aging non-Adventist university alumni, which concluded that "not only do persons with better health habits survive longer, but in such persons, disability is postponed and compressed into fewer years at the end of life" (Vita et al., 1998).

The information presented below shows that Adventists are perhaps the longest-lived population that has yet been formally described. In addition to longevity, it is instructive to consider the causes of death among Adventists as compared with others, to evaluate comparative life expectancy for different age groups, to note the sex-ratio of Adventists who survive to older ages, and to evaluate time trends in life expectancy.

LIFE EXPECTANCY IN ADVENTISTS AND OTHERS

We will examine the evidence in support of the fact that Adventists live longer than others. All of our calculations use the current life table method, in which we form a population of "synthetic lives," those that would be observed if the actual mortality rates for different age groups during the limited calendar period of the study were those of the synthetic population as they all passed from young adulthood to old-age and death. This is a useful means of summarizing the lifetime effects of mortality rates currently being observed, for the purpose of comparison with another population whose data are being examined in the same way. One measure derived from such life tables is the predicted average age of people at death, or life expectancy. Life tables also allow for the construction of a survival curve showing the proportion of a population predicted to survive to particular ages.

Life expectancies were calculated in two of the smaller studies of European Adventists and then compared with the concurrent national experience. In the Netherlands, for Adventists already surviving to the age of 26.8 years (the average age for joining the Adventist church in this study group), the predicted average ages at death were 79.1 and 79.3 years, respectively, for men and women (Berkel and deWaard, 1983). These were 8.9 and 3.6 years greater, respectively, than the predicted ages for other Dutch men and women at that time (1968–1977). In Norway, the predicted average ages at death for Adventists already surviving to 20 years of age were 76.4 and 79.7 years, respectively, for men and women, these being 3.0 years ($p < .001$) and 0.7 years, respectively, greater than for other Norwegians (Fønnebø, 1992). If the analysis is limited to Norwegian Adventists who joined the church before the age of 19, and who then theoretically experienced the full benefit of the Adventist lifestyle, the additional Adventist life expectancy is 5.2 years ($p < .001$) for both men and women.

A comparison of survival between 47,000 California Adventists enrolled in the Adventist Mortality Study (AMS) and other Californians was made by using Adventist Mortality Study statistics (1960–1962) and California State life tables (1959–1961) (Lemon and Kuzma, 1969). For those already surviving to the age of 35, predicted average ages at death were 77.4 and 80.1 years for Adventist men and women, exceeding values for other Californians by 6.2 and 3.7 years, respectively. Even at the age of 65, the Adventists had greater remaining life expectancy by 3.2 and 1.9 years in men and women.

It is possible that a healthy-volunteer effect in the Adventist study group could distort the comparison with other Californians. Chronically ill individuals, while being fully represented in California state statistics, are less likely to join a research program such as the AMS. This can perhaps improperly reduce calculated mortality in the research group during the early follow-up period. However, during the follow-up, a proportion of enrolled Adventist study subjects will become chronically ill, and a proportion of those Adventists who chose not to enroll, because of chronic illness, will die. Thus the study population and the total Adventist population become more and more similar with regard to the proportion of chronically ill subjects, and any biases preventing a fair comparison will finally disappear. Whether the delay of two years from 1958, when Adventist subjects entered the study, to 1960, when mortality statistics were first used, was sufficient for a healthy-volunteer bias to disappear is not certain, but based on later Adventist Health Study (AHS) data (noted below), this should have taken care of most of the problem.

We have also compared survival data for the more recent Adventist Health Study cohort and for other Californians (Fraser and Shavlik, 2001). Unless otherwise stated, analyses for both Adventists and non-Adventists shown here are for persons who have already survived to the age of 30. Mortality rates in infancy, childhood, and young adult years are thus excluded. An advantage of the data in the Adventist Health Study population over that of many other cohorts is that there was no upper age limit and deaths were observed through the oldest ages. Between 1980 and 1988, there were 1657 deaths observed in men and 2808 in women. Of these decedents, 17% of men and 24% of women were over the age of 90.

The survival curves in Figures 4–1 and 4–2 clearly show a greater survival rate at any particular age, and hence greater life expectancy, for both Adventist men and women. Predicted average ages at death are 81.2 years (men) and 83.9 years (women) in Adventists, and 73.9 and 79.5 years, respectively, for other Californians. Thus, there is a difference of 7.28 years (95% confidence interval, 6.59–7.97) for men and 4.42 years (95% confidence interval, 3.96–4.88) for women.

Adventist men, on average, live even longer than non-Adventist California women, and their survival rate exceeds that of the non-Adventist women throughout life (compare Figures 4–1 and 4–2). Vegetarian Adventist men and women had even greater longevity, with predicted ages at death of 83.3 years (95% confidence interval, 82.39–84.25) and 85.7 (95% confidence interval, 84.89–86.42) years, differences of 9.5 and 6.1 years as compared with non-Adventists.

A healthy-volunteer bias is again possible in these analyses. It had previously been established that there was a gradual increase in age-standardized mortality rates during the first three years of the follow-up period for the Adventists, and this was ascribed to the resolution of a healthy-volunteer

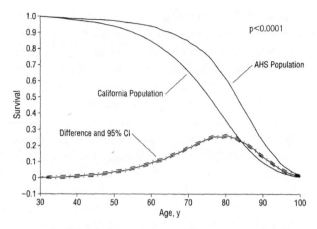

Figure 4–1 Survival of California versus Adventist Health Study population (males). *Source:* Reproduced by permission from Fraser GE, Shavhik DJ, Ten years of life: is it a matter of choice? *Arch Int Med* 161:1645–1652, 2001. Copyright 2001, American Medical Association.

effect. However, beyond this time the upward trend disappeared (Lindsted et al., 1996). Thus, our recent life table comparison using mortality statistics from the Adventist Health Study included only data from follow-up years four to twelve (1980–1988),[1] and compared these with mortality data for California non-Hispanic whites for 1985 (Center for Health Statistics, 1999).

To place these results in a broader perspective, Table 4–1 adds results for all Adventists, and for vegetarian Adventists, to previously published international life expectancy results that pertain to the same calendar pe-

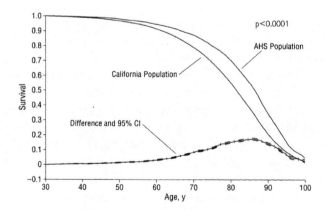

Figure 4–2 Survival of California versus Adventist Health Study population (females). *Source:* Reproduced by permission from Fraser GE, Shavhik DJ, Ten years of life: is it a matter of choice? *Arch Int Med* 161:1645–1652, 2001. Copyright 2001, American Medical Association.

Table 4–1. Expected Length of Life (Years) at Birth and at Age 65: California Adventists Compared with International Populations

Country (Year)	Men		Women	
	At Birth	At Age 65	At Birth	At Age 65
Australia (1990)	73.9	15.2	80.0	19.0
Canada (1985–1987)	73.0	14.9	79.7	19.1
Denmark (1989–1990)	72.0	14.1	77.7	17.9
Finland (1989)	70.9	13.8	78.9	17.7
Iceland (1989–1990)	75.7	16.1	80.3	19.3
Japan (1990)	75.9	16.2	81.8	19.9
New Zealand (1987–1989)	71.6	14.1	77.6	17.8
Norway (1990)	73.4	14.6	79.8	18.6
United Kingdom (1985–1987)	71.9	13.4	77.6	17.3
United States (1990)	73.0	14.9	79.7	19.1
California Adventists (1980–1988)[a]	78.5	19.1	82.3	21.6
Vegetarian California Adventists (1980–1988)[a]	80.2	20.3	84.8	22.6

[a]Mortality hazards for ages 0–29 are those from California State data, as data for these ages are not available for Adventists.

Source: Reproduced by permission from Fraser GE, Shavlik DJ, Ten years of life: is it a matter of choice? *Arch Int Med* 161:1645–1652, 2001. Copyright 2001, American Medical Association.

riod or a somewhat later period. In this table results are given for life expectancy at birth. As can be seen, life expectancies are greater among the Adventists, this being especially so for men. The Adventist vegetarians show the greatest longevity (see also Table 4–3), substantially exceeding that of other populations.

DIFFERENCES IN LIFE EXPECTANCY AT DIFFERENT AGES

When a population lives longer, one may wonder whether the greater life expectancy is seen at all ages. Another question is whether the usually observed differences in survival between men and women are also seen in the low-risk population.

As expected, the additional Adventist life expectancy diminishes with an increasing baseline age, consistent with suggestions in previous chapters that in regard to chronic disease, the beneficial effects of being Adventist are more pronounced in younger and middle-aged subjects. Hence the years of life saved for Adventists are particularly those years of the younger and more productive periods. When comparing Adventists with other Californians, predicted life expectancies (remaining years of life) for those who have already survived to particular ages are found in Table 4–2.

Table 4–2. Life Expectancy (95% Confidence Intervals) Given Survival to Different Ages: California Adventists (1980–1988) and Other Californians (1985)

Age	Men			Women		
	Adventists	Other Californians	Difference	Adventists	Other Californians	Difference
30	51.15	43.87	7.28	53.94	49.52	4.42
40	41.78	34.78	7.00	44.12	30.93	4.19
50	32.25	25.96	6.29	34.72	30.71	4.01
60	23.22	18.15	5.07	25.89	22.21	3.68
70	15.14	11.71	3.43	17.52	14.81	2.71
80	8.61	7.20	1.41	10.12	8.79	1.33
85	6.36	5.69	0.67	7.44	6.51	0.93
90	4.69	4.53	0.16	5.35	5.02	0.33
95	3.46	3.42	0.04	3.97	3.96	0.01
100	2.06	2.74	-0.68	2.25	3.06	-0.81

Source: Adventist data from Adventist Health Study. California data from Center for Health Statistics. California Deaths, 1985. Sacramento, California: Dept of Health Services, 1999.

There is much interest in the mortality of the oldest group (people 85 and over), as this is a rapidly growing group that takes a disproportionate share of health-care dollars (vanWeel and Michels, 1997). The results in Table 4–2 include those who have already survived to advanced ages. Even at the age of 85, Adventists have slightly but significantly better survival rates ($p < .001$ males, $p < .0001$ females).

Another way of making these comparisons is to compare Adventist and other populations (1982 data) with respect to both the proportions surviving to the age of 65 or of 85, and the proportion who, having already survived to age 65, live until at least age 85 (see Table 4–3). A much greater proportion of Adventists survive to these ages, and this is particularly so for the vegetarians. For instance, 19.5% of U.S. men survive to the age of 85, whereas this is so for 48.6% of Adventist vegetarian men. Similar figures for U.S. women are 39.3% and for vegetarian Adventist women, 60.1%. Only Japanese women survive to the age of 65 with frequency similar to that of the Adventist women, but they appear to do less well over the next 20 years of life. The results for vegetarian Adventists probably make them the longest-lived population that has yet been formally described.

It is well known that mortality rates in the elderly are substantially higher in men than in women. The effect of this in the United States (Suzman et al., 1992, p. 25) is that for the age groups 85–89 and 95–99, only 29.6% and 21.3%, respectively, of the population are men (1990 data). The percentage of men in the population at different ages is shown in Table 4–4, which compares Adventists with other Californians.

As can be seen, the percentage of males in the population of non-Hispanic white non-Adventist Californians is a little higher than that cited here for the whole United States, but there is a consistent trend in which the percentage of men in the elderly Adventist California population is 20% to 25% higher than that of other Californians. This was expected, given that additional years of survival for Adventist men exceeded those for Adventist women, when they were compared with the non-Adventist population. Expressed differently, while the difference between men and women in the predicted average age at death for non-Adventist, non-Hispanic white Californians was 5.65 years, that for the Adventists was only 2.79 years. Adventist couples can expect to have several more years of life together.

COMPRESSION OF MORTALITY

There is an ongoing debate among demographers as to whether increases in life expectancy will or will not result in compression of mortality. What does this mean? Mortality can become compressed if there exists a genetically determined upper age limit, say, Q_i, to the life of individual i, that

Table 4-3. Proportions of Life Table Subjects Surviving to 65 Years, 85 Years, and from 65 to 85 Years

Country	Percentage of Males Surviving			Percentage of Females Surviving		
	To Age 65	To Age 85	From Age 65 to Age 85[a]	To Age 65	To Age 85	From Age 65 to Age 85[a]
Australia	74.7	17.6	23.6	86.4	38.4	44.5
Canada	75.1	19.6	26.1	86.3	40.0	46.3
Germany, Fed. Rep.	73.4	14.2	19.3	85.8	31.7	36.9
Hungary	60.9	8.2	13.4	79.3	21.0	26.5
Japan	80.8	23.6	29.2	89.5	41.1	45.9
Sweden	78.7	20.4	25.9	88.4	39.8	45.0
United Kingdom	75.0	14.5	19.3	84.6	32.7	38.6
United States	72.0	19.5	27.1	84.1	39.3	46.7
California Adventists	86.7	41.0	47.2	89.3	54.4	60.9
California Adventist Vegetarians	89.2	48.6	54.4	94.1	60.1	64.6

Note: Non-Adventist data in this table refer to survival probabilities of a child born in 1982 and continuing to experience age-specific mortality conditions as estimated from life tables for 1982. Adventist data are for the years 1980–1988, using California state mortality hazards from the year 1985; for ages 0–29, as the available Adventist data starts at 30 years of age.

[a]Of those having survived to 65 years, the proportion alive at 85 years.

Source: Life tables for non-Adventists prepared by the Center for Demographic Studies, Duke University, based on World Health Organization computer tape transcripts.

Table 4–4. Predicted Percentages of the Population That Are Men, at Different Ages: Adventists (1980–1988) Compared to Other Non-Hispanic White Californians (1985)[a]

Age (Years)	Percentage of Men		Ratio of Adventists Versus Other Californians
	Adventists	Other Californians	
30	0.50	0.50	1.0
50	0.50	0.49	1.02
70	0.49	0.46	1.06
80	0.47	0.39	1.20
90	0.40	0.32	1.25
100	0.31	0.25	1.24

[a]This analysis starts with an equal number of men and women at age 30, in both populations.

will not be exceeded even if the subject has subscribed to the most advantageous health habits and experienced the least noxious environmental exposures. This upper limit is sometimes called the life span. If this is a correct model, any greater life expectancy for the population that is achieved by improving health habits will result in a higher proportion of the population living closer to their individual upper age limits, followed by a very high mortality rate as these limits are approached. Thus, the average survival curve becomes more "squared" at the top end, and we then say mortality is compressed. The extreme, and some may think ideal, compressed situation would be zero mortality till ages Q_i, with everyone then experiencing sudden death! However, if most are not yet even approaching their Q_i ages at death, people at all ages can benefit from improved health habits and fewer hazardous environmental exposures. If this is the case, increases in life expectancy will not cause the survival curve to become bunched up or squared at the oldest age levels. There is then little compression of mortality, or perhaps none at all.

As the Adventist population, particularly the vegetarians, live longer than others, is their curve more squared, or is life expectancy among the very elderly also extended, the shape of the curve being unchanged? The shape of a survival curve can be economically described by a statistic called the entropy function (Vaupel, 1986); this takes the value of zero if the curve is perfectly squared, and the value of 1.0 for a negative exponentially shaped survival curve, which represents the opposite extreme when the force of mortality is a constant—the same for every age. The entropy values for Adventist and California men are 0.187 and 0.259, respectively ($p < .025$ for the difference). The values for Adventist and California women are 0.176 and 0.214 ($p = .001$ for the difference). Thus, the curve is a little more squared for the Adventists. This suggests that beneficial lifestyle differences cause at least some compression as they increase life expectancy. Adventists, particularly those who are younger or middle-aged, are able to live closer to their genetic potential, but it is unclear how close they actually are to this potential.

CAUSES OF DEATH IN CALIFORNIA ADVENTISTS AS COMPARED WITH OTHERS

The differences in longevity between Adventists and others may be due to a somewhat uniform reduction in mortality rates from all common causes or, more likely, may result from different reductions in risks for particular causes of death. If the former is true, the proportion of different causes of death for Adventists would be quite similar to that for others, but those events would just be delayed till later ages; if the latter is true, a large reduction in one cause of death would save more individuals to be at risk in regard to other competing causes of death. Then the proportions dying from particular causes will change. Does lifestyle determine not only how long we live, but also what diseases we die from?

Although it is easy to enumerate the proportions of deaths due to particular causes actually observed in the cohort during the follow-up period, this may not fairly reflect the actual cause-specific forces of mortality at work in the Adventist population. The volunteer nature of the cohort may distort the data for the proportions of subjects found at particular ages and of each sex, as compared to a theoretical underlying Adventist population that begins with the same risk characteristics, but is then followed completely across the whole life span with no losses to the follow-up (the life table approach). Fortunately, distortions in the proportions of subjects at different ages that are due to volunteerism do not interfere with the ability to estimate age- and sex-specific risks, or hazards of mortality, that are necessary to properly construct a life table.

For both Adventists and non-Adventist, the age- and sex-specific distributions of deaths, by cause, are calculated from a series of multivariate life table analyses, each having a particular cause of death as the endpoint of interest, but allowing other causes of mortality to compete (see Table 4–5). These analyses use a recently described nonparametric hazard rate model that accounts for competing causes of death and is exponential in exposures (Fraser and Shavlik, 1999). The results include only deaths of people over 30 years of age, and are compared with the predicted distribution of causes of death for people beyond age 30 who are among the other Californians (Center for Health Statistics, 1999), with the same death certificate ICD codes being used to define the causes. For Adventists, the

Table 4–5. Percentages Dying from the Named Causes and Average Ages at These Fatal Events: California Adventists[a] in Specified Risk Groups[b] and Non-Adventist Californians[c]

	All Californians		All Adventists		Low-Risk Adventists		High-Risk Adventists	
	%	Age (Years)	%	Age (Years)	%	Age (Years)	%	Age (Years)
MEN								
Cause of death (%)								
Disease of the heart	39.0	75.7	40.4	82.9†††	30.7	88.0	44.8**	75.5***
Malignant neoplasms (cancer)	23.4	71.2	19.0†††	77.9†††	29.9	85.3	13.8***	73.5***
Cerebrovascular disease (stroke)	6.6	79.4	8.7††	85.8†††	11.0	91.0	8.2	78.9***
Unintentional injuries	2.9	59.5	3.5	69.6†††	4.7	82.5	3.4	68.3
COPD and allied conditions	5.6	76.3	2.5†††	82.6†††	0.4	74.6	3.3*	77.7
Pneumonia and influenza	4.5	81.8	6.1†	87.8†††	10.4	89.1	3.6*	84.2
Diabetes	1.1	73.0	1.3	81.6††	0.3	80.8	1.3	76.8
WOMEN								
Cause of death (%)								
Disease of the heart	38.6	83.1	38.1	86.9†††	36.0	92.0	41.4	81.1***
Malignant neoplasms (cancer)	21.4	71.6	17.2†††	75.8†††	18.5	80.2	18.0	73.2**
Cerebrovascular disease (stroke)	10.9	83.9	12.2†	87.0†††	16.2	92.7	7.9**	81.5***
Unintentional injuries	1.8	69.4	2.1	73.4	3.1	84.7	1.3	71.4
COPD and allied conditions	4.2	76.4	1.4†††	81.3†††	1.9	96.7	0.9	80.8*
Pneumonia and influenza	5.5	86.2	4.4††	90.4†††	4.8	94.4	3.2	88.8
Diabetes	1.4	76.9	1.3	81.1†	0.4	74.8	2.3*	84.1

COPD, chronic obstructive pulonary disease.

[a]All results are from multiple decrement current life table analyses, using Adventist data for follow-up years 1976–1988 and data for the year 1985 for California non-Adventists.

[b]Low risk is meat ≤1/monthly, exercise vigorously three times weekly, nuts ≥5/week, BMI in medium tertile; Medium risk is meat <1/week, exercise vigorously occasionally at work or leisure, nuts 1–4/week, BMI medium tertile; High risk is meat ≥1/week, never exercise vigorously, nuts <1/week, BMI high tertile.

[c]Asterisks refer to the comparisons between high-risk Adventists and low-risk Adventists. Daggers refer to comparisons between all Californians and all Adventists.

*$p \leq .05$, **$p \leq .01$, ***$p \leq .001$

†$p \leq .05$, ††$p \leq .01$, †††$p \leq .001$

predicted effects of two different risk behavior profiles on the causes of death are also compared. In the first profile all subjects have low-risk values for vegetarian status, nut consumption, body mass index (BMI), and physical activity; and in the second all subjects have high-risk values for these variables (see footnote b to Table 4–5).

When we compare the causes of death for all Adventists with those for other Californians, a number of differences emerge. Although the percentage of deaths ascribed to heart diseases is similar for Adventists and non-Adventists, death from cancer is less common among the Adventists. Note, however, that the average age for both of these types of events is substantially higher among the Adventists. Death from stroke is a little more likely among Adventists, but these stroke deaths occur at much greater ages. Death from chronic obstructive pulmonary disease (COPD) is much less common among Adventists, no doubt due to the absence of cigarette smoking. Death from pneumonia or from flu is a little less likely among Adventist women and a little more likely among Adventist men but, on average, occurs at much more advanced ages than it does among the non-Adventists. Finally, death ascribed to diabetes is less likely among the Adventists, and, as discussed later, this is probably at least partially dependent on lifestyle differences.

In summary, Adventists are more likely to die from stroke; about equally likely to die from heart disease; and less likely to die from cancer, unintentional injuries, COPD, or diabetes—but all of these deaths occur at much older ages.

Equally interesting is the comparison of the predicted cause of death among Adventists who choose different lifestyles (see Table 4–5). The focus thus sharpens from the effects of simply being Adventist to the effects of particular combinations of lifestyle components and how they may influence the causes of death. The Adventists with high-risk behavior show results that are often closer to those of non-Adventist Californians, though deaths still often occur 2 to 4 years later among the high-risk Adventists. As compared with low-risk-behavior Adventists, a greater proportion of high-risk Adventist men die from heart disease and fewer die from cancer, but both types of death occur at ages about 12 years younger among the high-risk group.

The low-risk Adventists allow us to explore the causes of death and ages at death in a very low-risk population. Does their pattern of causes of death differ from that for others? Again the main difference is in the age at death, which is deferred by 12 to 14 years among men for the common causes of death, and by about 9 years among women, when they are compared to non-Adventists.

These results add some insights to the relative risk statistics found frequently in the medical literature and in other parts of this book. People in low-risk populations have lower rates for most causes of death at any year of their lives, but they will finally die. The analyses described in this chapter apparently show that the main effect of a prudent lifestyle is to delay death from most causes. The major causes of death among Adventists, even low-risk Adventists, are the same as those observed in other populations, and their relative proportions are only modestly altered.

TIME TRENDS IN MORTALITY AND LIFE EXPECTANCY FOR CALIFORNIA ADVENTISTS

There have been substantial gains in life expectancy seen at birth in the United States between the years 1900 and 1985 (29.32 years for females and 24.74 years for males), but much of this success was due to marked reductions in infant mortality. For those already surviving to age 50, the gains have been smaller at 9.40 and 5.00 years, respectively (Olshansky et al., 1991).

Over the more recent period between 1960 and 1986, in California, life expectancy at birth increased 4.9 years for both males and females, and in those already surviving to age 65, the increases were 2.5 years (for males) and 2.9 years (for females) (Barnhouse, 1988).

Have California Adventists also experienced these modest gains in adult life expectancy? There is good evidence that in the twentieth century, the major contributors to improved public health were social and lifestyle factors (Berkman and Breslow, 1983). If these factors are still important, California Adventists may have benefited less than others due to their relatively favorable health habits and socioeconomic profile, even in 1960. However, continuing improvements in standards of living, social circumstances, and medical progress are potentially available to all members of society. To the extent that these factors affect longevity, some improvements in Adventist life expectancy between 1960 and 1988 may be expected.

As reported above, the earlier AMS results (1960–62) predicted average ages at death of 77.4 and 80.1 years in Adventist men and women who had already survived to 35 years of age. The equivalent data in the more recent AHS are 81.8 and 84.5 years. Hence our best estimates indicate 4.4 years of greater life expectancy between the early 1960s and the early 1980s among both Adventist men and women who had survived to age 35. This is very similar to the 4.9-year increase in life expectancies (at birth) of both non-Adventist men and women during the same time period. Apparently the long-lived Adventist population has also benefited from forces in modern society that continue to extend life expectancy.

SUMMARY

1. Adventists live longer than others. This is especially true for men. In the mid-1980s, for those surviving to age 30, California Adventist men lived 7.28 years longer and women 4.42 years longer than other Californians. California Adventist vegetarian men and women lived 9.5 and 6.1 years longer than other Californians and are probably the longest-lived population that has been formally described. Our data cannot directly evaluate differences in quality of life.
2. The years of life saved among Adventists are particularly those in the productive middle years of life. This pattern leads to a mild compression of mortality. Whether there is a genetically determined life span and how close the population may be to such a limit are unclear.
3. The difference in predicted ages at death between Adventist men and women is much less than that seen between non-Adventist men and women.
4. Adventist men and women generally die of the same causes as others. A typical Adventist has a slightly greater chance of dying from stroke and about the same chance of dying from heart disease, but is less likely to die from cancer, diabetes, or chronic obstructive lung disease than a non-Adventist. For all endpoints the Adventists die at considerably older ages.
5. Differences in cause of death among Adventists who subscribe to different behaviors are sometimes superficially surprising until we also consider the different ages at predicted death. Adventists with low-risk behaviors, as compared with other Californians, are more likely to die from cancer (men only), stroke, or unintentional injuries. They are less likely to die from heart disease, chronic obstructive lung disease (men), or diabetes. Deaths in the low-risk group occur at much older ages than in the high-risk group, whatever the cause of death.
6. For the common causes of death, low-risk Adventist men die at ages about 13 years older and women about 9 years older than other Californians.
7. Despite their greater life expectancy in the 1960s, Adventists also seem to have benefited from influences that have led to greater longevity in the whole population over the more recent decades.

NOTES

1. Removing person-years from the analysis before the years 1978, 1979, . . . , or 1986, in turn, resulted in estimated life expectancies (for men and women combined) of 83.23, 83.22, 83.13, 83.18, 83.28, 83.30, 83.36, 83.29, and 83.46 years. Thus there is very little evidence of any healthy-volunteer bias that may affect these results.

5

Diet and the Risk of Coronary Heart Disease

Adventist men, and at least younger and middle-aged Adventist women, experience fewer fatal and nonfatal heart attacks than non-Adventists at a given age (see Chapter 2). This observation demands explanation, so in this chapter dietary associations with coronary heart disease (CHD) that may partially explain the lower risk among Adventists are sought. Detailed information on diet and other health habits was collected in the Adventist Health Study. Since no non-Adventists were included as a comparison group, the contrasts were between the CHD experience of different groups of Adventists defined by their dietary habits. One benefit of looking only within the Adventist group is that there is less risk that differences in other lifestyle, psychological, educational, or even genetic factors may interfere with the interpretation of comparisons.

This chapter is the first of three dealing with the possibility that individual foods or food groups can influence the risk of chronic disease. It is confusing to the public and to health professionals that well-designed dietary epidemiologic studies often seem to produce conflicting results when specific dietary factors are evaluated. Few foods or nutrients have not been claimed, on the basis of some study, to be either hazardous or beneficial in regard to cardiovascular disease or cancer. As this book focuses on diet and health and uses epidemiologic data as its main basis, an attempt at clarification is in order.

An important problem that potentially interferes with the interpretation of all studies in dietary epidemiology is that of measurement errors. These occur when we do not measure exactly what we wish to measure. In dietary research this happens when subjects cannot remember accurately what they usually eat, or become tired with answering so many questions and less careful with their answers. The problem is that measurement errors flow through the analysis, often distorting the estimated effects of individual foods on the risk of disease and the statistical significance of the study findings (Fraser and Stram, 2001). This problem has undoubtedly produced many confusing results.

Fortunately, newer statistical methods can at least partially correct this problem in the analysis phase if future studies are correctly designed (Carroll et al., 1995; Thomas et al., 1993). Such studies should include a validation substudy probably containing at least 500 subjects (Fraser and Stram, 2001). In the meantime, it is best to interpret existing data cautiously as we try to draw conclusions. In this book, I have adhered to the following rules before concluding that a food or nutrient probably affects disease experience:

1. Similar results should be found in at least three well-designed large epidemiologic studies in the absence of convincing contrary results from other studies.
2. Epidemiologists should be particularly cautious about results of analyses where several correlated nutrients are included in the same analysis.
3. Some plausible biological mechanism that may account for the effect should be understood.
4. Results from prospective, rather than retrospective, case-control studies should be given precedence. In the latter, the existence of the disease in the cases at the time of the dietary measurement may distort their recall of dietary habits pertaining to the period before the diagnosis of disease.
5. The potential for uncontrolled or poorly controlled confounding of the analysis by other dietary or nondietary risk factors should be carefully considered.

Although measurement error problems also apply to foods, multivariate analyses where foods, rather than nutrients, are the risk factors are usually less prone to biases, which can in theory sometimes even exaggerate the estimated effects. This is because foods are usually less intercorrelated than nutrients. With this in mind, the epidemiologic results from Adventist studies that are presented below emphasize foods rather than nutrients.

WAYS THAT DIET MAY AFFECT CHD RISK FACTORS

Early epidemiologic research on coronary heart disease focused on biochemical, physiologic, and pathologic risk factors such as serum cholesterol, blood pressure, and diabetes, plus one behavioral factor, cigarette smoking. Diet was expected to play an important part by virtue of its influence on other risk factors. However, good research on its disease associations was delayed by the complexities of dietary measurement.

During the last 40 years, clear experimental evidence has accumulated on the link between diet and levels of serum LDL, VLDL, and HDL cholesterol. Saturated fats in the diet raise blood cholesterol, whereas mono- and polyunsaturated fats lower blood cholesterol (Howell et al., 1997). VLDL cholesterol is increased by intake of simple carbohydrates (Albrink et al., 1986; Hollenbeck, 1993), and HDL cholesterol is lowered by diets very low in fat and high in carbohydrates (Albrink et al., 1986; Howell et al., 1997)—and also by obesity (Fulton-Kehoe et al., 1992; Sowers and Sigler, 1999).

Dietary cholesterol will raise LDL levels in the blood, but in most people this is a relatively minor influence as compared to that of saturated fats. A higher intake of soluble dietary fiber decreases blood cholesterol modestly (Van Horn, 1997) and probably also reduces the risk of diabetes mellitus (Salmeron et al., 1997), itself a risk factor for CHD. We know that other cholesterol-lowering substances, aside from the unsaturated fatty acids and soluble dietary fiber, are present in particular plant foods (Howard and Kritchevsky, 1997). These include phytosterols (which chemically compete with dietary cholesterol and reduce its effect) and tocotrienols (relatives of vitamin E that have HMG CoA reductase inhibitor activity similar to but less potent than that of the statin cholesterol-lowering drugs.)

A vegetarian diet also appears to lower blood pressure levels and possibly levels of factor VII, a blood-clotting factor that some studies have related to the risk of CHD (see Chapter 12). There is good evidence that dietary unsaturated fats reduce platelet clumping (Fraser, 1994). It has been proposed that antioxidants in the diet prevent oxidation of LDL particles and that unoxidized particles are less likely to remain trapped in the artery wall and to then cause atherosclerosis (Witztum, 1994). Direct evidence from human studies that shows that dietary antioxidants such as vitamin E, carotenoids, flavonoids, and vitamin C are helpful in this regard is presently scant and inconsistent.

Much less is known about the statistical links between individual foods or food groups and their effects on risk factors such as blood lipids or platelet function, but certain deductions can still be made. It is clear that the nutrients expected to produce less favorable values for CHD risk factors are largely found in animal products. Meats generally contain a much higher percentage of saturated fats and cholesterol, no dietary fiber, and relatively small quantities of antioxidant vitamins. In contrast, fruits and vegetables—with their high content of dietary fiber, complex carbohydrates, antioxidants, and, sometimes, phytosterols and tocotrienols, and the absence of cholesterol—should be relatively beneficial. Certain nuts and fruits (e.g., avocados) contain fats that are mostly unsaturated and they may also be expected to reduce risk. Nuts are probably the best natural source of the antioxidant vitamin E, and many whole grains also contain substantial quantities of this vitamin. It is widely known that oats modestly lower blood LDL cholesterol, probably due to their relatively high content of soluble dietary fiber (Brown et al., 1999a).

Cold-water fish are a probable exception to the less favorable profile of animal foods. These fish contain a particular type of polyunsaturated (omega-3) fat, perhaps because these tissue fats remain relatively fluid at the low temperatures found in the ocean. Good evidence indicates that consumption of omega-3 fatty acids will decrease platelet clumping, although they do not appear to affect blood LDL cholesterol levels (Leaf, 1990).

Thus, much is known about links between diet and physiologic risk factors such as blood lipids, platelet function, and perhaps LDL oxidation. It might be expected, then, that epidemiologic research could clearly indicate that persons subscribing to certain dietary habits, or preferring particular foods, would experience correspondingly lower or higher risks of CHD.

NONDIETARY RISK FACTORS AND CORONARY HEART DISEASE IN ADVENTISTS

It is instructive to very briefly review associations between traditional nondietary risk factors and the frequency of CHD among Adventists to check whether these results reliably duplicate the well-established epidemiology of coronary heart disease observed in non-Adventists. If so, this will give more confidence in the general applicability of the dietary results found in the Adventist cohort.

There are clear associations between a number of traditional risk factors and the risk of CHD among Adventists. As might be expected, strong positive associations were found in the Adventist Health Study (see Table 5–1 which shows these for fatal CHD) between the risk of both fatal and nonfatal CHD events and diabetes, hypertension, past cigarette smoking, physical inactivity, and obesity (nonfatal events only) (Fraser et al., 1992a). These associations are indicated by hazard ratios (a form of relative risk) that are much greater than 1.0, and mostly with confidence intervals that do not include 1.0. Blood lipid results were not available for this data set.

Thus, most of the usual CHD risk factor associations from studies of non-Adventists are also found among Adventist populations. There is no reason to suspect that Adventists develop a different form of CHD or respond differently to biochemical and physiological risk factors than other people.

Table 5-1. Proportional Hazards Analysis Associating Traditional Coronary Risk Factors with Risk of Definite Fatal Coronary Heart Disease: The Adventist Health Study[a]

Variable	Hazard Ratio (95% Confidence Interval)		
	Men	Women	Total
Sex (M, 1; F, 0)			1.67*** (1.26–2.21)
Age (years)			
25–44	0.07 (0.01–0.34)	0.28 (0.06–1.31)	0.13 (0.04–0.44)
45–64	1.00***	1.00***	1.00***
65–79	7.71 (4.58–12.97)	13.95 (6.63–29.33)	9.17 (6.02–13.95)
80+	16.71 (9.23–30.26)	79.68 (37.86–167.67)	36.20 (23.53–55.69)
Diabetes	2.05** (1.18–3.55)	1.71* (1.06–2.76)	1.86*** (1.30–2.67)
Hypertension	2.22*** (1.49–3.29)	1.50* (1.07–2.09)	1.78*** (1.37–2.30)
Cigarette smoking			
Never	1.00	1.00***	1.00**
Past	1.48 (1.01–2.16)	1.82 (1.05–3.17)	1.57 (1.15–2.14)
Current	0.71 (0.10–5.16)	8.05 (3.26–19.90)	3.12 (1.37–7.10)
Physical activity			
Low	1.00	1.00***	1.00***
Medium	0.75 (0.46–1.22)	0.64 (0.40–1.01)	0.66 (0.48–0.92)
High	0.60 (0.39–0.93)	0.46 (0.30–0.70)	0.50 (0.37–0.68)
Quetelet index			
Low	1.00	1.00	1.00
Medium	0.77 (0.44–1.36)	0.74 (0.49–1.11)	0.74 (0.54–1.02)
High	1.11 (0.65–1.90)	0.89 (0.60–1.32)	0.98 (0.72–1.33)

[a] *$p < .05$, **$p < 0.01$, ***$p < 0.001$, likelihood ratio test of null hypothesis that all exposure categories have equal effects.

Source: Fraser GE et al., Effects of traditional coronary risk factors on rates of incident coronary events in a low risk population, *Circulation* 86:406–413, 1992, by permission. Copyright by Lippincott, Williams and Wilkins, 1992.

SPECIFIC DIETARY ITEMS AND CORONARY
HEART DISEASE AMONG ADVENTISTS

Surprisingly little is known, even with only a reasonable degree of certainty, about the relationship of diet to the frequency of coronary heart disease events in either Adventist or non-Adventist populations. The effect of diet on a number of risk factors is established, but the direct link to disease experience, a slightly different—though related—question, is much harder to prove. It is theoretically possible for a dietary factor to modestly change a risk factor that is measured with considerable accuracy, but it is also possible for this magnitude of change to have a biologically insignificant effect on disease experience. It is also possible for a dietary factor to modify one risk factor toward a beneficial direction but to counterbalance this by having a reverse effect on some other risk factor. Hence, it is necessary to evaluate the direct links between diet and heart attack, such as those presented in the next pages, before drawing conclusions.

For each food, food group, or nutrient discussed below, the Adventist data are presented as a focus for discussion and are then placed in the context of similar research from non-Adventist study groups. This is important because the consistency of results across different prospective studies of different populations is one requirement for concluding that a causal relationship is probably present.

Foods and Food Groups

Vegetarian status and CHD events

The first report that meat consumption may increase the risk of fatal CHD came from the earlier Adventist Mortality Study (Snowdon et al., 1984). Overall, the age-adjusted relative risk in nonvegetarians (meat consumption one or more times per week) was 1.51 for men (95% confidence interval, 1.3–1.7) and 1.37 for women (95% confidence interval, 1.2–1.6), as compared to the vegetarians. The results were essentially unchanged when only those subjects with no history of heart disease at the study baseline were included.

The apparent hazard associated with meat consumption was more evident among younger men, where relative risks are consistently elevated (see Table 5–2). In women the effect did not clearly differ at different ages, although small numbers of events at younger ages result in very wide confidence intervals. Adjustments for the intake of dairy products, coffee, and eggs and for obesity, marital status, and smoking history did not significantly change these results.

Table 5-2. Age-Specific Relative Risks of Fatal Ischemic Heart Disease, 1960–1980: Nonvegetarians versus Vegetarians in the Adventist Mortality Study

Age	Relative Risk for Nonvegetarians[a] (95% Confidence Interval)		No. of Deaths (Nonveg./Veg.)		Person-Years (Nonveg./Veg.)	
	M	F	M	F	M	F
45–54	4.02 (1.6–9.9)	0.93 (0.4–2.4)	20	9	20,077	34,899
			5	8	20,186	28,723
55–64	1.79 (1.2–2.6)	1.40 (0.8–2.4)	67	35	19,159	35,297
			39	23	19,909	32,478
65–74	1.68 (1.3–2.2)	1.40 (1.1–1.8)	131	112	13,054	27,451
			99	96	16,538	32,970
75–84	1.28 (1.1–1.6)	1.38 (1.2–1.6)	163	256	6,837	16,950
			234	302	12,591	27,503
Age-adjusted (45–84)	1.51 (1.3–1.7)	1.37 (1.2–1.6)	381	412	59,127	114,597
			377	429	69,224	121,674

[a]The reference category for each relative risk is the group of vegetarians (Veg.)—those consuming meat less than one day per week.

Source: Reprinted with permission from Snowden DA et al., Meat consumption and fatal ischemic heart disease, Prev Med 13:490–500, 1984.

Breaking down the level of meat consumption into finer categories (<1, 1–2, 3–5, or 6+ days of use per week) produced relative risks (95% confidence intervals) of 1.00, 1.44 (1.2–1.7), 1.60 (1.3–2.0), 1.62 (1.2–2.1), with a p (trend) < .001, in men; and 1.00, 1.38 (1.2–1.6), 1.25 (1.0–1.5), 1.58 (1.3–2.0), with a p (trend) < .001, in women. The p statistics indicate that the observed trend of an increased risk resulting from increased meat consumption is unlikely to result simply from chance fluctuations.

Further support for such an association is found in the more recent Adventist Health Study (Fraser et al., 1992b). Analyses (see Table 5–3) indicate that the risk of fatal CHD more than doubles for men who eat beef at least three times each week (relative risk is 2.31), but no significant overall association is seen for women, although the confidence intervals for women are again wide. When the event of interest was a case of incident myocardial infarction, no clear effects were observed. These results are adjusted for traditional risk factors and for the consumption of nuts, cheese, fish, coffee, legumes, fruit, and type of bread.

Further evaluation of the apparent lack of effect of beef on the risk of fatal CHD among women (see Fig. 5–1) indicates that there is in fact an age-dependent relationship (p < .05 for effect modification by age), such that younger and middle-aged nonvegetarian Adventist women do have a higher risk than vegetarians, but this effect is not seen in older women (Fraser et al., 1999a). As most events among women occur at the older ages, the result here predominates in the above summarization given for all ages. By contrast, among men, nonvegetarians have a higher (but diminishing) risk at all ages.

Evidence from studies of non-Adventists has lent support to these observations. Three other cohort studies have included a high proportion of vegetarians (Chang-Claude et al., 1992; Key et al., 1996; Thorogood et al., 1994). In each case, vegetarians experienced a lower mortality rate from CHD than non-vegetarians. Although these cohorts were rather small, and adjustments for other risk factors were not always possible, the results are consistent with the CHD mortality rate findings for California Adventists and will be described in more detail in Chapter 10.

The only reported results relating meat consumption to incident myocardial infarction come from the study of California Adventists, and the lack of any obvious effect in either sex (see Table 5–3) is difficult to interpret. Confidence intervals are wide and allow the possibility of at least moderate effects that have not been detected. Alternatively, it may be that meat is less important for the occurrence of myocardial infarction, which nearly always involves a coronary thrombosis, than for fatal events that are often caused by cardiac arrhythmias, often without clear evidence of recent myocardial infarction.

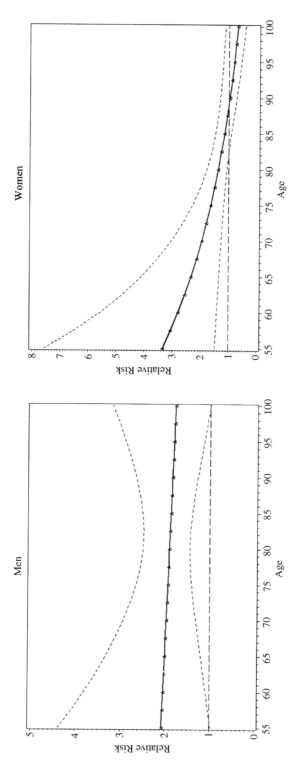

Figure 5–1 Hazard ratios (solid lines) for fatal CHD (95% confidence intervals, dotted lines) that compare omnivore to vegetarian (eat meat, fish, poultry less than once monthly) men and women: Change in this effect with age.

Table 5–3. Proportional Hazard Analyses Associating Consumption of Selected Foods with Risk of Coronary Heart Disease (CHD) Endpoints[a]

Food Item	Frequency of Use	Relative Risk (95% Confidence Interval)	
		Definite Nonfatal Myocardial Infarction[b]	Definite Fatal CHD[b]
Nuts	<1/wk	1.00	1.00
	1–4/wk	0.78 (0.51–1.18)	0.76 (0.56–1.04)
	≥5/wk	0.49 (0.28–0.85)**	0.52 (0.36–0.76)****
Bread	White	1.00	1.00
	Mixed	0.59 (0.32–1.07)	0.96 (0.60–1.54)
	Whole wheat	0.56 (0.35–0.89)**	0.89 (0.60–1.33)*
Beef index (men only)	Never	1.00	1.00
	<3/wk	1.00 (0.56–1.80)	1.93 (1.12–3.33)
	≥3/wk	0.71 (0.32–1.59)	2.31 (1.11–4.78)***
Beef index (women only)	Never	1.00	1.00
	<3/wk	0.92 (0.36–2.04)	0.81 (0.50–1.32)
	≥3/wk	0.86 (0.22–2.59)	0.76 (0.37–1.56)
Fish	Never	1.00	1.00
	<1/wk	1.07 (0.67–1.70)	1.08 (0.77–1.51)
	≥1/wk	1.09 (0.53–2.24)	0.82 (0.44–1.50)
Fruit	<1/day	1.00	1.00
	1–2/day	1.24 (0.70–2.20)	1.41 (0.91–2.19)
	>2/day	1.28 (0.73–2.26)	1.09 (0.70–1.69)

[a]Adjusting for nondietary risk factors and consumption of nuts, bread, beef, fish, fruit, all as appropriate, also for cheese, coffee, and legumes. All food variables are entered simultaneously into the Cox model, along with age, sex, smoking, exercise, relative weight, and high blood pressure.

[b]International diagnostic criteria (Gillum et al., 1984).

*Overall χ^2 $p < 0.05$, **overall χ^2 $p < .01$, ***overall χ^2 $p \leq .001$, ****overall χ^2 $p < .0001$.

Source: First four variables published in Fraser et al. (1992b).

Other recent studies show that diets emphasizing more fruits and vegetables and less meat have been associated with less CHD. For example, in the Health Professionals Study (Hu et al., 2000), subjects with higher scores on a scale that measures a dietary pattern characterized by more vegetables, fruit, legumes, whole grains, fish, and poultry had progressively less risk, whereas the opposite was true with increasing levels of a pattern emphasizing red meat, processed meat, refined grains, sweets and desserts, french fries, and high-fat dairy products. Those participants in the Women's Health Study with higher intakes of fruit and vegetables also showed a lower CHD risk rate, but this was only of borderline statistical significance (Liu et al., 2000a). Broadly similar findings have been noted in the Nurses' Health Study, which evaluated the CHD experience of a group of women with a pattern of low-risk health habits (dietary and others) (Stampfer et al., 2000).

Nut consumption and CHD events

That the frequent consumption of nuts results in a lower risk of CHD events was first shown by analyses in the Adventist Health Study (Fraser et al., 1992b) (see Table 5–3). Even after adjustments for differences in traditional risk factors and in other dietary variables (including use of beef), those who consumed nuts at least five times per week had only half the risk of a nonfatal CHD event (relative risk $= 0.49$, $p < .005$) or a fatal one (relative risk $= 0.52$, $p < .001$), as compared with Adventists who ate nuts less than once per week.

An important additional observation was the consistency of this finding within different subgroups of the study population (see Fig. 5–2). Whether we limited the analysis to men, women, those who were younger or older, who had or never smoked, who were normotensive or hypertensive, vegetarian or nonvegetarian, relatively thinner or fatter, relatively inactive or active Adventists, or those preferring either white or whole-grain breads, the advantage of higher nut consumption is always seen and is statistically significant in 14 of 16 of these subgroups. Multiple-decrement life table analyses demonstrate that Adventists who eat nuts at least five times each week had an approximately 40% ($p < .05$) lower lifetime risk of a coronary event (Fraser et al., 1995) than those who avoid nuts.

Many risk factors become much less important in very elderly subjects (Fraser et al., 1999). However, the apparent effect of eating nuts was largely retained (Fraser and Shavlik, 1997a) even among those Adventists who reached the age of 85. Adjusting for traditional risk factors as well as for the intake of several common foods, the relative risks for fatal CHD among those eating nuts at least five times weekly were 0.66 for men (95% confidence interval, 0.38–1.14) and 0.61 for women (95% confidence interval, 0.42–0.88) (p trend $< .001$, for both sexes combined), when they were compared with those who eat nuts less than once weekly.

A protective effect of frequent nut consumption has now been demonstrated in several other cohort studies, including the Nurses' Health Study (Hu et al., 1998), the Iowa Women's Health Study (Kushi et al., 1996; Prineas et al., 1993), the Physicians' Health Study (Albert et al., 1998b), and the control group of men with established CHD in the CARE trial (Brown et al., 1999b). In all of these studies those consuming nuts frequently had relative risks in the range 0.50–0.65, consistent with the Adventist data. The Oxford Vegetarian Study notes a less impressive relative risk of 0.87 for those eating nuts at least five times per week; how-

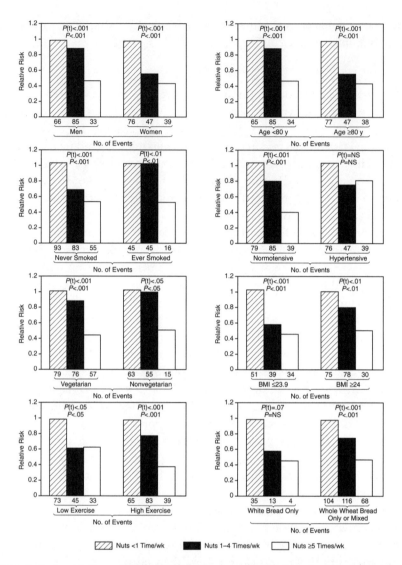

Figure 5–2 Associations (Mantel–Haenszel summary stratified analysis) between the consumption of nuts and definite coronary heart disease events in different subgroups of the population in the Adventist Health Study. *P*(t) is the *p* value for a test of trend; *P* is the *p* value for the overall test of difference between categories. NS indicates not significant; BMI, body-mass index. *Source:* Fraser GE et al., A possible protective effort of nut consumption on risk of coronary heart disease, *Arch Int Med* 152:1416–1424, 1992, by permission. Copyright 1992, American Medical Association.

ever, the 95% confidence interval included a relative risk that is possibly as low as 0.45 (Mann et al., 1997).

One explanation for this effect of nuts is that regular nut consumption results in a 5% to 15% lowering of LDL cholesterol levels, in comparison to the effect of more typical sources of fat in the diet (Abbey et al., 1994; Berry et al., 1991, 1992; Colquhoun et al., 1996; Curb et al., 2000; Rajaram et al., 2001; Jenkins et al., 2002; Durak et al., 1998; Sabate et al., in press; Sabate et al., 1993; Spiller et al., 1990, 1992, 1998; Zambon et al., 1998). These results are in accord with expectations based on the fatty acid profile of nuts. Their high content of unsaturated fatty acids would indeed be expected to lower blood cholesterol if we use formulae based on the extensive human fat consumption studies of Keys, Anderson, and Grande (Jacobs et al., 1979).

However, the important but modest reduction in blood cholesterol levels predicted by the consumption of 1 to 1.5 oz of nuts daily cannot alone account for the 40% to 50% reduction in CHD risk demonstrated by the epidemiologic studies. A blood cholesterol lowering of 13%, for instance, is predicted to lower CHD risk by only about 20% (Gould et al., 1998). Thus mechanisms other than lipid-lowering ones almost certainly play a role. Effects on oxidation of LDL particles, endothelial function, and possible cardiac rhythm control (Durlach and Rayssiguier, 1993) are contenders for this additional unexplained risk reduction. It may be relevant that nuts have the highest concentration of the antioxidant vitamin E that is to be found naturally and are an excellent source of both potassium and magnesium (Fraser, 1999b).

The aforementioned results form an impressive body of detailed and consistent evidence in support of a causal association between nut consumption and CHD events (Fraser, 1999b).

Consumption of whole grains and risk of CHD

The risk for fatal and, particularly, nonfatal CHD events is significantly lower among those Adventists who preferred whole-grain rather than white breads (see Table 5–3). This association remains significant after an adjustment for vegetarian status, traditional risk factors, and consumption of nuts, fruit, beef, fish, coffee, and cheese.

Others have also found evidence suggesting that whole-grain bread consumption, or fiber from grain-based cereal, is associated with lower risk of CHD events, and they have speculated on the mechanisms involved (Key et al., 1996; Morris et al., 1977; Pietinen et al., 1996; Slavin et al., 1997). The content of fiber, vitamin E, magnesium, modest amounts of polyunsaturated fat, and, in some grains, tocotrienols, or lignans, are all possible active agents that may decrease risk of CHD.

Specific examples of other large-cohort studies that found apparent protection from a higher intake of grains are the Iowa Women's Health Study and the Nurses' Health Study. In the Iowa study, there was a graded reduction of relative risks of 1.0, 0.92, 0.69, 0.61, and 0.70 ($p = .02$) across increasing categories of intake of whole grains after an adjustment for multiple coronary disease risk factors (Jacobs et al., 1998). Interestingly, this was only slightly attenuated by an adjustment for fiber intake, which suggests that constituents of the grains, aside from fiber, also had important effects in reducing risk. By contrast, the study found no association of risk with the intake of refined grain products. In the Nurses' Health Study (Liu et al., 1999), a multivariate analysis found a relative risk of 0.75 for CHD when comparing the upper to the lowest quintiles of whole-grain intake ($p = .01$ for the trend). Even stronger associations were found, in the same study, with the risk of ischemic stroke (Liu et al., 2000b).

Consumption of other selected dietary items and risk of CHD

Fish consumption may protect against CHD (Daviglus et al., Dolecek, 1992; Kromhout et al., 1985; Rissanen et al., 2000; Rodriguez et al., 1996 [heavy smokers only]) and against stroke (Gillum et al., 1996; Iso et al., 2001; Keri et al., 1994); however, some apparently well-designed studies could not demonstrate these effects (Ascherio et al., 1995; Curb and Reed, 1985; Lapidus et al., 1986; Morris et al., 1995; Orencia et al., 1996; Vollset et al., 1985). There have been two randomized clinical trials of either fish consumption or omega-3 fatty acid supplementation in subjects with established heart disease (Burr et al., 1989; GISSI-Prevenzione Investigators, 1999; Brown, 1999). Both suggested that there was benefit to the intervention although neither provided conclusive evidence. It has been suggested that the protective effect occurs at very low amounts of fish, such as one serving per week (Kromhout et al., 1995), and this is the range that the study of California Adventists could address, as more than 3000 in the cohort consumed fish about this frequently. No significant association could be demonstrated (see Table 5–3), although confidence intervals were wide (Fraser et al., 1992b). The effect may be specific for cardiac death (Gissi Prevenzione Investigators, 1999; Oomen et al., 2000) or even for sudden death (Gissi Prevenzione Investigators, 1999; Albert et al., 1998a), rather than for myocardial infarction, and this idea needs further investigation. It may also be true that a protective effect is found only with fatty, omega-3, acid-rich, rather than lean, fish (Oomen et al., 2000).

Consumption of fruit may reduce the risk of CHD, and the epidemiologic evidence for this has been recently reviewed (Ness and Powles, 1997). Of the 16 prospective studies reviewed by Ness and Powles, 6 found results consistent with protection. It is known that the dietary fiber of fruits can modestly lower LDL cholesterol, and fruits also contain substantial quantities of folate, and of antioxidant phytochemicals such as flavonoids, as well as vitamin C and beta-carotene. These facts provide possible mechanisms for any protective effect. On the basis of ecologic arguments, Powles et al. (1996) hypothesize that seasonal reductions in the availability of fresh fruits and vegetables may elevate the risk of CHD.

The lack of significant associations for the latter two food groups in the Adventist data is of interest. Specifically, we could find no evidence of any protective association with more frequent consumption of fish or fruits (see Table 5–3). However, very few Adventists eat fish more than once per week, and very few eat fruits less than once daily. Thus, the extremes of a comparison are poorly represented. Such "negative" results must always be interpreted carefully when the confidence interval is relatively wide, as is sometimes the case in these data. Indeed, a nonsignificant result should not be considered a "negative" one when the wide confidence interval readily allows the possibility of a biologically important effect.

That we did see strong protective associations between fruit consumption and several cancers (see Chapter 6) suggests that our measurement of fruit intake was adequate (and there is other, more direct evidence to support this). It is possible that the year-round abundance of fruits in California places most California Adventists in our cohort above a threshold that delivers the maximum possible CHD protection from the consumption of fresh fruits. In support of this, a protective association between fruit consumption and cardiovascular disease (myocardial infarction, death due to CVD, coronary angioplasty, or bypass surgery) was observed in the large Women's Health Study (Liu et al., 2000a). However, the greatest change in effect appeared to occur for those eating small and moderate quantities of fruit and there was little difference among the higher three quintiles of intake. More evidence is thus necessary to reach a firm conclusion.

Drinking water may prevent fatal heart attacks (Chan et al., 2002). This result from the Adventist Health Study was striking in that consumption of water appeared to be protective, but a greater intake of "fluids other than water" was associated with increased risk, at least in women. Drinking five or more glasses of water per day, as compared to one to two glasses per day, was associated with a relative risk of 0.33 for men (95% confidence interval, 0.17–0.62; p trend of $<.001$), and a risk of 0.57 (0.29–1.11) for women (p trend $= .17$). This was adjusted for traditional risk factors and for intake of "fluids other than water." For intake of "fluids other than water," again comparing the apparent effect of five or more to that of one to two 8-oz cups per day, we found no effect in men (a relative risk of 1.00) but a wide, 95% confidence interval (0.45–2.22). In women, however, there was an important effect with a relative risk of 2.79 (95% confidence interval, 1.03–7.62, p trend = .04). This was also adjusted for traditional risk factors and intake of water.

Hypohydration may be associated with low water intake, and this is widely known to cause measurable shifts in the hematocrit and hence blood viscosity (Dvilansky et al., 1979; Kristal-Boneh et al., 1988). In contrast, the intake of hyperosmolar fluids such as juices and sodas can elevate blood viscosity by causing fluid shifts from the circulation to the intestinal lumen (Maughan and Leiper, 1999; Shi et al., 1995). Such carbohydrate-rich fluids are also associated with acute rises in blood triglyceride levels (Kurowska et al., 2000; Stein et al., 1999), which may increase risk of CHD (Karpe et al., 1999; Schaefer et al., 2001; Stone, 1990). Our epidemiologic findings need confirmation by others but suggest some interesting new avenues for prevention.

A recent study of a large U.S. cohort described a protective association between intake of legumes and CHD incidence (Bazzano et al., 2001). This was such that, when comparing a legume consumption of four or more times each week to that of less than once per week, the relative risk was 0.79 (95% confidence interval, 0.69–91) after adjustments for energy, traditional risk factors, and other dietary variables. However, the validity of the measurement of legumes was not stated (in our experience this is a problem), and the investigators, properly from a botanical perspective, included peanuts and peanut butter as legumes. The latter are nutritively quite different from other legumes. As peanuts have been associated with a lower CHD risk (Hu et al., 1998), it would be interesting to know the effect, if any, of legumes apart from peanuts.

Selected Nutrients, Minerals, and Vitamins

We have preferred to work with foods rather than nutrients in the Adventist Health Study, as foods probably involve less measurement error. However, some associations between CHD risk and nutrient intake in these data are interesting and are now reported with caution. These results include both traditional analyses based on food frequency questionnaire data, and regression calibration analyses (Rosner et al., 1990). The latter should provide estimates of effects that are closer to those that we would have obtained had diet been measured with no error. This, however, is obtained at the cost of some loss in statistical power and a widening of confidence intervals. The Adventist Health Study was not designed in 1974 for regression calibration, but the Special Nutrition Substudy (see the Appendix), although much smaller than what would be ideal, has provided data necessary for these analyses.

Fats

Among the variables available to us in the Adventist Health Study, saturated and unsaturated fats are especially interesting with respect to risk of fatal CHD. This is because saturated fats raise, and unsaturated fats lower, blood cholesterol levels. Table 5–4 shows the results of logistic regression analyses with and without regression calibration, when adjusting for age and sex. All nutrients are energy-adjusted using the residual method (Willett, 1998a). This ensures that a higher intake of fat, for instance, is not simply due to this being a larger person who eats more of most nutrients; rather, the fat intake is set in the context of a person's total energy intake. The effects are calculated by comparing the CHD experience of different subjects with values of the nutrients that are one unit apart (where the units are 100 g for the fats, 100 mg for magnesium, and 1 g for crude fiber).

Unsaturated fatty acids show a protective effect in regard to fatal CHD that is either statistically significant or nearly so, in different analyses, whereas saturated fat has a nearly significant hazardous effect on risk. Although not shown in Table 5–4, there was no evidence that total fat con-

Table 5–4. Apparent Effects of Fats, Fiber, and Magnesium on Risk of Incident Fatal Coronary Heart Disease Events (1976–1988), Using Logistic Regression with and without Regression Calibration[a]

Variable (Unit)	Per-Unit Change Relative Risk (95% Confidence Interval)	
	Traditional	Regression Calibration
"UNIVARIATE" RESULTS		
Saturated fat (10 g)	1.12 (0.97–1.30)	1.15 (0.96–1.37)
Unsaturated fat (10 g)	0.86 (0.76–0.98)	0.77 (0.60–1.00)
log [crude fiber] (1 unit)[b]	0.85 (0.73–1.00)	0.76 (0.58–1.01)
Magnesium (100 mg)	0.81 (0.69–0.96)	0.74 (0.56–0.97)
MULTIVARIATE MODELS[c]		
Model 1		
Saturated fat (10 g)	1.14 (0.99–1.32)	1.18 (0.96–1.45)
Unsaturated fat (10 g)	0.85 (0.75–0.97)	0.75 (0.57–0.99)
Model 2		
Magnesium (100 mg)	0.81 (0.68–0.97)	0.73 (0.52–1.03)
Saturated fat (10 g)	1.07 (0.91–1.25)	1.08 (0.84–1.39)
Unsaturated fat (10 g)	0.84 (0.74–0.95)	0.81 (0.61–1.09)

[a]All analyses age and sex adjusted, and all nutrients are adjusted for energy (residual method); $N = 774$ events. Regression calibration calibrates to the mean of five 24-hour recalls.

[b]The unit here is a change of 1.0 in log (crude fiber) expressed in grams.

[c]Severe collinearity between fiber and saturated fat limits the ability to draw conclusions for these variables in a regression calibration model, so such a model is not reported.

sumption had any effect, perhaps because the positive and negative effects of the saturated and unsaturated fats approximately cancel each other. As might be expected, the regression calibration method always suggests a stronger effect per unit of intake than the traditional analyses. This is because dietary measurement errors in univariate analyses always cause effects to the underestimated, and this is also most often the case in a multivariate analysis.

The assumption is that the regression calibration analyses are giving, on average, more accurate results. In fact, both forms of analysis suggest that higher consumption of unsaturated fats is probably protective, although multivariate regression calibration produces wider confidence intervals that inject a little more uncertainty. Specifically, Adventists consuming 10 g/day more of unsaturated fat have, at the same level of total energy intake, an estimated 30% lower risk of a fatal heart attack (see Table 5–4). This is independent of saturated fat, but a larger study is required to clearly establish independence from the effects of fiber and magnesium.

Other well-known large-cohort studies have also found associations between different dietary fats and the risk of CHD events, usually in directions expected from their effects on blood lipids. However, it should be noted that none of this work employs any means of bias correction, such as regression calibration. These results come from the Western Electric Study (Shekelle et al., 1981), the Seven Countries Study (Keys, 1980), the Ireland–Boston Diet–Heart Study (Kushi et al., 1985), the Health Professionals Follow-up Study (Ascherio et al., 1996), and the Nurses' Health Study (Hu et al., 1997). Although some prospective studies do not demonstrate significant associations with dietary fats (Esrey et al., 1996; Gordon et al., 1981; Pietinen et al., 1997), it is typically the more recent, larger studies, especially designed to evaluate diet, that have found associations in the expected directions. Perhaps the most impressive confirmation comes from the Nurses' Health Study (Hu et al., 1997).

Trans-fatty acids appear to increase risk of CHD (Hu et al., 1997; Pietinen et al., 1997; Willett et al., 1993), although there are some questions about the adequacy of adjustment for possible confounding factors. Studies of the effects of serum levels of trans-fatty acids have not proven conclusive (Aro et al., 1995; Roberts et al., 1995). However, there seems little doubt that dietary trans-fatty acids raise LDL levels and may decrease HDL cholesterol levels (Kris-Etherton, 1995; Nestel, 1995). Another fatty acid that is especially interesting is linolenic acid, which is the only omega-3 acid found in any meaningful quantities in vegetable products. The relative risk of fatal CHD reported in the Nurses' Health Study was 0.55 ($p = .01$) for the highest quintile as compared to the lowest quintile of linolenic intake, after adjustment for standard risk factors and the intake of omega-6 linoleic acid and other nutrients (Hu et al., 1999).

Randomized trials have also been used to evaluate the effect of changes in the pattern of fat intake on the risk of a first CHD event. Typically, these trials have involved diets lower in saturated and total fat or higher in unsaturated fats (Dayton et al., 1969; Hjermann et al., 1981; Rinzler, 1968; Turpeinen et al., 1979). All of these earlier trials have their weaknesses but in total leave little doubt that changes in the quality or quantity of fat plays an important role in the prevention of CHD. Further support for this is provided by a cluster analysis of dietary patterns in the Italian section of the Seven Countries Study, where there was markedly lower CHD risk in the group (or cluster) of subjects who all had relatively similar diets characterized in part by the inclusion of greater amounts of polyunsaturated fat (Farchi et al., 1989).

There are also indications that changing dietary fat intake in patients with known coronary disease may reduce risks of subsequent heart attack or death. These studies have often been small and underpowered, but despite this one randomized trial of the Mediterranean diet (which includes a higher intake of omega-3 fatty acids and vegetables but less red meat) found a large and significant benefit for the dieting group (De Lorgeril et al., 1994). Oliver (1997) reviewed a number of dietary fat trials, and others that incorporated additional interventions, and concluded, correctly in my view, that the present evidence is in keeping with the benefits of increasing unsaturated fats rather than lowering total fat intake. It is also very likely that future research will continue to strengthen the case that higher intake of saturated fat is, by contrast, a cause of heart attacks.

The relative strength of evidence for unsaturated fats may seem superficially inconsistent with the fact that dietary saturated fats raise blood cholesterol twice as powerfully as unsaturated fats lower blood cholesterol, gram for gram (Jacobs et al., 1979). Dietary effects on risk factors, however, should not be equated directly with their effects on the risk of clinical events. Dietary fats affect risk not only by changing blood cholesterol levels but also by changing platelet function, the resistance to LDL oxidation (Fraser, 1994), and probably endothelial function (Tomaino and Decker, 1998).

Fiber in the diet

We found that increasing the intake of crude fiber by the multiple of 2.7, when energy intake remained fixed, was associated with a reduction in fatal CHD risk of about one-quarter (see Table 5–4). Our data could not clearly establish that this was independent of the effects of the fats and magnesium, however.

The work of others provides some support for an effect of fiber. However, usually (Humble et al., 1993; Khaw and Barrett-Connor, 1987; Kromhout et al., 1982; Kushi et al., 1985; Morris et al., 1977; Pietinen et al., 1996; Rimm et al., 1996a), the association weakened or was lost in a multivariate adjustment, or it was not adequately adjusted for the potentially confounding effects of dietary fats. A recent report from the Nurses' Health Study found a lower risk, though of borderline significance, in those consuming most fiber, and it was cereal fiber that showed the strongest association (Wolk et al., 1999). Thus, the modest lowering of LDL cholesterol, or other effects produced by dietary fiber, may result in reduced event rates, but doubts remain.

Dietary magnesium

An increase in intake of magnesium by 100 mg per day, at a fixed energy level, was associated with a reduction in risk of fatal CHD of about one-quarter in the Adventist Health Study (see Table 5–4). This moderately strong association persisted after adjustments for age, sex, total energy, and dietary fats, using traditional and regression calibration analyses. As the mean intake of magnesium was 223 mg per day and the energy-adjusted standard deviation was 45.75 mg per day, this implies that subjects in extreme quintiles of energy-adjusted magnesium intake would have CHD mortality rates that differ by 30%. Magnesium is widely distributed in foods but is found in its highest concentrations in nuts, legumes, and whole grains. That these are foods that show some evidence of reducing risk may be no accident.

The epidemiologic literature that describes associations between magnesium consumption and CHD event rates is quite small. An earlier literature somewhat inconsistently related drinking water hardness to risk of CHD, this being possibly due to the calcium or magnesium content of hard water. Marx and Neutra (1997) and Purvis and Movahed (1992) have provided detailed reviews. A recent Swedish report from a case-control study of myocardial infarction found a multivariate odds ratio of 0.64 (95% confidence interval, 0.42–0.97), when comparing those in the highest quartile of magnesium intake from drinking water with the other three quartiles (Rubenowitz et al., 2000). Others have found associations between magnesium levels in red blood cells and CHD risk (Lassere et al., 1994), lower myocardial magnesium levels at the time of an autopsy in cardiac patients (Chipperfield and Chipperfield, 1973; Elwood and Beasley, 1981; Johnson et al., 1979), and possible therapeutic benefits from an intravenous infusion of magnesium in coronary patients (Casscells, 1994).

More recently, the Atherosclerosis Risk in Communities (ARIC) Study (Liao et al., 1998) reported negative associations between serum magnesium levels and risk of CHD, but in men only. The same study (Ma et al., 1995) found significant inverse associations between serum magnesium and mean carotid artery wall thickness in women, but not so clearly in men. The National Health and Examination Survey (NHANES) I Epidemiologic Follow-up Study also found a significant protective association between serum magnesium, CHD, and all-cause mortality, although not between magnesium and CHD incidence (Ford, 1999). It has been suggested that the magnesium content of nuts may be an important cause of their apparent beneficial effects (Durlach and Rayssiguier, 1993). Hence, a possible protective effect of dietary magnesium has some support, and this is a variable that deserves further attention.

Antioxidant vitamins

A strong protective association between the risk of fatal CHD and dietary vitamin E, but only in men, was found in the Adventist Health Study (Pribiš, 1996). However, this weakened considerably and lost statistical significance when it was adjusted for the consumption of polyunsaturated fat. As foods rich in vitamin E usually also contain a good deal of polyunsaturated fat, there may be confusion as to whether vitamin E or polyunsaturated fat, or both, are protective. Our data cannot clarify this, although they suggest that most of the effect comes from the polyunsaturated fat.

The recent interest in antioxidant vitamins has resulted in many reports of the possible effects of dietary vitamins C and E, and beta-carotene on rates of heart disease. Some data suggest that vitamin C may be protective (Bolton-Smith et al., 1992; Enstrom et al., 1992; Knekt et al., 1994a; Losonczy et al., 1996; Sahyoun et al., 1996), although the adjustment for important dietary and nondietary risk factors is usually incomplete or the validity of the dietary data is not reported. Other good studies have found no significant associations (Kushi et al., 1996; Manson et al., 1992; Rexrode and Manson, 1996; Rimm et al., 1993; Stampfer et al., 1992). A recent large British study did find a consistent protective association between plasma ascorbic acid (vitamin C) levels and risk of CHD mortality (Khaw et al., 2001) that was somewhat more powerful in men. To what extent plasma ascorbic acid may act as a surrogate for other important phytochemicals from fruits and vegetables is unclear.

The situation for beta-carotene is not promising—much good prospective observational data have not supported any significant association with CHD (Knekt et al., 1994a; Kushi et al., 1996; Sahyoun et al., 1996). A few studies have suggested protection (Kardinaal et al., 1995; Morris et al., 1994; Pandey et al., 1995; Rimm et al., 1993), but there was either inadequate adjustment for other potential confounders, such as the fatty acids or vitamin E, or the association was found only in subgroups such as nonsmokers, or current/former smokers, or when adipose levels of polyunsaturated fats were high. More conclusively, for this vitamin, there is clinical trial evidence that any effect is either absent or very small (Alpha-Tocopherol Beta Carotene Cancer Prevention Study Group, 1994; Hennekens et al., 1996; Omenn et al., 1996).

The evidence for a protective effect of vitamin E is overall quite weak. Several good observational studies have found apparently protective associations—two for supplementary use of vitamin E only (Losonczy et al., 1996; Stampfer et al., 1993), two for dietary use of vitamin E only (Knekt et al., 1994a; Kushi et al., 1996), and one for both (Rimm et al., 1993). Aside from the reports by Rimm et al. and Stampfer et al., the adjustment for other potentially important dietary factors, such as other vitamins and unsaturated fat, was incomplete. A smaller study of elderly subjects found no associations for either dietary intake or serum tocopherol, after adjusting for other dietary factors (Sahyoun et al., 1996).

Again there is clinical trial evidence, with one study showing a small and nonsignificant decrease in first-event rates with a small supplementary use of vitamin E (Virtamo et al., 1998), but another study (Stephens et al., 1996) of subjects with established CHD (using either a 400- or an 800-IU supplement of vitamin E) found a significant reduction in nonfatal, but not fatal, myocardial infarction. Yet other, larger trials recently found no discernible effect of 400 IU of vitamin E on a variety of cardiovascular outcomes over a period of 4.5 years (Heart Outcomes Prevention Evaluation Study Investigators, 2000), or 300 IU over 3.5 years in heart attack survivors (GISSI Prevenzione Investigators, 1999). Thus, some of the previously mentioned evidence suggests an effect, but overall, this seems unlikely.

Other vitamins and phytochemicals

A few other dietary factors are currently of interest to researchers as they may prevent CHD, but the Adventist studies did not include the necessary information regarding these factors. Higher blood levels of homocysteine have been associated with a higher risk for CHD in some cohort studies (Arnesen et al., 1995; Bostom and Selhub, 1999; Chason-Taber et al., 1996; Robinson et al., 1998; Stampfer et al., 1992), although others did not find this (Alfthan et al., 1994; Evans et al., 1997; Kuller and Evans, 1998). It has been reported that diets higher in fruits and vegetables and lower in fat are associated with lower serum homocysteine levels, and this effect is particularly associated with their folate content (Appel et al., 2000).

As both folate and pyridoxine supplementation can lower levels of blood homocysteine, there is some interest as to whether higher intakes of these vitamins protect against CHD events. At present, the number of studies that investigate associations between the dietary intake of these vitamins and CHD risk are relatively few (Folsom et al., 1998a; Rimm et al., 1998; Voutilainen et al., 2001), and one of these did not show clear protection from a higher intake. However, three prospective studies do link serum folate to CHD risk (Chason-Taber et al., 1996; Morrison et al., 1996; Voutilainen et al., 2000). Other prospective studies have not been so clearly supportive (Ford et al., 1998; Giles et al., 1998; Loria et al., 2000). As yet, there are no intervention trials using these vitamins.

Flavonoids are polyphenolic compounds widespread among fruits, leaves, nuts, seeds, green tea, and wine. They are of interest because many are potent antioxidants, and some may lower blood cholesterol, in animals at least (Ursini et al., 1999). Although wine is widely recognized as a source of certain flavonoids, it has also been pointed out that many vegetables and fruits contain higher quantities of common flavonoids, such as quercetin, than an equal amount of red wine (Trichopoulou et al., 1999).

There is little direct epidemiologic evidence linking consumption of flavonoids to lower rates of CHD. However, those subjects in the Dutch Zutphen Elderly Study who consumed amounts in the upper tertile of flavonols (mainly from apples and onions, but also from tea and wine) had about one-half the rate of new CHD than those in the lower tertile of intake (Hertog et al., 1993, 1997a). No adjustment was made for other possibly protective components of fruits and vegetables, such as folate and antioxidant vitamins, in this analysis. In support of the Dutch findings, a Finnish cohort (Knekt et al., 1996) also showed significantly reduced risk in the highest quartile of consumption of flavonoids as compared with the lowest quartile of intake. The flavonoid intake is much lower in Finland and comes largely from apples and onions (but also from fruits and berries). The association lost some strength after an adjustment for intake of fatty acids and antioxidant vitamins.

In marked contrast, a British cohort showed a positive association between risk of CHD and intake of flavonols (mainly from tea in this population) after an adjustment for traditional risk factors and intake of energy, fat, and antioxidant vitamins (Hertog et al., 1997b). The American Male Health Professional Study found no association between intake of flavonoids and CHD after an adjustment for traditional risk factors and vitamin E consumption (Rimm et al., 1996b). Again the major flavonoid consumed was quercetin.

Thus the evidence remains unclear. This is probably due to inconsistent adjustments for other dietary constituents for which use of flavonoids could be a marker, or possibly to inaccurate flavonoid nutrition tables, or, finally, to the fact that different populations consume quite different proportions of the various flavonoids.

Phytoestrogens are another group of compounds that some have speculated may reduce the rates of CHD. While soybean products (containing phytoestrogen isoflavones, genistein and daidzein) do lower blood cholesterol (Erdman, 2000), there is as yet no direct evidence that they affect rates of CHD. Lignans are another class of phytoestrogens whose precursors are found particularly in seeds, cereals, berries, and some vegetables. They are predictably found at much higher levels in the body fluids of vegetarians (see Chapter 12). One prospective nested case-control study has reported a 60% to 65% lower risk of an acute coronary event for men whose serum levels of enterolactone (a lignan) were in the upper quartile, as compared with subjects with levels in the lower quartile (Vanharanta et al., 1999).

SUMMARY

1. Because of the very large number of foods that people eat, and the reliance on memory, dietary assessment is relatively inaccurate. This presents many difficulties for dietary research. However, newer analytic techniques, the insistence on a validation study for dietary assessment, and appropriate multivariate adjustments should reduce the frequency of false "positive" and "negative" results in the future.

2. Consistent evidence from studies of non-Adventists suggests that broad dietary patterns favoring more fruits and vegetables are associated with a better profile of risk factors and with lower rates of CHD events. However, proving that individual foods or, particularly, individual nutrients or vitamins, are either hazardous for or protective against disease, is more difficult.

3. Vegetarians clearly have a lower risk of fatal CHD, and data on California Adventists suggest that the absence of red meat accounts for at least part of this effect. This evidence forms an important part of a larger body of material confirming such an effect (see Chapter 10). Insofar as there are clearly contrasting groups of Adventists who do or do not eat red meat, this question could be addressed with unusual clarity. It is of interest that the evidence for a particularly marked reduction in CHD events among younger Adventists, as compared with younger non-Adventists (reported in Chapter 2), is closely mirrored by the greater effect of red meat consumption in younger than in older Adventists. Thus, younger vegetarians among Adventists are probably at least partially responsible for their age-dependent much lower risk when compared with non-Adventists (see Figs. 2–1 to 2–3).

4. The Adventist Health Study has provided strong evidence that daily consumption of a small quantity of nuts provides protection against a heart attack. This is now supported by other epidemiologic work, and also by evidence that nuts lower blood cholesterol levels. Probably this effect of nut consumption explains part of the Adventist vegetarian advantage, as Adventist vegetarians eat more nuts than nonvegetarians (see Table 1–5).

5. Adventists who preferred whole-grain bread experienced significantly fewer heart attacks. This is consistent with a moderate body of other evidence from non-Adventists.

6. It is also likely that dietary fatty acids affect the risk of CHD events. At present, the evidence seems strongest for a protective association with unsaturated fats, although it is probable that saturated and *trans*-unsaturated fats are also independently hazardous.

7. Analysis of the Adventist data on CHD revealed a protective association with dietary magnesium. This needs further support from other studies, but as nuts and whole-grain breads are good sources of magnesium, this is consistent with results pertaining to these apparently protective foods.

8. The consumption of small amounts of fatty fish may protect against cardiac death, and especially sudden death, but more research is necessary. The evidence is strongest in those with established disease. Adventist data did not provide further support for such an effect, although only intake of all, rather than just fatty, fish was measured.

9. The current evidence that dietary fiber, cholesterol, linolenic acid, flavonoids, vitamin E, vitamin C, carotenoids, folate, flavonoids, phytoestrogens, oats, and fruits affect risk of CHD is interesting but incomplete. It is quite likely that the named antioxidant vitamins may be mainly acting as markers for other (possibly unidentified) active factors in fruits and vegetables.

6

Diet and the Risk of Cancer

Cancers that occur in different organs of the body and in different tissues are not one disease, but many different diseases. Although they share some features, they also exhibit differences. This complicates the epidemiologic picture since different cancers have different sets of causal factors, although some may be important for several cancers.

Cancers as a group are common, but cancer of a particular organ is much less so. Even the more frequent cancers, such as breast, colon, and prostate, are less common than cardiovascular disease. Thus statistical power is often a problem in prospective studies because it is difficult to find sufficient numbers of new cases of a particular cancer.

Until recently, cancer epidemiology relied mainly on retrospective case-control studies, which could identify large numbers of cancers at a specific site much more efficiently than prospective studies. But unfortunately, retrospective studies may not be so well suited to dietary epidemiology. The cases in a case-control study are those that already have cancer. These persons may well have altered their diet as a result of the disease and, further, may not be able to accurately recall what they ate before developing cancer. Nonetheless, given the focus of this book, it is worth mentioning a meta-analysis that combined a number of case-control studies in Italy (Tavani et al., 2000) and showed significantly increased risks in those eating more meat for cancers of the stomach, colon, rectum, pancreas, bladder, breast, uterus, and ovaries.

A person's accurate dietary recall must be the goal in this kind of preventive research, as we need to identify dietary habits that make a difference *before* cancer is diagnosed. The measurement error problem that pervades nutritional epidemiology is pertinent to studies of cancer and is potentially worsened when retrospective data are used. Thus, the Adventist studies described here are all prospective ones and, where possible, attention is also confined to prospective studies of non-Adventists when they are cited for comparison.

As in Chapter 5, the studies of Adventists cited in this chapter will compare those within the group who have different dietary habits, rather than using non-Adventists as an external reference. The advantage of this design is that the major cultural or nondietary differences between groups that may confuse dietary comparisons are less intrusive.

The effect of a dietary variable on the risk of cancer is usually expressed as a relative risk. In the context of this chapter, a relative risk means the risk of a cancer (usually over a one-year period) in a person who eats the diet of interest, divided by the corresponding risk in a person who eats a comparison diet but does not differ with regard to age, sex, or other factors for which adjustment has been made in the analysis. For instance, a relative risk of 2.0 implies that the exposed person has twice the risk of the corresponding unexposed subject, and a relative risk of 0.5 would imply that the exposed person has only half the risk of the unexposed subject, both risks existing over a defined time period.

HOW DIET MAY AFFECT THE RISK OF CANCER

Dietary factors may influence cellular function in two broad ways—either by direct contact with cells or by changing the cellular biochemical environment, even though the cells never come in contact with the foods. The direct contact mechanism is most obviously possible for cells of the gastrointestinal tract. As many dietary chemicals are digested and metabolized at or soon after absorption, they cannot thereafter directly make contact with other internal tissues, but a few (e.g., dietary fiber) are not absorbed and pass through to the lower gastrointestinal tract.

Eating more dietary fiber reduces the time that stool is in contact with the lining of the colon by decreasing the stool transit time. Thus hazardous dietary factors or metabolites have less opportunity to interact with cells. Fiber also alters the chemistry of the colonic fluid by changing the metabolic activities of colonic bacteria. Then larger amounts of short-chain fatty acids, such as butyrate, are produced in the colon, and concentrations of secondary bile acids are reduced—changes that reduce the rate of cell proliferation (Boffa et al., 1992; Reddy et al., 1994). Conversely, a high-fat diet tends to increase the formation of secondary bile acids.

Other chemicals in foods, such as flavonoids, vitamins, minerals, certain polycyclic hydrocarbons, and heterocyclic amines, may be absorbed largely intact (or with minor metabolic changes) and so can make direct contact with the cells of internal organs via the bloodstream. Some of these compounds promote cancer and are thus called carcinogens (or procarcinogens if they need just a little chemical alteration to become activated). Possible dietary carcinogens include nitrosamines—heterocyclic amines that may be formed when meat is heated to a high temperature—and polycyclic aromatic hydrocarbons that are formed if meat is intensely heated or burned. The effects of most of these chemicals in humans are still considered hypothetical (Bingham, 1999; Layton et al., 1995), although there is good support for a cancer-producing role when they are applied to laboratory tissue cultures or are fed to animals (Potter, 1997).

The second mechanism by which dietary substances may affect risk of cancer does not require them to be in direct contact with cells but may either cause cells to be, or prevent cells from being, bathed in fluids that contain new types of chemicals, perhaps metabolites of the dietary factor. The interrelations may be complex, as some foods contain substances that stimulate liver enzymes that convert procarcinogens to active carcinogens, but other foods may stimulate detoxifying enzymes that neutralize cancer-causing chemicals.

Cruciferous vegetables (e.g., broccoli, cabbage, brussels sprouts) contain indoles and isothiocyanates—chemicals that stimulate the production of detoxifying enzymes (Jongen, 1996) or reduce the activity of other liver enzymes that convert environmental chemicals from weaker to stronger carcinogens (Wang et al., 1997). There is some evidence that these vegetables may protect against a variety of cancers (Verhoeven et al., 1996). Vegetables of the onion family are good sources of the sulfur-containing allium compounds, which are also shown to have anticancer effects in laboratory studies (Fukushima et al., 1997).

Vegetables and fruits contain a number of antioxidants, such as vitamin C, beta-carotene, other carotenoids, vitamin E, and flavonoids. These can neutralize oxidizing substances that are produced naturally in the body and that may also cause damage to the DNA, which controls cell division and multiplication. Thus in theory, dietary antioxidants may protect against cancer, as cancers always involve a loss of control of cellular multiplication. Vitamin C also reduces the production of nitrosamines—cancer-causing substances formed from nitrites and nitrates in the diet. Folate deficiency may impair DNA stability, replication, and repair, as folate is essential for the biosynthesis of purines and thymidylate, both important components of DNA (Giovannucci et al., 1993a).

Since some tumors and tissues are sensitive to the influence of sex hormones, plant estrogens (phytoestrogens), such as lignans (which are found in some grains and seeds) and isoflavones (which are found in beans, particularly soybeans), can alter tissue growth. Breast and prostate tissues, and often tumors in these same organs, may grow or shrink in response to sex hormones. Obesity alters the metabolism of important sex hormones in postmenopausal women (Potishman et al., 1996), increases their blood levels, and hence may accelerate the growth of breast tumors.

Another hormone, insulin, is a cancer cell promoter in the laboratory (Giovannucci, 1995), and levels of insulin are influenced by both diet and obesity. Foods with a lower glycemic index (e.g., beans, nuts, whole grains) are associated with lower insulin levels (Jenkins et al., 1985, 1987), but obesity promotes higher insulin levels (Mayer-Davis et al., 2001). Higher blood levels of vitamin D metabolites (Blutt and Weigel, 1999; Lipkin and Newmark, 1999) reduce the rate of cell division in many tissues. Dietary vitamin D will influence blood levels and may thus affect the rate of new cancers in animals and perhaps humans.

Finally, there is evidence that some of these mechanisms are much more potent in some individuals than in others. People possessing common, genetically determined enzymatic abnormalities may be at higher risk than others when eating certain foods, either if their detoxifying enzymes are only weakly active or if their enzymes that convert procarcinogens to carcinogens are overactive (Lin et al., 1998; London et al., 2000; Probst-Hensch et al., 1997; Slattery et al., 1999). Folate deficiency may be particularly detrimental in those with certain polymorphisms of the enzyme methylenetetrahydrofolate reductase (Kim, 2000). Thus the optimal dietary recommendations for one individual will not necessarily be the same as those for another. Unfortunately, our ability to easily distinguish these different types of individuals, and so establish their different susceptibilities, is still rudimentary, but is being actively researched.

The epidemiologic evidence summarized next can be thought of as applying to an average individual. At present, everyone must consider themselves average, given that individual genetic information is not readily available.

EPIDEMIOLOGIC EVIDENCE ASSOCIATING SPECIFIC FOODS WITH RISK FOR CANCERS

The sections below, organized by cancer site, first describe the data from the Adventist Health Study as a focus for discussion and then briefly cite the relevant evidence from other work. The numbers of cancers detected in the Adventist Health Study can be found by reference to the Appendix (see Table A–7). The results presented here will largely describe associations between risk and the intake of foods rather than of nutrients.

Multivariate associations between cancer risks and intake of nutrients, vitamins, or minerals are not presented from the Adventist data due to our inability to effectively use bias correction techniques, such as regression calibration (see Chapter 5), with the smaller number of cases available for individual cancer sites. The events that we observed were indeed too small in number to provide adequate statistical power for regression calibration, as has usually also been the case in non-Adventist studies. Results of traditional multivariate analyses of the effects of nutrients and vitamins in studies of non-Adventists will sometimes be mentioned, but these data must be interpreted cautiously, as nutrients and vitamins measured by food frequency questionnaires are often correlated and usually contain important errors. Consistency of findings between different prospective studies allows greater confidence in such results.

Colon Cancer

Colon cancer is one of the more common cancers in the United States. It was estimated, for example, that about 107,300 new cases would be diagnosed in 2002, and that there would be 48,100 deaths from this type of tumor (Jemal et al., 2002). The five-year survival rate is only 62% in white subjects. A number of dietary associations with this cancer were found in the Adventist Health Study (Singh and Fraser, 1998).

The risk of colon cancer increased as meat consumption increased ($p = .01$) (see Fig. 6–1). These results, and the others for colon cancer that follow, are adjusted for any differences between dietary groups in age, sex, obesity, amount of physical activity, parental history of colon cancer, smoking and alcohol history, and the frequency of the use of aspirin.

We wanted to determine whether the increased risk from meat was confined to consumers of red meat, or if white meats (poultry and fish) were also hazardous. As Adventists who ate more red meat often also ate more white meat ($r = .77$), multivariate analyses may not easily distinguish between effects of these two classes of meat. Fortunately, the unique characteristics of this population enabled us to make further progress. We found quite large subgroups of the population that preferred one or the other meat, despite the general tendency for nonvegetarian Adventists to eat both red and white meats.

Thus, among Adventists who rarely ate white meat (less than once each week), increasing consumption of red meats was associated with an increasing risk of colon cancer (see Fig. 6–1). Analyzing the intake of red meat in more specific categories (no meat, less than once, 1–4 times, greater than 4 times per week) produced relative risks of 1.00, 1.38, 1.77, and 1.98, respectively. Similarly, among Adventists who rarely ate red meats (less than once per week), increasing consumption of white meat was associated with an increasing risk of colon cancer (Fig. 6–1). Again, using

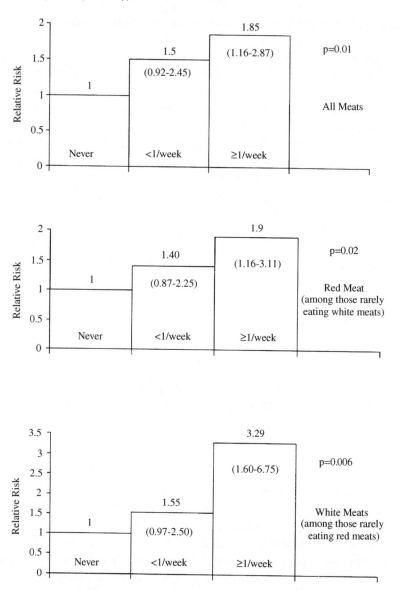

Figure 6–1 Consumption of red and white meats and risk of colon cancer (adjusted for age, sex, obesity, exercise, parental history of colon cancer, smoking, alcohol, and aspirin use). *Source:* Singh PN, Fraser GE, Dietary risk factors for colon cancer in a low risk population, *Am J Epidemiol* 148:761–774, 1998, by permission of Oxford University Press.

the same finer categories of consumption for white meats produced relative risks of 1.00, 1.55, 3.37, and 2.74.

Thus there appear to be independent effects of red and white meats that we isolated by analyzing data within subgroups that had a wide variation in the intake of the meat of interest but kept the other meat at low, relatively constant levels of intake. The results strongly suggest an effect of meats in increasing risk, and it appears that white meats may be just as hazardous as red in this regard.

The effect of meat consumption on risk of colon cancer has been evaluated in many other studies. Most case-control studies have found relative risks of colon cancer that are greater than 1.0 (often substantially greater) among those who have high meat intakes (Potter, 1997), and this is true for four of nine prospective cohort studies (Giovannucci et al., 1994; Singh and Fraser, 1998; Tiemersma et al., 2002; Willett et al., 1990) and in the preliminary reports from two others (Sweet, 2002). Those cohort studies showing an effect include the Physicians' Health Study (Willett et al., 1990) and the Nurses' Health Study (Giovannucci et al., 1994)—two large-cohort studies managed at Harvard University, where special attention has been given to the validity of dietary data. That several other cohort studies (Appleby et al., 2002; Bostick et al., 1994; Goldbohm et al., 1994; Knekt et al., 1994b; Phillips and Snowdon, 1985) did not find an effect has no clear explanation but may relate to measurement errors, and perhaps to a small range of meat consumption, a situation that can seriously limit statistical power (White et al., 1994). In fact, two of these studies did find strong associations but only with processed meats.

The natural constituents of meat—including fat, nitrates, nitrites (Rowland et al., 1991), and carcinogens formed during cooking (Jagerstad et al., 1991; Yang and Silverman, 1998)—may explain an increased risk among meat-eaters. Meat consumption has also been recently shown to result in higher levels of fecal N-nitroso compounds, which are well-known carcinogens (Bingham, 1997). These factors could also explain why the cells of the colonic lining (epithelium) of Adventist vegetarians are less actively dividing or proliferating than those of non-Adventists (Lipkin et al., 1985).

The one food that showed a protective association with the risk of colon cancer in the Adventist Health Study was legumes. Overall, the association was such that dividing the population into those subjects who ate legumes less than once per week, 1–2 times per week, and more than twice weekly produced relative risks (95% confidence intervals) of 1.00, 0.71 (0.49–1.02), and 0.53 (0.33–0.86) (p for the trend = .03).

However, multivariate analyses that also included meats in the model revealed an unexpectedly complex situation (see Fig. 6–2). It was found that meat consumption is only hazardous in those who rarely eat legumes, yet legume consumption is only protective in meat-eaters. This suggests that a hazardous ingredient in meat is neutralized by the legumes. The effect of the interaction between legumes and meat on the risk of colon cancer is statistically significant ($p = .03$). Nonvegetarians who ate legumes

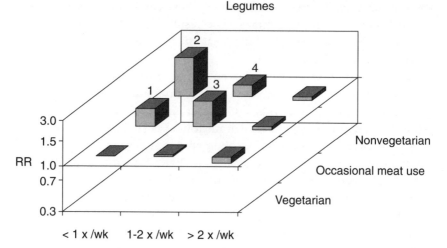

Figure 6–2 Risk ratios (RR) from a model relating nine categories of total meat (vegetarian, no meat intake; occasional meat use, 0–<1 time/week (wk); nonvegetarian ≥1 time/week) by legume (categories as indicated in the figure) intake to the risk of colon cancer. Risk ratios are expressed relative to vegetarians with a legume intake of <1 time/week and are adjusted for age, sex, and parental history of colon cancer: Adventist Health Study, California, 1976–1982. Relative Risks for the numbered bars of the figure are 1–1.55; 2–2.54; 3–1.84; 4–1.33; p (interaction) = 0.03. Source: Singh PN, Fraser GE, Dietary risk factors for colon cancer in a low risk population, Am J Epidemiol 148:761–774, 1998, by permission of Oxford University Press.

less than once weekly had a relative risk of 2.54 (95% confidence interval, 1.20–5.37), when compared with vegetarians who ate legumes less than once per week.

Legumes contain several potentially protective factors, although none is definitely known to neutralize carcinogenic compounds in cooked meat. These factors include dietary fiber that binds bile acids, may decrease the formation of secondary bile acids, and also speeds stool transit time; protease inhibitors that inhibit absorption and increase excretion of ingested proteins; and saponins that bind to bile acids. These possible mechanisms have been extensively discussed by others (Cummings, 1983; Fleming et al., 1985; Kennedy, 1998; Yavelow et al., 1983) and may explain the protection that legumes appear to give meat-eaters in the Adventist study.

Few other cohort studies have looked for associations between legumes and risk of colon cancer. The Iowa Women's Health Study did not find any significant effect (Steinmetz et al., 1994), although the range for legume consumption was small. Those Japanese men in Hawaii who ate more legumes, seeds, and nuts had a reduced risk (Heilbrun et al., 1989), although this was not statistically significant. Case-control evidence is also not consistent and has been reviewed by Potter (1997).

Obesity was significantly related to risk of colon cancer in Adventist men (Singh and Fraser, 1998), with relative risks, for BMI tertiles 2 and 3, of 2.67 (95% confidence intervals, 1.16–6.13) and 2.63 (95% confidence intervals, 1.12–6.13), when compared with tertile 1. There was no hint of a similar effect of BMI on risk among Adventist women. Much other epidemiologic evidence supports an obesity–colon cancer association, and a review by Giacosa et al. (1999) also notes that the association of the cancer with body mass index is stronger in men, but that waist/hip ratio is an important predictor of risk in women.

Giovannucci (1995) has proposed that higher blood insulin levels increase the risk of colon cancer by stimulating cell proliferation. Any dietary or other factors that promote insulin resistance or a higher glucose load would lead to increased levels of blood insulin, and to increased risk, under this hypothesis. Examples would include male-pattern obesity and the consumption of more meat and fewer legumes (legumes promote lower blood sugar levels than many other foods; Jenkins et al., 1985).

Such men were indeed at a high level of risk in our data. The relative risk of nonvegetarian men who consume low amounts of legumes and are men above the median body mass index, was 5.10 (95% confidence interval, 1.48–17.5), as compared with vegetarian men below the median body mass index who rarely ate legumes.

Higher folate intake may protect against colon cancer (Glyn and Albanes, 1994; Sellers et al., 1998), perhaps in keeping with adverse effects of folate deficiency on DNA synthesis and repair (Kim, 2000). There is also evidence that higher calcium intake may protect against this cancer, although associations sometimes lost significance following multivariate adjustment (Bostick et al., 1993; Garland et al., 1985; Kearney et al., 1996; Martinez et al., 1996). The Adventist studies could not provide evidence on these suggestive, but as yet unproven, associations.

Greater physical activity has often (Colditz et al., 1997; Martinez et al., 1997; McTiernan et al., 1998; Slattery et al., 1999), but not always (IM Lee et al., 1997), been reported as being preventive against colon cancer. Our data did not find a significant relationship with exercise, but confidence intervals were wide enough so that an important effect could have been missed by chance.

Prostate Cancer

Prostate cancer is also one of the more common cancers, and it was estimated that in 2002 in the United States, 189,000 new cases would be diagnosed and 30,200 deaths would occur (Jemal et al., 2002). This male genital cancer is one of those that is responsive to sex hormones, and hence possibly phytoestrogens; phytoestrogens are chemicals found in some plants that have a similar chemical structure to human estrogens and weak estrogenic activity when consumed. Dietary associations with the risk of prostate cancer have been revealed by several studies, including the Adventist Health Study (Jacobsen et al., 1998; Mills et al., 1989a).

Our initial analyses of apparent effects of various animal products, fruits, and vegetables on risk of prostate cancer were adjusted only for age. Two foods showed a statistically significant or a marginally significant link with increased rates of prostate cancer: meats ($p = .07$), and fish ($p = .02$). Several other foods showed significant protective trends: dried fruits ($p = .01$), citrus fruit ($p = .03$), nuts ($p = .02$), tomatoes ($p = .05$), and legumes ($p = .02$).

As some of these foods are correlated with each other, it is important to conduct multivariate analyses in an attempt to isolate the effects of individual foods. When all the foods mentioned above were placed together in a model, they produced the results that are shown in Table 6–1. Most of the dose–response trends of the previously mentioned univariate analy-

Table 6–1. Multivariate Relative Risks (RR) for Prostate Cancer According to Consumption of Selected Foods[a]

Food	RR (95% Confidence Interval)	Food	RR (95% Confidence Interval)
Meat, fish, poultry		Dried fruit	
Never	1.00	<1 × wk	1.00
<Daily	1.15 (0.79–1.69)	1–4 × wk	1.17 (0.82–1.66)
≥Daily	1.41 (0.79–2.51)	≥5 × wk	0.62 (0.36–1.06)
Fish		Nuts	
Never	1.00	<1 × wk	1.00
<1 × wk	1.37 (0.95–1.96)	1–4 × wk	0.86 (0.59–1.24)
≥1 × wk	1.57 (0.88–2.78)	≥5 × wk	0.79 (0.51–1.22)
Legumes		Tomatoes	
<1 × m	1.00	<1 × wk	1.00
1–2 × wk	0.74 (0.46–1.08)	1–4 × wk	0.64 (0.42–0.97)
≥3 × wk	0.53 (0.31–0.90)	≥5 × wk	0.60 (0.37–0.97)
Citrus fruit			
<1 × wk	1.00		
1–4 × wk	0.93 (0.65–1.32)		
≥5 × wk	0.88 (0.52–1.47)		

[a]Cox proportional hazards model includes terms for age; education; current use of fish, meat, poultry; legumes; citrus fruits; dried fruits; nuts; and tomatoes.

Source: Mills PK et al., Cohort study of diet, lifestyle, and prostate cancer in Adventist men, Cancer 64(No. 3):598–604, 1989. Adapted and reprinted by permission of Wiley-Liss, Inc., a subsidiary of John Wiley and Sons, Inc.

ses remain evident in these new analyses. Confidence intervals for the high level category of consumption of legumes, and categories of medium and high levels of consumption of tomatoes, do not include the null, or "no-effect," value of 1.0. Nevertheless, when all three consumption categories for these foods are taken together, none of the response trends is statistically significant, although several are close to it. Data from larger studies are required to give greater confidence in these findings.

A subsequent study of Adventists in 1995 (Baldwin et al., 1997) evaluated diet in relation to prostate problems, and measured prostate-specific antigen (PSA) in the blood of 940 men from the Adventist cohort, but 19 years after the first study of this cohort had begun. It was again found that those who reported a high consumption of tomatoes on both the 1976 and 1995 questionnaires had a 37% lower risk of current prostate enlargement ($p = .02$), and a 41% lower risk of either a PSA level greater than 4.0 ng/mL or a past history of prostate cancer ($p = .03$).

A link between meat consumption and prostate cancer has been reported by others (Gann et al., 1994; Giovannucci et al., 1993b; Le Marchand et al., 1994), but little relevant information seems to be available from other cohort studies about any effect of fish consumption. Few other studies have evaluated the effects of legumes on the risk of prostate cancer, but one case-control study reported a weak protective effect (Schuman et al., 1982), and a large Netherlands cohort study found a protective association with greater consumption of pulses (Schuurman et al., 1998). The associations with fruit or nut consumption that others have described have not been consistent, although subtypes of fruit were usually not evaluated.

A hazardous association between fat consumption and prostate cancer was not demonstrated in the Adventist Health Study (unpublished data). However, this does not strongly argue against this possibility as confidence intervals were wide. In fact, some other large studies have found significant associations (Giovannucci et al., 1993b; Graham et al., 1983; Le Marchand et al., 1994; Whittemore et al., 1995), and although others have not (Schuurman et al., 1999; Severson et al., 1989; Veierod et al., 1997), fat intake may turn out to increase risk. Several of the earlier studies did not adjust for energy intake, and this may confuse some results.

Tomato consumption is also found to protect against this type of cancer, according to one other large cohort study of health professionals (Giovannucci et al., 1995). These researchers also found that higher blood levels of an antioxidant carotenoid, lycopene, (which gives tomatoes their red color) are associated with a lower risk of prostate cancer, particularly the more aggressive cancers ($p = .05$). If attention is confined to the placebo group of this trial (the others received beta-carotene supplements), com-

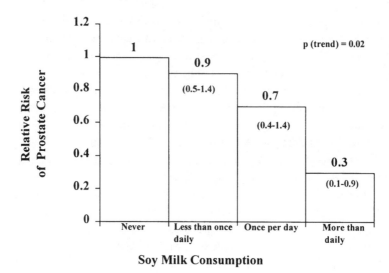

Soy Milk Consumption

Figure 6–3 Association between soy milk consumption and risk of prostate cancer in California Adventist men. (Adjusted for age, BMI, coffee, milk, eggs, citrus fruits, and age at first marriage. Further adjustment for a variety of other variables, including meats, dairy products, different fats and calcium, one at a time, did not substantially change these results.) *Source:* Jacobsen B, Knutsen SF, Fraser GE, Does high soy milk intake reduce prostate cancer incidence? The Adventist Health Study (United States). *Cancer Causes Control* 9:553–557, 1998, with kind permission of Kluwer Academic Publishers.

paring the risk of aggressive prostate cancer for subjects in the highest to the lowest quintiles of blood lycopene levels produced an odds ratio of 0.4 (p trend = .006) (Gann et al., 1999).

Soy milk may protect against prostate cancer. Many soy products contain high levels of genistein and daidzein, which are isoflavones that have weak estrogenic activity. An evaluation of the relative risk of prostate cancer among Adventist soy milk drinkers produced interesting results (see Fig. 6–3) (Jacobsen et al., 1998). Those who consumed soy milk more than once daily were substantially protected against prostate cancer (relative risk, 0.3; 95% confidence interval, 0.1–0.9; p = .02). Although the numbers of cases in the high-consumption soy milk subgroup were very small, the effect remained even when it was adjusted individually for the intake of a wide variety of other foods and possible risk factors. The only other prospective study of a soy product and prostate cancer is of Japanese men in Hawaii: those who ate tofu (a soy product) five or more times per week had a relative risk of 0.4 (95% confidence interval, 0.1–1.4), when compared with others (Severson et al., 1989). These provocative results need further support.

Some have suggested that a higher level of calcium intake increases the risk of prostate cancer, possibly by decreasing blood levels of vitamin D, and a little epidemiologic support for this idea comes from a large prospective study (Giovannucci et al., 1998a). As mentioned, vitamin D may reduce cellular proliferation in many tissues. Dairy products have often been associated with increased risk, and it is not clear whether this is due to their calcium or fat content, or both (Chan et al., 2001; Le Marchand et al., 1994; Michaud et al., 2001; Schuurman et al., 1999). More evidence is necessary.

Breast Cancer

This common cancer in women can occur either before or after menopause, and causal factors may differ somewhat in these two instances. It was estimated that in 2002 in the United States, 203,500 new cases of breast cancer would be diagnosed, with 39,600 deaths ascribed to this cause (Jemal et al., 2002). This is a cancer that has been extensively studied and its nondietary epidemiology is widely known.

As is true for ischemic heart disease, the epidemiology of breast cancer in Adventists is very similar to that of non-Adventist populations. Table 6–2 shows that the effects of a woman's mother having had breast cancer, age at cessation of menses, age at first childbirth, and years of education all give results as expected when based on research among non-Adventists. Specifically, breast cancer is more common in those whose mothers had breast cancer, in those who gave birth to their first child at later ages, and in those who experienced menopause at later ages. Better-educated women have a higher risk, probably because they often defer their first childbirth to a later age. These typical results for well-established risk factors give more confidence that dietary and other associations found in Adventists can also properly represent the broader community.

In contrast to most other cancers that we have evaluated, there were few significant associations between diet and risk of breast cancer in our data (Mills et al., 1989b). This does not necessarily indicate that diet has no influence on risk but, rather, that if such effects exist, we did not find them. As compared to vegetarian Adventists (defined as those who eat meat less than once each month), nonvegetarians had an increased but nonsignificant relative risk of 1.25 (95% confidence interval, 0.87–1.80) when adjusted for age. Adjustment for other risk factors did not substantially change these results (Mills et al., 1989b).

One dietary variable, consumption of cheese, did have a significant association with risk after adjusting for traditional risk factors, where relative risks of 1.00, 1.30, and 1.43 (p trend = .03) were associated with con-

Table 6–2. Age-Adjusted Effects of Traditional Risk Factors on Relative Risk (RR) of Breast Cancer in Adventists

Variable	Category	RR (95% Confidence Interval)	p (Trend)
Maternal breast cancer	No	1.00	
	Yes	1.91 (1.15–3.18)	.008
Age at first live child (years)	≤20 y	1.00	
	21–24	1.24 (0.82–1.88)	
	25–30	1.51 (0.99–2.29)	
	31+	1.95 (1.17–3.24)	.005
Age at menopause (years)	≤44	1.00	
	45–49	1.14 (0.75–1.72)	
	50–54	1.19 (0.81–1.77)	
	55+	1.69 (1.02–2.81)	.06
Education	8th grade or less	1.00	
	Some high school	1.62 (0.89–2.94)	
	High school grad.	1.55 (0.78–3.08)	
	Some college	2.05 (1.18–3.56)	
	College grad.	2.66 (1.42–5.00)	.003

Source: Mills PK et al., Dietary habits and breast cancer incidence among Seventh-day Adventists, *Cancer* 64(No. 3):582–590, 1989. Adapted and reprinted by permission of Wiley-Liss Inc., a subsidiary of John Wiley and Sons, Inc.

sumption frequencies of less than once each week, 1 to 2 times per week, and at least three times per week. However, in view of the multiple testing involved in these analyses and the lack of a clear a priori or prespecified hypothesis, this could be a chance finding. Support from other studies would be necessary before we draw conclusions, and at present this cannot be found.

Ecologic studies comparing average dietary habits with rates of disease in different countries have often found that countries with lower intakes of fat and animal products are those with lower rates of breast cancer. This has been interpreted to suggest that the consumption of dietary fats and animal products increases the risk of breast cancer. Such comparisons cannot lead to strong conclusions, however, as there are many cultural, dietary, and environmental differences among different countries. To settle on one variable, such as differences in dietary fat, as the cause of differences in breast cancer rates is rather presumptuous. Thus, studies of individuals within a single population are preferable.

In fact, an analysis of seven cohort studies combined (of which the Adventist Health Study was one) could find no evidence that eating more fat (Hunter et al., 1996), meat, or dairy products (Missmer et al., 2002) changed the risk of breast cancer. There was little indication that meat consumption influences risk of breast cancer, as there was conflicting evidence from individual cohort studies (Gaard et al., 1995; Hirayama, 1986; Kinlen, 1982; Toniolo et al., 1994; van den Brandt et al., 1993; Willett et al., 1992).

Diets high in fruit and vegetables may protect against breast cancer, but most of the reported effects are modest and usually not statistically significant (Hunter et al., 1993; Rohan et al., 1993; Shibata et al., 1992). One prospective study (Toniolo et al., 2001) has found quite strong associations between the serum carotenoids—lutein, β-cryptoxanthin, α-carotene, and β-carotene—and total carotenoids and breast cancer risk. This is interesting as serum carotenoids are usually good indicators of fruit and vegetable consumption. As there were no adjustments for other dietary factors, it is possible, however, that correlated noncarotenoid components of fruits and vegetables were the active principles.

It is still possible that meat may increase risk, but only in those with certain genetic traits. One study found that consumption of well-done meat markedly increased the risk of breast cancer (relative risk, 7.6; 95% confidence interval, 1.1–50.4), but only among those with rapid or intermediate N-acetyl transferase activity (Deitz et al., 2000). This enzyme is necessary to transform heterocyclic amines formed in well-done meat to active carcinogens. The investigators found, in addition, an odds ratio of 3.6 in those preferring well-done meat, but this was seen only in the presence of yet another genetic attribute, the sulfotransferase *1A1* genotype, that leads to greater rates of both inactivation of estrogens and activation of heterocyclic amines (Zheng et al., 2001). These results suggest that the way we eat and live does not always have the same consequences in different people.

As soy products contain isoflavones with weak estrogenic activity, they may protect against breast cancer, another cancer responsive to hormones (Beckmann et al., 1998; Hansen and Bissell, 2000), and, although all the details are not clear, soy consumption does have effects on ovarian hormone levels (Lu et al., 2000; Wu et al., 2000). There is research support for a connection between soy consumption and reduced risk of breast cancer—at present, largely from ethnically Asian populations. With one exception (Nomura et al., 1978), where data on soy consumption were quite rudimentary, this evidence is based on case-control studies (Lee et al., 1991; Shu et al., 2001; Wu et al., 1996).

We have also looked for associations in the California Adventist data and find that women who drink soy milk at least daily have a relative risk for breast cancer of 0.74 (95% confidence interval, 0.36–1.50), when compared with those drinking less soy milk. The number of frequent soy milk consumers was small, and thus the confidence intervals are wide. Consequently the Adventist data do support a protective effect from soy products, but provide only weak evidence. Although Adventists commonly eat other soy-containing foods, particularly commercial meat analogues, the 1976 dietary questionnaire did not include them as a separate item.

Adventist women who exercised vigorously for at least 15 minutes, three times weekly, had a relative risk of breast cancer of 0.68 (95% confidence interval, 0.52–0.90), as compared with others (Fraser and Shavlik, 1997b). Moreover, life table analyses showed that the predicted age of onset of breast cancers that did develop in the exercising women occurred, on average, 6.6 years (95% confidence interval, 2.22–10.93 years) later. This effect appeared to be stronger in younger women and was independent of obesity status. Others have also found similar evidence of protection (Bernstein et al., 1994; Gammon et al., 1998; McTierran et al., 1998; Sesso et al., 1998; Thune et al., 1997), although it is not clear from all studies whether the effect of exercise is stronger for those with pre- or with postmenopausal breast cancers.

Lung Cancer

It was estimated that 169,400 new cases of lung cancer would develop in the United States in 2002, and that there would be 154,900 deaths from this cause (Jemal et al., 2002). The five-year survival rate, after this cancer has been diagnosed, is only 15% (derived from 1992–1997 statistics). Lung cancer is widely known to be closely associated with cigarette smoking, which dramatically elevates risk. This does not preclude the possibility that other factors, including dietary factors, may add to or subtract from the risk of smoking for smokers or may operate alone for nonsmokers.

The Adventist population provides both advantages and disadvantages in the study of causes of lung cancer. A great advantage is the virtual absence of cigarette smoking in this population, as this allows the evaluation of other factors without the interference of a large smoking subgroup. The lack of smokers also means, however, that the number of cases that develop in an Adventist study cohort is comparatively lower, and statistical power is a greater problem.

The study of lung cancer among those in the Adventist cohort (Fraser et al., 1991) was indeed limited by the relatively few cases ($N = 61$) that occurred during the six years of the follow-up period. Nonvegetarians had a relative risk of 1.16 (95% confidence interval, 0.56–2.38), when compared with Adventist vegetarians who ate meat less than once per month. Such a wide confidence interval does not allow any conclusion.

However, the effect of one food stood out, and that was fruit. Analyses of the effects of other foods suggested small-to-moderate effects, if any, but the size of the estimated effect of higher levels of fruit consumption

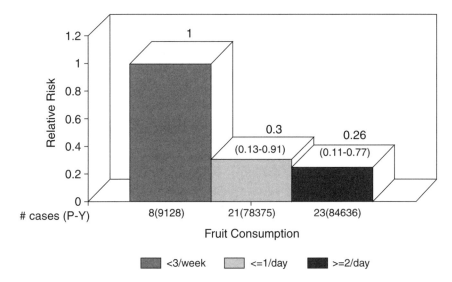

Figure 6–4 Association between fruit consumption and incident lung cancer stratified by age, sex and cigarette smoking history in California Seventh-day Adventists, 1977–1982. *Source:* Fraser GE et al., Diet and lung cancer in California Seventh-day Adventists, *Am J Epidemiol* 133:683–693, 1998, by permission of Oxford University Press.

(see Fig. 6–4) was sufficiently large to achieve statistical significance ($p =$ .006). Specifically, subjects who ate fruit at least twice daily experienced only 25% (95% confidence interval, 10%–70%) of the risk for those eating fruits less than three times each week. The effect appeared similar for both past smokers and those who had never smoked, and for both squamous cell carcinomas and adeno-carcinomas.

We note that the expected effect of smoking on the risk of this cancer was seen even in this population. As compared with those who had never smoked, past smokers had a relative risk of 3.39 (95% confidence interval, 1.75–5.96) and the few current smokers (usually non-Adventist spouses living in Adventist households) had a relative risk of 12.24 (95% confidence interval, 5.06–26.5).

That diets high in fruit and vegetables are protective against lung cancer was one of the very few diet–cancer associations for which the evidence was considered "convincing" by the expert panel reporting to the World Cancer Research Fund and the American Institute for Cancer Research (Potter, 1997). Among the seven cohort studies they reviewed, all gave some evidence of protection, as the great majority of relative risks reported for individual fruits and vegetables were less than 1.0, although many of these were not statistically significant. Case-control studies are also supportive of a protective association.

The effect of carotenoids contained in fruit and vegetables on risk of lung cancer is controversial. Results from combined observational data for 46,974 men and 77,283 women found that an index of intake of alpha-carotene and lycopene was associated with a lower risk. Results for beta-carotene, while nonsignificant, did suggest a lower risk at a higher intake level (Michaud et al., 2000). It is rather confusing that another large cohort of 58,279 Dutch men produced evidence that a different group of carotenoids—lutein and zeaxanthin (combined), and β-cryptoxanthin—was protective, and that this was not true for alpha-carotene, beta-carotene, or lycopene (Voorrips et al., 2000). For lung cancer, there is also clinical trial evidence that for smokers a daily supplement of 20 mg of beta-carotene for 5 to 8 years was associated with a significant 18% *increase* in risk of lung cancer (Alpha-Tocopherol Beta Carotene Cancer Prevention Study Group, 1994). Aside from carotenoids, the Dutch results also suggested that greater intakes of both folate and vitamin C were associated with a lower risk.

Some evidence suggests that cruciferous vegetables (cabbage, broccoli, etc.) protect against this cancer. This may be due to the pungent isothiocyanates and other chemicals released from their cells when they are chewed. Moreover, it may be only those with particular genetically determined metabolic traits that gain protection (London et al., 2000; Spitz et al., 2000; Zhao et al., 2001). Thus, while fruits and vegetables do protect, the identity of the protective component(s) is much less clear. Whether the active principles involved are indeed the carotenoids, other vitamins, isothiocyanates, or some associated phytochemical(s) is uncertain. Any effects of vitamins may also be different for smokers, as smoking can affect their metabolism (Hunter, 1998).

Cancer of the Pancreas

As is true for lung cancer, cancer of the pancreas has a high mortality rate, with an even poorer five-year survival rate of only 4% (1992–1997). It was predicted that 30,300 new cancers of the pancreas would be diagnosed in the United States during 2002 and essentially the same number of deaths (Jemal et al., 2002). This is a much less common cancer than those that we have already considered. Over a six-year follow-up period, in the Adventist Health Study cohort, only 40 of the study's participants died of pancreatic cancer (Mills et al., 1988). In view of this small number of cases, confidence intervals for relative risks are quite wide, and for multivariate analyses it was necessary to divide subjects into just two levels of intake of a particular food.

Table 6–3. Relative Risks (RR) of Fatal Pancreas Cancer among Adventists as Derived from Cox's Proportional Hazards Regression Models: Selected Dietary Factors

Exposure	High	Low	Multivariate-Adjusted Predicted RR	95% Confidence Interval
MODEL 1[a]				
Current meat, poultry, or fish	≥3/wk	<1/wk	2.26	0.72–7.12
Current eggs	≥3/wk	<1/wk	3.42	0.72–16.26
Current coffee	≥daily	Never	2.21	0.61–7.99
MODEL 2[b]				
Vegetarian protein products	≥3/wk	<1/wk	0.15	0.03–0.89
Beans, lentils, and peas	≥3/wk	<1/wk	0.03	0.003–0.24
Raisins, dates, and dry fruit	≥3/wk	<1/mo	0.19	0.04–0.86
Current use of meat, poultry, or fish	≥3/wk	<1/wk	1.00	0.28–3.61

[a]Variables simultaneously included in the proportional hazards model include age, sex, smoking status, and the primary exposure variable of interest (i.e., meat, eggs, or coffee consumption).

[b]Variables simultaneously included in the proportional hazards model include age; sex; smoking status; meat, poultry, or fish; and the primary exposure variable of interest (i.e., vegetarian products, beans, or dried fruit).

Source: Mills PK et al., Dietary habits and past medical history as related to fatal pancreas cancer risk among Adventists, Cancer 61(No. 12):2578–2585, 1988. Reprinted by permission of Wiley-Liss Inc., a subsidiary of John Wiley and Sons, Inc.

The results of multivariate analyses, adjusting for age, sex, past smoking habits, and use of meats (where appropriate), are shown in Table 6–3. As can be seen, despite the wide confidence intervals, many of the effects are apparently quite dramatic. It appears that greater intakes of legumes, dried fruits, and vegetarian meat analogues (usually based on soy, nut, or gluten protein) may have a protective effect. It is interesting that the apparent elevation in risk for those who eat more meat (see model 1 of the table) is probably explained by the meat-eaters smaller intake of important vegetable foods rather than the meat itself. When the plant-based foods are included in the statistical model, the apparent effect of meat disappears completely (relative risk, 1.00 in model 2 of the table). A cautionary note is appropriate so as to indicate that the very broad grouping of dietary habits into only high- and low-intake levels allows the possibility of incomplete control of confounding that may occur between the different foods. Nevertheless, apparent strong effects for several of these foods suggests that at least some of them are indeed protective.

Other cohort studies have experienced the same difficulty with small numbers as did the Loma Linda investigators. Nevertheless, the other two cohort studies that have examined this cancer and its associations with diet both find evidence of increased risk from meat consumption (Hirayama, 1989; Zheng et al., 1993). Whether the effect persisted after a multivariate adjustment for other foods is not clear. These same studies found only nonsignificant associations with various fruits and vegetables. Case-control studies (which, despite other methodologic weaknesses, can enroll large numbers of cases) have generally supported the finding of a hazardous effect for meats and of some protection from a diet high in fruits and vegetables (Potter, 1997).

Cancer of the Bladder

It was estimated that in 2002, there would be 56,500 new cases of bladder cancer and 12,600 deaths from this cancer in the United States (Jemal et al., 2002). Again, this is a somewhat less common cancer, and we documented 52 new cases in the Adventist cohort during the follow-up period (Mills et al., 1991). When compared with those who had never smoked, past smokers (relative risk, 2.44; 95% confidence interval, 1.26–4.74), and current cigarette smokers (relative risk, 5.67; 95% confidence interval, 1.73–18.61) have much higher risk in the Adventist data. Significant trends were also found, showing that those with a greater maximum number of cigarettes smoked each day ($p = .001$) or a greater number of years of smoking ($p = .0006$) had a much greater risk of bladder cancer. This is similar to the findings of many others (Silverman et al., 1992).

Those who eat more meat may have a greater risk of bladder cancer. In view of the relatively small number of cases in the Adventist Health Study, foods were again divided into only two categories of consumption. A multivariate proportional-hazards model found that Adventists who ate meat three or more times per week had a relative risk of 2.38 (95% confidence interval, 1.23–4.61, $p = .01$), as compared with those eating meat less frequently. Even when evaluating this association separately among either nonsmokers or the combination of past and current smokers, the estimates of a meat effect were substantial, with relative risks of 1.52 and 2.40, respectively. However, the confidence intervals were relatively wide. In view of the small numbers and the possibility of residual confounding, these results can only suggest an effect, and this needs to be examined further in larger data sets.

A few other cohort studies have examined dietary associations with bladder cancer (Chyou et al., 1993; Michaud et al., 1999; Shibata et al., 1992; Steineck et al., 1988). Two of these have described a hazardous effect of meat consumption on risk of bladder cancer. A Swedish study (Steineck et al., 1988) found a relative risk of 2.2 (1.1–4.4) with a greater intake of pork and beef, and a study in Hawaii (Chyou et al., 1993) reported a relative risk of 1.5 (0.8–3.2) when meat was consumed five or more times per week as compared to one time or less. Thus, these results are compatible with the findings for Adventists.

The large Health Professionals Follow-up Study (Michaud et al., 1999) found a protective association between consumption of all vegetables and the risk of bladder cancer. Although this lost significance in a multivariate adjustment, the association with cruciferous vegetables remained statistically significant ($p = .008$), with a relative risk of 0.49, when comparing those eating five or more servings to those eating one serving or less per week. Thus, it is possible that meat is hazardous and, at the same time, certain vegetables are protective. Either way, a vegetarian should gain protection.

Epithelial Cancers of the Ovaries

It was estimated that in 2002 there would be 23,300 new cancers of the ovaries in the United States and 13,900 deaths from this cause (Jemal et al., 2002). During a follow-up period between 1976 and 1988, and from 1988 to 1994 in a smaller subgroup, we detected 71 cases of epithelial ovarian cancer in the Adventist cohort.

Both fatal and nonfatal cases were found between 1976 and 1982 and 1988 and 1994. However, we searched for fatal cases only in the middle years of the follow-up period (1983–1988). To achieve a consistent means of analysis, the assumption was made that fatal cases detected then had first been diagnosed 1.8 years before. This was the average survival time for those cases where we knew both time of diagnosis and of death. Fortunately, changing this assumption across a range of 1.0 to 3.0 years altered the results in only trivial ways. We also would not have detected an estimated 8 to 10 cases of those who were diagnosed but did not die between 1983 and 1988. However, unless these were very atypical cases, erroneously counting them as noncases, among a group of more than 20,000 women, should not affect relative risks in any discernible way.

The results (Kiani et al., 2001) were quite striking (see Table 6–4). Age-adjusted relative risks were close to 2.0 for those who ate more meat or cheese. By contrast, risk was decreased 40% to 75% in those eating more tomatoes, and greater fruit consumption was also possibly protective. When attention is restricted to the 60 postmenopausal cancers, the trends were stronger and the statistical significance was greater. Because there were relatively few cases of ovarian cancer for analysis, it was not appropriate to include all foods in the statistical model simultaneously. However, when pairs of foods were included in the analysis (e.g., tomatoes and

Table 6–4. Foods Associated with Risk of Ovarian Epithelial Cancers in the Adventist Health Study: Age-Adjusted Relative Risk (95% Confidence Intervals)

Dietary Variable	Level	All Cases (N = 71)	Postmenopausal (N = 60)[a]
Meat	Never	1.00	1.00
	<1/wk	1.39 (0.67–2.89)	1.59 (0.69–3.68)
	≥1/wk	1.75 (0.93–3.27)	2.30 (1.12–4.70)
Cheese	Never	1.00	1.00
	1–2/wk	1.43 (0.79–2.60)	1.45 (0.76–2.78)
	>2/wk	1.81 (0.97–3.38)	2.10 (1.08–4.09)
Tomatoes	≤1/wk	1.00	1.00
	<5/wk	0.72 (0.36–1.44)	0.55 (0.27–1.13)
	≥5/wk	0.32 (0.14–0.76)	0.32 (0.13–0.75)
Fruit	≤5/wk	1.00	1.00
	1–2/day	1.24 (0.58–2.69)	1.37 (0.58–3.21)
	>2/day	0.59 (0.27–1.28)	0.53 (0.22–1.26)

[a]Adjusted for use of postmenopausal hormones.

meat, fruit and cheese, tomatoes and fruit), there did not appear to be important pairwise confounding, as results were broadly similar to those in the univariate analyses. An exception is the fact that, when controlled for meat intake, the apparent effect of cheese diminished somewhat.

With three exceptions, other published data on diet and ovarian cancer appear to come from case-control or retrospective studies. Of the three prospective studies, the Iowa Women's Health Study (Kushi et al., 1999) found only one statistically significant association between ovarian cancer risk and certain foods, and that was a protective effect from a higher intake of green leafy vegetables. Meat and fruit consumption was not associated with risk, although the lowest level of meat consumption was nine servings per week, which is probably greater than the highest level in the Adventist study. Results for tomatoes were not reported. Another large prospective study, from Japan, did find a positive association with meat consumption (Hirayama, 1981). The Nurses' Health Study analyzed associations between the intake of various vitamins and food groups (including fruit) and the risk of ovarian cancer (Fairfield et al., 2001) but did not find significant relationships. Associations with meat and tomato intakes were not reported, although the intake of lycopene (an important constituent of tomatoes) did not predict risk in their data (confidence intervals were wide, however).

Results from case-control studies have shown significant positive associations between saturated fat and cholesterol intake (Risch et al., 1994), a protective association with monounsaturated fat intake but no association here with saturated fat intake (Tzonou et al., 1993), a positive association with red meat intake (Tavani et al., 2000), and a protective association with the consumption of the carotenoids lutein and zeaxanthin (Bertone et al., 2001). All of these findings need confirmation and do not occur consistently enough to either confirm or deny the Adventist results.

Other Cancers

A number of cancers are not included among those discussed here. With one exception, these are relatively uncommon, and dietary hypotheses cannot be effectively examined prospectively, even in a relatively large data set. The exception is cancer of the uterus, of which we detected 124 new cases. Preliminary analyses in the Adventist data do not suggest any strong dietary effects for this cancer.

The other relatively rare cancers—nevertheless common enough to cause significant morbidity and mortality—include those of the kidney, cervix, and stomach. Cancers of certain other organs or tissues are quite common as a group but comprise a number of relatively rare and different histologic types that probably all have their own distinct causal factors. Examples are cancers of the brain (astrocytomas, gliomas, meningiomas, ependymomas, etc.) or of the lymphatic and hemopoietic tissues (Hodgkin's disease, non-Hodgkin's lymphoma, chronic and acute myelogenous and lymphocytic leukemias, etc.), where the rarity of specific histologic types makes prospective epidemiologic research quite difficult. Nevertheless, the large Nurses' Health Study has recently published results suggesting that non-Hodgkin's lymphoma is significantly less common in women who eat more vegetables, particularly cruciferous vegetables, and possibly fruit (Zhang et al., 2000).

In the Adventist data, the numbers of cases of these uncommon subtypes are very small and preclude any useful analyses. Although results are published in regard to the epidemiology of kidney cancer (Fraser et al., 1990), all hemopoietic cancers (Mills et al., 1990) and all brain cancers (Mills et al., 1989a), the emphasis in these publications has not been on dietary risk factors.

SUMMARY

1. Exploring dietary associations with the risk of specific cancers presents the same challenges that we face when investigating similar associations with cardiovascular disease. In addition, there is usually a problem of small numbers in prospective studies involving individual cancer sites. Despite these hurdles, strong associations with risk of cancer can be detected and are probably causal when they are observed in several diverse

populations and when the mechanisms are understood. The Adventist Health Study is one of a relatively small number of cohort studies of cancer that have focused on dietary associations.

2. The known nondietary epidemiology of breast cancer, and the associations of past and present smoking habits with bladder and pancreatic cancer that have been documented in many studies of non-Adventists, were also found in this population, giving greater confidence that dietary associations found in the Adventist data will also have applications to the general population.

3. No convincing associations were detected between diet and breast cancer.

4. We have found evidence that meat consumption (both red and white meats) significantly increases the risk of colon cancer and probably also that of prostate, bladder, and ovarian cancers.

5. More frequent consumption of legumes was associated with lower rates of pancreatic, colon (among nonvegetarians only), and possibly prostate cancers.

6. Higher levels of fruit consumption predicted much lower risk of lung cancer, probably lower rates of prostate and pancreatic cancers, and possibly less ovarian cancer.

7. Higher consumption levels of tomatoes may protect against prostate and ovarian cancers.

8. Men drinking soy milk more than once per day had a much-reduced risk of prostate cancer.

9. Cheese consumption may be associated with higher risk of breast and ovarian cancers in Adventists, though more evidence is necessary.

10. Regular physical activity has been associated with reduced risk for both colon and breast cancer, although in the Adventist data, we could detect an effect only for breast cancer.

11. Although most of the results reported for Adventists are statistically significant at traditional levels, the confidence intervals are often quite wide. Thus it is important to compare these results with those of other studies (which, unfortunately, often suffer from the same problem).

7

Diet, Other Risk Factors, and Aging

People may develop a variety of diseases as they age. These include disorders of the blood vessels (usually atherosclerotic), cancers of many different organs, diseases of the joints, and gradual loss of lung tissue and brain cells. Many of these diseases have well-understood pathological mechanisms, the effects of which become more prominent in later years.

This age-dependency aspect of disease can simply result from an older person's longer exposure to harmful environmental influences. Older subjects indeed have the possibility of longer exposure to a poor diet, cigarette smoking, physical wear and tear on joints, ultraviolet and gamma radiation, and other hazards. If the effects of these factors are cumulative over time, disease will be more common in the elderly. There may also be cohort effects, whereby elderly subjects in earlier periods of their life had less adequate medical care and less knowledge of preventive medicine, and therefore lived less healthfully. Many more older men than younger men, for instance, are past smokers or past consumers of diets heavy in animal fat.

Our health is affected in a complex way by interactions between environmental factors, health habits, and genetic predisposition. In certain strongly familial forms of Alzheimer's disease, or in the hereditary neurological disorder Huntington's chorea, for instance, the characteristic clinical abnormalities due to genetic defects are displayed only by middle age. This introduces the idea that genes affecting aging may also be programmed to turn on at particular times during the life cycle.

A fundamentally different pathologic process is also associated with advanced age but does not target particular bodily organs or severe dysfunction of isolated metabolic systems, such as those that may underlie cancer or atherosclerosis. Rather, this process involves a general decline in the functioning of most tissues and metabolic processes. Thus, those fortunate individuals who avoid the major organ-specific diseases will nevertheless ultimately die from the gradual deterioration, or aging, of multiple organs. This appears to be a genetically programmed sequence of events and may conceivably be amenable to genetic manipulation in the future. It is referred to here as "mandatory aging." Whether its rate is affected by environmental exposures and health habits remains unknown. These questions were also discussed in Chapter 4.

We saw in that chapter that Adventists live longer than other groups. In this chapter we attempt to discover why this is so. Can the components of the Adventist lifestyle that contribute to this increased longevity be identified? Younger and middle-aged Adventist women, and Adventist men at all ages, have lower mortality rates in coronary heart disease. Adventists also have a lower overall rate of risk for cancer, when compared to the general population. This is particularly true for smoking-related cancers, but the risk for several nonsmoking-related cancers is also lower, probably because of dietary and other lifestyle factors (see Chapter 3). Thus the greater longevity of Adventists is due at least in part to their lower risk of two major classes of disease that are very common in older persons. Whether Adventists also experience a different mandatory aging rate is unknown but possible.

Ideally, we should separately consider the contributions that both specific diseases and the mandatory aging process make to total mortality, but the latter is not yet easily measured in individuals. Thus, an evaluation of the effects of health habits on life expectancy must combine possible effects from both causal pathways.

DIET AND ALL-CAUSE MORTALITY

Traditional cardiovascular risk factors predict the rate of mortality from all causes as well as CHD mortality. Norrish et al. (1995) found that cigarette smoking, higher systolic blood pressure, higher body mass index (BMI), and lower HDL cholesterol were all significantly related to the risk of dying from any cause. Japanese men in the Honolulu Heart Program cohort have one of the longer life expectancies in the world: 79 years. The most consistent predictors of healthy aging (defined as the avoidance of major physical illness and of cognitive dysfunction) for this group were low blood pressure, low blood glucose, avoidance of cigarettes, and avoidance of obesity (Reed et al., 1998). In a cohort of Italian men, deaths from all causes were predicted by smoking habits, diabetes, and high blood pressure (Menotti and Seccareccia, 1988). Several well-designed cohort studies have also found that physical inactivity is associated with a higher mortality rate for all causes (Kaplan et al., 1987; Lantz et al., 1998; Leon and Connett, 1991; Paffenbarger et al., 1986; Pekkanen et al., 1987; Sandvik et al., 1993).

Whether diet has a role in determining the all-cause mortality rate is not quite so clear, as dietary epidemiology has most commonly focused on specific diseases. When effects of diet are evaluated, it is important to not also include traditional risk factors in the statistical model that may causally intervene between diet and mortality. For instance, if vegetarian status influences the risk of hypertension and hence mortality, to place hypertension and vegetarian status together in the model would confuse the results. This is because the effect of hypertension on mortality will contain some of the effect of vegetarian status, and the effect then ascribed to vegetarian status, being the remainder, will be inappropriately diminished. In the analyses given below, terms for hypertension or BMI are not included in the models.

During the period 1976–1988 we found 3293 deaths (1293 men and 2000 women) among Adventists in the Adventist Health Study who had no history of CHD or cancer in 1976. Subjects with such a history were excluded as they may have made recent dietary changes in response to their health problems, thus confusing the picture. Associations between exercise habits, 11 dietary variables, and all-cause mortality were explored using proportional-hazards regression analyses. Only those variables showing significant effects—that is, with confidence intervals that exclude 1.0—are noted (see Table 7–1). The magnitudes of most of the statistically significant effects are modest and often involve the same foods that are significantly associated with cardiovascular mortality. The implication is that they mainly affect the overall mortality rate by way of their effects on these diseases. The three foods with statistically significant effects—meat, nuts, and doughnuts—are all relatively fatty and are either known to affect blood cholesterol or have the potential to do so. Greater physical activity is also associated with a 20% reduction in the rate of all-cause mortality.

Total energy intake may also be related to mortality. Four broad dietary patterns were identified for subjects who were part of an Italian study (Farchi et al., 1989). Those adhering to a dietary pattern involving greater caloric and alcohol intake had a substantially higher mortality rate from all causes over a 20-year follow-up period. The widely known work done on many animal species shows that moderate calorie restrictions result in much greater longevity for the animals and in improved health at all ages (Hopkin, 1995). The moderately lower estimated caloric consumption of Adventists, as compared with their neighbors (see Table 1–2), could thus play a causal role in their greater longevity.

Table 7-1. Multivariate Analysis of Dietary Habits, Exercise, and All-Cause Mortality: Subjects of All Ages in the Adventist Health Study[a]

Variable	Level	Men		Women	
		Relative Risk	95% Confidence Interval	Relative Risk	95% Confidence Interval
Exercise	Low	1.00		1.00	
	Medium	0.81	0.68–0.96	0.82	0.71–0.95
	High	0.81	0.69–0.95	0.81	0.72–0.92
Meat	Vegetarian	1.00		1.00	
	Semivegetarian	1.00	0.85–1.17	1.07	0.95–1.21
	Nonvegetarian	1.16	1.00–1.34	1.12	0.99–1.27
Nuts	<1/wk	1.00		1.00	
	≥1/wk, <5/wk	0.79	0.69–0.91	0.87	0.78–0.98
	≥5/wk	0.67	0.57–0.79	0.85	0.75–0.97
Doughnuts	<1/wk	1.00		1.00	
	≥1/wk	1.12	0.96–1.30	1.17	1.03–1.33

[a]Adjusted for diabetes and age. Also adjusted for differences in consumption of cheese, whole, low-fat and nonfat milk, green salads, fruit, and bread type, none of which were close to statistical significance. Subjects with past coronary heart disease or cancer are excluded. The low exercise category excludes those with chronic diseases that may preclude physical activity.

There is little information relating dietary fat consumption to all-cause mortality, but a large study of men at a high risk level for CHD, the Multiple Risk Factor Intervention Trial, measured diet carefully, using five or six structured 24-hour dietary recalls given by each subject. The analyses (Dolocek and Grandits, 1991) suggested that a decreased risk of death from any cause resulted from a greater intake of either omega-6 linoleic acid ($p < .07$) or two omega-3 polyunsaturated fatty acids, linolenic acid ($p < .01$) and eicosapentaenoic acid ($p < .02$). These analyses were adjusted for differences in age, race, smoking habits, blood pressure, and high- and low-density lipoprotein blood cholesterol levels. An analysis of data from all of the communities in the Seven Countries Study treated whole communities, rather than individuals, as the units providing information. Although this is a less satisfactory study design, it was found that the higher the average percentage of daily calorie intake from saturated fats in a community, the higher the rate of all-cause mortality. More calories from monounsaturated fats predicted lower mortality rates (Keys et al., 1986).

Further evidence that dietary patterns influence mortality rates is provided by a study of 42,254 women involved in a breast cancer screening project (Kant et al., 2000). Among the 23 foods recommended by current dietary guidelines (different fruits, vegetables, whole grains, lean meat and poultry, and low-fat dairy products), a score was constructed that corresponded simply to the number of these foods eaten at least once per week. Women who scored in the upper quartile of this dietary index had a highly significant 30% to 35% reduction in mortality rates when several different models were used, even after adjustment for differences in a variety of co-variates. Moreover, the effects seemed to be of similar magnitude for deaths from cancer, coronary disease, stroke, or other causes.

Perhaps in keeping with the likely effect of fruit and vegetables to re-duce mortality rates, a recent analysis of a British cohort found a strong protective association between the total mortality rate and plasma vitamin C levels (Khaw et al., 2001). Indeed, highly significant reductions of 24% (men) and 20% (women) in the mortality rate occurred for each 20 μmol/L rise in plasma vitamin C. As usual, with a limited adjustment for other di-etary covariates or their biological counterparts, it is still possible that vit-amin C was not the active principle.

Different Effects of Diet on All-Cause Mortality at Different Ages

The great majority of epidemiologic studies show just one relative risk as-sociated with each risk factor, although perhaps separately for men and women. Age is nearly always included as a covariate in these analyses. This means that if more older subjects than younger ones happen to eat food X, and of course also die more frequently due to their age, this does not distort the estimated effect of food X. However, there is generally no al-lowance made for the fact that the effect of food X may actually be very different at different ages. The usually reported single relative risk would then amount to a weighted average of the effects at different ages. If the age range of the subjects enrolled in the study is rather narrow, this prob-lem is minimized, but then the ability to generalize the results to other ages is limited.

Hence we have used proportional-hazards regressions, which include a product term (e.g., meat $\times$ age) between each risk factor and age, to in-vestigate whether or not relative risks are indeed constant across different ages. If they are not, such differences should be reported. Indeed, we have already seen the results of one such (univariate) analysis in Figure 5–1, where the effect of being a nonvegetarian on the risk of CHD was much greater for younger than older women. The results of further multivariate analyses of this sort for vegetarian status and other risk factors are shown in Table 7–2. Each entry in the table is the relative risk—it compares risks when the particular variable is present with when it is absent. The multi-variate model always includes terms for vegetarian status, nut consump-tion, physical activity, body mass index, and for smokers versus those who have never smoked. When diabetes or hypertension are the variables of in-

Table 7-2. Do the Effects of Traditional Risk Factors on Coronary Heart Disease (CHD) and All-Cause Mortality Vary by Age? Multivariate Analysis[a] in the Adventist Health Study

Risk Factor	At Age 52.5	At Age 82.5	At Age 92.5	p[b]
	Relative Risks			
ALL-CAUSE MORTALITY[c]				
Men				
Nonvegetarian	1.67	1.12	0.98	.004
Diabetes	2.25	1.66	1.50	.18
Hypertension	2.05	1.53	1.38	.03
Women				
Nonvegetarian	1.38	1.14	1.07	.08
Diabetes	3.63	1.76	1.38	.0001
Hypertension	1.44	1.35	1.33	.55
CHD MORTALITY				
Men				
Nonvegetarian	2.19	1.71	1.57	.49
Low nut consumption	1.96	1.32	1.15	.35
High BMI	2.80	1.27	0.97	.05
Diabetes	3.22	1.79	1.47	.27
Hypertension	3.30	1.61	1.26	.04
Women				
Nonvegetarian	2.65	1.16	0.88	.02
Low nut consumption	0.54	1.39	1.92	<.02
Low BMI	1.87	1.34	1.20	.39
High BMI	4.45	1.51	1.05	.004
Diabetes	8.26	2.63	1.79	<.002
Hypertension	6.00	2.16	1.54	.001

BMI, body mass index.

[a]Reference group is low-risk status for each variable in turn, which for BMI is low BMI in men but medium BMI in women. All variables (including medium risk values) were included in the statistical model.

[b]Test of whether the differences by age are statistically significant.

[c]Selected variables—those where effect modification by age was statistically significant, or nearly so, for either men or women.

terest, they are also added to the model, so their effects are described independently of other correlated risk factors.

Although younger nonvegetarians had a greater all-cause mortality rate than younger vegetarian Adventists, this difference largely disappeared by the oldest ages. As most deaths occur during old age, this explains why there is only a modest overall protective effect for vegetarianism (see Table 7–1). A similar situation was found in the earlier Adventist Mortality Study, in which nonvegetarian men, when compared with vegetarians, showed a relative risk of dying, from any cause, of 3.09 at age 50, but corresponding results at ages 80 and 90 were 1.54 and 1.22. Nonvegetarian women showed a 53% increase in risk at age 50 (although not statistically significant), but little suggestion of any effect at age 80 or older (data are from an unpublished analysis). This pattern does mean that premature deaths are the ones prevented, as they are the deaths that occur at younger ages.

Diabetes is a particularly important risk factor for both CHD and all-cause mortality, and Table 7–2 shows that it also has a much greater effect in younger subjects, particularly younger women. In addition, the hazardous effects of high BMI and hypertension are much greater in younger subjects.

Different Effects of Diet on CHD Mortality at Different Ages

We have just seen that important differences were often found in the effect of risk factors on all-cause mortality rates at different ages. Similar differences by age, when risk of CHD is analyzed, are even more striking in magnitude (see the lower part of Table 7–2).

Indeed, there is clear evidence of major differences, by age, in the effect of most of these factors on the risk of CHD in women, but in men, aside from a high BMI and diabetes, similar trends do not achieve statistical significance. Relative risks for CHD that are associated with nonvegetarianism, high BMI, diabetes, and hypertension are between three and eight in younger women, but are much lower in older women.

However, the protective effect of nut consumption for women appears to be greater at older ages. Indeed, it appears at first that low levels of nut consumption may protect younger women, but more detailed modeling shows that the few events among younger women result in very wide confidence intervals here. Thus this unexpected result is easily compatible with a chance fluctuation that might occur with a neutral or even a moderately hazardous true effect.

Surprisingly little detailed data are available from other sources concerning age-dependency as it relates to the effects of risk factors on either CHD or all-cause mortality. The Honolulu Heart Program noted that cigarette smoking was a greater risk for those who are less than 60 as compared with those who are older (Benfante et al., 1989). Other factors showed little variation in their effects at the two age groups. However, the average ages of the two groups differed by only 7.6 years, so differences in the risk-factor effects would be difficult to detect. An analysis of Framingham Heart Study data (Psaty et al., 1990) has demonstrated a marked decline in the effects of smoking and higher blood cholesterol on risk of CHD as age increased from 35 and 84 years, and probably a decline (though not statistically significant) in the effect of higher blood pressure with age. In another very large study (Stevens et al., 1998), the effect of obesity in increasing all-cause or cardiovascular mortality declined significantly from ages 35 to 85, and was essentially absent by age 75 in women and age 85 in men. Thus these results, broadly speaking, agree with those found for the same, or related, variables in Adventists, but the Adventist data extend the age range of the results and pertain mainly to behavioral variables.

RISK FACTORS, CHD, AND ALL-CAUSE MORTALITY IN THE OLDEST-OLD

The information from Adventists cited in the preceding section comes from statistical modeling of the effects at different ages, and suggests that effects were often much weaker at the oldest ages. As the very elderly population is rapidly increasing in many economically developed countries, a high proportion of all chronic diseases in communities are found in this age group. Thus associations of mortality with lifestyle in the very elderly deserve special scrutiny. The discussion that follows gives a close look at associations when analyses are restricted to Adventists aged 85 and older.

The Adventist Health Study did not impose an upper limit to the age at entry, and indeed there were men who enrolled in the study at the age of 99 and women who enrolled at the age of 100. However, during the follow-up (1976–1988), we observed men and women, over the age of 84, for a total of 3445 person-years (men) and 8383 person-years (women), respectively, and also recorded 451 and 936 deaths within this age range for men and women, respectively. This is perhaps the largest published data set of very elderly subjects that includes detailed dietary and lifestyle information.

Important protective effects (see Table 7–3) in this age group are seen for greater exercise and nut consumption, and hazardous effects are seen for greater doughnut consumption and the presence of diabetes mellitus (Fraser and Shavlik, 1997a). Men who ate more beef had a greater risk of CHD, but there is no evidence for this in the oldest women. Similar analyses for legumes, green salads, cheese, milk, sweet desserts, fish, bread, past smoking habits, and vitamin E supplementation did not suggest any significant effects on either CHD mortality or all-cause mortality in this age range. As shown in Table 7–2, when the focus is on a behavioral variable, hypertension and diabetes are omitted as they may be intervening variables between diet and mortality.

Different effects of red meat on the risk of CHD in men and women are particularly evident in this age range. As suggested by the analyses in the whole cohort (see Table 7–2), harmful effects of red meat on all-cause or CHD mortality in women have probably disappeared at these oldest ages, but this is not so for men. Further, the apparent protective effects of

Table 7–3. Multivariate Proportional Hazards Evaluation of the Effects of Selected Risk Factors and Foods on the Relative Risks (RR) of All-Cause and Coronary Heart Disease (CHD) Mortality: Adventists over Age 84[a]

	All-Cause Mortality		CHD Mortality	
Variable	RR	95% Confidence Interval	RR	95% Confidence Interval
Gender				
Female	1.00		1.00	
Male	1.39	1.21–1.59	1.03	0.73–1.46
Diabetes				
No	1.00		1.00	
Yes	1.48	1.28–1.72	1.98	1.42–2.76
Exercise				
Low[b]	1.00***		1.00***	
Medium	0.80	0.69–0.93	0.64	0.47–0.88
High	0.78	0.68–0.89	0.57	0.43–0.77
Nuts				
<1/wk	1.00**		1.00**	
1–4/wk	0.88	0.78–0.99	0.74	0.57–0.96
≥5/wk	0.83	0.73–0.94	0.59	0.44–0.79
Doughnuts				
<1/wk	1.00		1.00	
≥1/wk	1.21	1.06–1.37	1.39	1.06–1.83
Meat (Men)				
Never or rare	1.00		1.00*	
1–3/wk	0.97	0.79–1.18	1.59	1.02–2.49
≥4/wk	0.99	0.82–1.19	1.52	0.98–2.36
Meat (Women)				
Never or rare	1.00		1.00	
1–3/wk	1.00	0.87–1.15	1.03	0.75–1.41
≥4/wk	1.02	0.89–1.17	0.89	0.65–1.23

[a]All variables entered to the model plus specific year of age. Also adjusted for intake of cheese, nonfat, lowfat, and whole milk; green salads; and fruit and sweet desserts, none of which were statistically significant. Trend tests for variables at three levels: $^*p = .05$, $^{**}p \leq .01$, $^{***}p \leq .001$.

[b]Among those not suffering chronic disease at baseline that may prevent vigorous activity.

nut consumption persist unabated in this oldest group. Thus, these and other effects predicted at the oldest ages, by models applied to the whole cohort, are confirmed when the analyses are restricted to these ages.

Whether dietary factors affect mortality in other populations that are exclusively from the oldest groups has rarely been studied. However, some study groups over the ages of 65 to 70 have included those at the oldest ages, and it was found that the same variables important in younger individuals retain some effect in older subjects. A study of Greeks over age 70, living in three villages, found that adherence to a traditional Mediterranean diet (the details of which were defined before the analysis) was associated with decreased overall mortality (Trichopoulou et al., 1995). A group of subjects in Rome who were over 65 were studied prospectively, and those with greater intakes of citrus fruit, milk and yogurt, ascorbic acid, riboflavin, and linoleic acid had lower mortality risks. Greater consumption of meat (more than once weekly), however, was associated with greater mortality (relative risk, 1.82; 95% confidence interval, 0.91–3.60) (Fortes et al., 2000).

The continued importance of several traditional anthropometric and physiologic risk factors in old age is less certain. An investigation of British subjects over 70 years of age could find no significant association between survival time and height, body weight, blood pressure, or heart rate (Anderson and Cowan, 1976). A U.S. study of subjects over age 74 (the average age was 79.2 years) demonstrated that physical inactivity continues to be a risk factor for mortality in this age group (Langer et al., 1994), and that results were unchanged when an adjustment was made for health status at the study baseline.

A Danish cohort that had been studied for 26 years was used to show that baseline values for traditional risk factors measured at age 50 continued to strongly predict CHD events that occurred at ages 70 to 76 (Thomsen et al., 1995). There is a subtle distinction between this situation and that where risk factors are actually measured at the elderly ages, as then the possibility that habits were different at earlier ages is ignored. It is possible that the habits from earlier ages as well as current habits determine disease at the oldest ages. As habits are often relatively constant over many decades, the Adventist data (where lifestyle was measured at the oldest ages) cannot help make this distinction. Nevertheless, the suggestion from the Danish study is that risk factors have a long-lasting effect on health. Whether changes in behaviors or risk factors that occur at the oldest ages will still change risk is unclear.

Risk factor values measured at the oldest ages generally have smaller proportionate effects on mortality than at younger ages, but are still important. This is particularly so from the perspective of the number of events potentially saved by a better risk factor status. As there is a high absolute risk of dying at these ages, small proportionate reductions may save many lives.

HEALTH HABITS AND ALL-CAUSE MORTALITY IN A BLACK CALIFORNIA ADVENTIST POPULATION

The Adventist Health Study included a much smaller number of black members. The census questionnaire was completed by 3475 black Adventists and the lifestyle questionnaire by 1739 black Adventists (see the

Appendix, Table A–3). The latter group provided descriptive dietary data, and analyses based on these are contained in one of the very few published reports relating diet to mortality among black Americans. A summary of the frequency of consumption of selected foods by black Adventists was shown in Table 1–5. In comparison to white California Adventists, rather fewer black Adventists are vegetarians (meat less than once per week), and the black nonvegetarians eat proportionately more fish and poultry and less beef than white nonvegetarians.

We did not have information on the causes of death in this black population, but we could relate dietary habits and other characteristics to the sex-specific risk of all-cause mortality (see Table 7–4), adjusting for age, smoking habits, and physical activity (Fraser et al., 1997b). A powerful adverse effect of hypertension was found (relative risk, 2.5, $p < .001$), consistent with results from many other populations. However, we did not adjust for hypertension in the dietary analyses as it is possible that the dietary variables may act on mortality in part through their effects on blood pressure (see Chapters 8 and 12). There was not clear evidence of a hazardous effect of greater meat consumption among the black Adventists, although confidence intervals are wide and a sizable effect may have been missed by chance. Nevertheless, the only variables showing even a hint of increased risk from greater consumption were any meat, and cheese consumed at least three times weekly ($p = .15$).

By contrast, a consistent 30% to 40% reduction in the risk of dying is found for those who consumed nuts at least five times per week ($p < .05$), and there are also reduced risks for those eating more fruits ($p < .01$), salads ($p < .05$), and perhaps cooked green vegetables. These results do not arise simply because the greater consumers of nuts, fruits, or salads are more likely to be vegetarians, as inclusion of the consumption of meat, fish, and poultry as covariates in the model resulted in relative risks of 1.00, 0.60, and 0.55 for increased nut consumption; 1.00, 0.39, and 0.56 for increased fruit consumption; and 1.00, 0.57, and 0.66 for increased green salad consumption—all quite similar to those found in Table 7–4.

Our analyses were based on a relatively small study population, there being only 416 deaths recorded during the follow-up period. Nevertheless, results are broadly consistent with trends found among white populations, suggesting that black Americans are also wise to prefer fruits, nuts, and vegetables to animal products. The clear protective association seen again with greater nut consumption is noteworthy, this time in relation to all-cause mortality.

Another study of the mortality experience of black Adventists evaluated the 116 deaths among a group of 6002 members of the South Atlantic Conference of Seventh-day Adventists during the years 1980–1987

Table 7–4. Associations between Selected Foods and All-Cause Mortality in Black Respondents to the Lifestyle Questionnaire, Adjusted for Age, Smoking, and Exercise[a] ($N = 1668$)

Variable and Frequency of Use	Hazard Ratio (95% Confidence Interval)		
	Men	Women	Both Sexes
Meat, Fish, or Poultry			
Never[b]	1.00	1.00	1.00
<1×/wk	0.6 (0.2–2.0)	3.2 (1.4–6.9)	1.8 (1.0–3.4)
1–4×/wk	1.1 (0.5–2.6)	1.0 (0.4–2.8)	1.1 (0.6–2.1)
>4×/wk	1.4 (0.7–2.8)	1.3 (0.6–2.9)	1.3 (0.8–2.2)
Nuts			
<1×/wk[b]	1.00	1.00	1.00
1–4/wk	0.7 (0.4–1.4)	0.4 (0.2–0.9)	0.6 (0.4–0.9)
≥5×/wk	0.6 (0.2–1.3)	0.5 (0.2–1.2)	0.6 (0.3–1.0)
Legumes			
<1×/wk[b]	1.00	1.00	1.00
1–2×/wk	0.8 (0.4–1.4)	1.0 (0.5–1.9)	0.9 (0.6–1.4)
>2×/wk	0.6 (0.3–1.2)	1.4 (0.7–2.8)	0.8 (0.5–1.4)
Fruit			
<1×/wk[b]	1.00	1.00	1.00
1–14×/wk	0.3 (0.1–0.7)	0.5 (0.2–1.1)	0.4 (0.2–0.7)
>2×/day	0.6 (0.3–1.1)	0.6 (0.3–1.1)	0.6 (0.4–0.9)
Cooked green vegetables			
≤2×/wk[b]	1.00	1.00	1.00
3–6×/wk	0.5 (0.3–1.0)	0.7 (0.4–1.5)	0.6 (0.4–1.0)
≥1×/day	0.5 (0.2–1.0)	1.0 (0.5–1.9)	0.7 (0.4–1.1)
Salads			
<3×/wk[b]	1.00	1.00	1.00
3–6×/wk	0.7 (0.4–1.3)	0.4 (0.2–0.8)	0.5 (0.4–0.9)
≥1×/day	0.7 (0.3–1.3)	0.7 (0.3–1.3)	0.7 (0.4–1.1)
Tomatoes			
<1×/wk[b]	1.00	1.00	1.00
1–4×/wk	1.3 (0.6–2.6)	0.8 (0.4–1.5)	1.0 (0.6–1.6)
≥5×/wk	0.9 (0.4–2.2)	0.9 (0.4–2.1)	0.9 (0.5–1.6)
Cheese			
<1×/wk[b]	1.00	1.00	1.00
1–2×/wk	1.0 (0.5–2.0)	1.4 (0.7–2.7)	1.1 (0.7–1.8)
≥3×/wk	1.2 (0.5–2.8)	2.2 (1.1–4.3)	1.7 (1.0–2.9)

[a]Cox proportional hazard regression model always containing the food of interest, as well as age, smoking, and exercise.

[b]Reference category.

Source: Fraser GE et al., Epidemiology 8:168–174, 1997b, by permission. Copyrighted by Lippincott, Williams and Wilkins, 1997.

(Murphy et al., 1990). An unusual feature was a markedly increased proportion of deaths due to cardiovascular disease (77% of deaths), while cancers accounted for only 8% of deaths. This interesting pattern needs confirmation from a larger data set.

It is widely established that measures of socioeconomic status, such as education and family income, are important predictors of both CHD rates (Cassel, 1971; Cooper, 1993; Gillum et al., 1998) and all-cause mortality rates (Geronimus et al., 1996; Kaufman et al., 1998; U.S. Department of Health and Human Services, 1985) for black subjects. A few other studies have also demonstrated that the traditional nondietary risk factors for CHD operate in a similar fashion in black and in white populations (Cooper and Ford, 1992; Durazo-Arvizu et al., 1997; Folsom et al., 1998b; Gillum et al., 1998; Stevens et al., 1992).

EFFECT OF MODIFIABLE BEHAVIORS ON LIFE EXPECTANCY

Combinations of Risk Factors

Although we know a great deal about the effects of many risk factors in increasing or decreasing the proportionate risk of specific diseases and of all-cause mortality at a particular age, there is very little published information about how these factors may influence longevity, which is a related, but different, outcome.

The relationship between a relative risk for all-cause mortality of, say, 1.5 and its effect in reducing life expectancy is mathematically complex (Tsai et al., 1992; Vaupel, 1986). We have published the details of a statistical method to relate risk factors to life expectancy (Fraser and Shavlik, 1999) and have used this approach to provide the results that follow.

The variables chosen were behavioral factors that had clear associations with all-cause mortality in the cohort we examined. The exercise variable needed special handling in the analysis because in older subjects, an increasing proportion of the population exercises less frequently, not by choice, but because of the onset of a chronic disease. Thus, their poor outcome should not be ascribed only to their less frequent exercising but may be partly, at least, due to the chronic disease. In our analysis the less frequent exercisers were divided into those who had a past history of stroke, coronary heart disease, rheumatoid arthritis, rheumatism, or other forms of arthritis that might reduce exercise capacity and those free of these conditions. Thus, we could evaluate the effects of less frequent exercising among subjects without these conditions who presumably chose not to exercise. Our analytic model allowed subjects with these chronic diseases to remain in the analysis, however, and so contribute to estimates of the effects of other, nonexercise variables.

The effects of different combinations of values for several risk factors are shown in Figures 7–1 and 7–2 (Fraser and Shavlik, 2001). The bar on

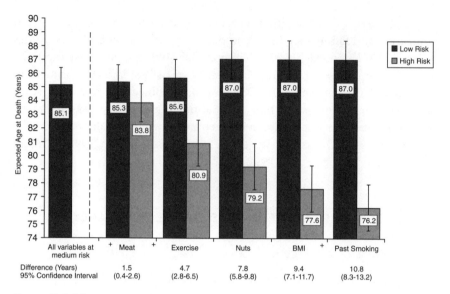

Figure 7–1 Men: expected ages at death (95% confidence interval) for subjects with jointly high or low risk values for the risk factor in a particular column and those to its left (other variables at medium risk values). (See Table 7–6 for definitions of high and low risk.) *Source:* Fraser GE, Shavlik DJ, Ten years of life: it is a matter of choice? *Arch Int Med* 161:1645–1652, 2001. Copyright 2001, American Medical Association.

the left shows the predicted life expectancy when all risk factors are set at medium risk values. Then moving from left to right, additional variables are set at either high risk values (lighter bars) or low risk values (darker bars). Thus, the solid bar for men labeled "nuts," for example, represents subjects having meat consumption, exercise, and nut consumption set at high risk values, while other variables to the right (i.e., BMI and smoking status) are still at medium risk values. This scheme means that the two bars at the far right contrast the life expectancies when all variables are set at either high- or low-risk values. In this last situation the differences in the predicted age of death are very large: 10.8 years (men) and 9.8 years (women).

The high-risk and low-risk groups on the right side of the figures may seem rather uncommon as these subjects have all high- or all low-risk values for the variables. However, 10.6% and 4.6% of the Adventist men and women in the study population either fit into the "lowest-risk" boxes of the figures or fail to meet only one of the necessary criteria, while 12.5% of the men and 9.3% of the women fit into the "highest-risk" boxes or fail to meet only one of their necessary criteria. As these risk factors are all behavioral in nature, their values and hence their consequences are matters

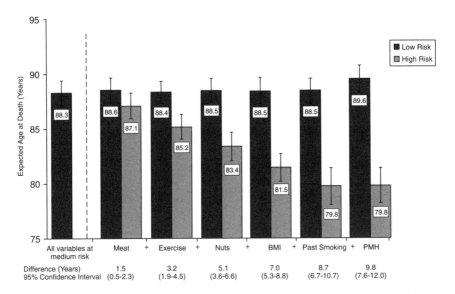

Figure 7–2 Women: expected ages at death (95% confidence interval) for subjects with jointly high or low risk values for the risk factor in a particular column and those to its left (other variables at medium risk values). (See Table 7–6 for definitions of high and low risk.) *Source:* Fraser GE, Shavlik DJ, Ten years of Life: it is a matter of choice? *Arch Int Med* 161:1645–1652, 2001. Copyright 2001, American Medical Association.

of individual choice. No doubt, the higher-risk combinations are more common in non-Adventist populations. Adding two pathophysiologic variables, hypertension and diabetes, to the simultaneous contrast of high- and low-risk values dramatically increases the difference in predicted ages at death to more than 20 years.

These analyses assume that the specified risk factors (except use of postmenopausal hormones) take the proposed values for all ages after 30. In fact, people's choices about behaviors such as these often remain relatively constant during their adult life. Those who become nonvegetarians, obese, or inactive at ages after 30 will undoubtedly experience somewhat lesser reductions in life expectancy than those shown in the figures. Notice that when all variables take medium-risk values (the bar on the left), there is a loss of only 1.9 years (men) and 1.3 years (women), as compared with the lowest-risk situation (the dark bar at the far right). Some may feel that it is not necessary to be too extreme!

This division of subjects into two or three categories for each of the variables defines 108 (in men) or 216 (in women) unique combinations of these factors, and only a subset is shown in the figures. By considering the frequency of particular combinations found in the study population, we

Table 7–5. Proportion of the Adventist Study Population Who Lost the Specified Number of Years of Life Expectancy Apparently Due to Their Lifestyle Choices[a]

	Percent of the Population	
Years Lost	Men	Women
One or more	97.5	94.8
Two or more	82.6	87.6
Three or more	68.7	71.5
Four or more	53.5	51.0
Five or more	40.0	34.2
Six or more	29.7	19.0
Seven or more	15.0	9.9
Eight or more	7.5	4.2
Nine or more	3.8	1.3
Ten or more	1.5	0.4

[a]Does not penalize subjects possibly unable to exercise above low levels due to existing coronary heart disease, stroke, rheumatoid arthritis, other arthritis, or rheumatism.

Source: Fraser GE, Shavlik DJ, Ten years of life: is it a matter of choice? Arch Int Med 161:1645–1652, 2001, by permission. Copyright 2001, American Medical Association.

calculated the proportion of Adventist subjects who lose a given number of years of life expectancy, apparently due to their lifestyle choices. For the purposes of this analysis, low exercisers, who also have one of the chronic illnesses, are scored as medium exercisers, to satisfy the requirement that an exercise choice is possible. This is a conservative approach, as some of these subjects would have chosen low exercise even if they had not been disabled. The results are shown in Table 7–5: more than 80% of both the California Adventist men and women lose two years or more, apparently due to their choices. About half lose four years or more, and about 10% lose seven to eight years.

To put this in proper perspective, it has been estimated that eliminating all CHD and cancers in the United States would increase life expectancy by only 7.02 years in females, and 8.1 years in males (Olshansky et al., 1990). Yet we find that the differences due apparently to choice of lifestyle exceed these numbers. Moreover, although rates of cardiovascular disease and of certain cancers are reduced in Adventists, sometimes substantially, a significant risk of these diseases still remains. Through most of the twentieth century the gains in adult life expectancy for the general population aged 50 years were reportedly only 9.4 years for women and 5.0 for men (Olshansky et al., 1991). It has been suggested that average "life expectancy should not exceed 35 years at age 50, unless major breakthroughs occur in controlling the fundamental rate of aging" (Olshansky et al., 1990, p. 638). Yet, many of the subgroups of Adventists defined in Figures 7–1 and

7–2 have a life expectancy that exceeds 85 years. This suggests the possibility that Adventists subscribing to lower risk behaviors are also experiencing a slower progression of the mandatory aging or "fundamental rate of aging" described by Olshansky et al. (1991).

Individual Risk Factors

A natural question that arises is, How many years' difference in life expectancy may be associated with moving only one risk factor from a high-risk to a low-risk category, while leaving other factors constant? A possible difficulty here is that the change in life expectancy produced by changing one variable may in theory depend on values of other variables. However, in our data at least, this interactive effect seems small, and the effects of a single variable are fairly similar whether other variables take average- or high-risk values.

This is illustrated by the results in Table 7–6 (Fraser and Shavlik, 2001), where contrasting values of individual variables are considered, with all other variables remaining at either average or high risk values. As "high risk" for an Adventist (i.e., a nonvegetarian, who rarely exercises or eats nuts, has a BMI of more than 25.9 [for males] or more than 25.2 [females], and is a past or present smoker), involves a combination of factors seen more commonly in the general population, these results may have a more accurate application to non-Adventists when other variables are set at "high-risk" levels.

Individual factors typically contribute 1.1 to 2.7 years' difference in life expectancy (Table 7–6). Thus each variable appears to make a modest contribution to longevity, but their combined effects are substantial. The size of these differences is consistent with the idea that the greater life expectancy experienced by Adventists (see Chapter 4) is largely related to their unusual dietary and other behaviors.

A few other investigators have predicted the effects of different risk factor values on life expectancy. Tsevat et al. (1991) used data from U.S. Vital Statistics and the Framingham Heart Study to estimate extensions in longevity that occurred when those who initially had elevations of a particular risk factor changed the elevation to an ideal value. This method involved making some approximations and assumptions about effects that occurred above age 85, but predicted that men and women smokers would gain 2.3 and 2.8 years, respectively, from quitting smoking; men and women hypertensives would gain 1.1–5.3 and 0.9–5.7 years, respectively, (depending on the severity of the hypertension) by reducing diastolic levels to 88 mm Hg; men and women with high cholesterol values would gain

Table 7-6. Estimates of the Effects of High- versus Low-Risk Values of Individual Risk Factors: Covariates All at Either Medium-Risk or High-Risk Values

Contrasts		Difference (Low Risk − High Risk) in Life Expectancy (95% Confidence Interval)	
Low Risk	High Risk	Males	Females
COVARIATES AT MEDIUM RISK			
Vegetarian	Nonvegetarian	1.53 (0.41, 2.65)	1.51 (0.53, 2.50)
High exercise[a]	Low exercise[b]	2.73 (1.41, 4.06)	1.88 (0.86, 2.90)
High nut consumption[c]	Low nut consumption	2.74 (1.60, 3.88)	1.87 (0.72, 3.02)
Medium tertile BMI	High tertile BMI	1.41 (0.34, 2.49)	2.25 (1.27, 3.23)
Never smoker	Past smoker	1.25 (0.44, 2.07)	1.80 (0.56, 3.04)
PMH ever	PMH never		1.06 (0.27, 1.86)
COVARIATES AT HIGH RISK			
Vegetarian	Nonvegetarian	2.38 (1.12, 3.63)	1.65 (0.65, 2.65)
High exercise[a]	Low exercise[b]	2.14 (0.43, 3.85)	2.19 (0.92, 3.45)
High nut consumption[c]	Low nut consumption	2.87 (1.64, 4.11)	1.18 (0.06, 2.29)
Medium tertile BMI	High tertile BMI	1.51 (0.35, 2.68)	1.90 (1.03, 2.76)
Never smoker	Past smoker	1.33 (0.44, 2.22)	1.49 (0.40, 2.58)
PMH ever	PMH never		0.82 (0.14, 1.50)

BMI, body mass index; PMH, postmenopausal hormone.

[a]Vigorous activity three times each week, at least 15 min on each occasion.

[b]Among individuals not limited in their ability to exercise by existing coronary heart disease, stroke, rheumatoid arthritis, rheumatism, or other arthritis.

[c]Five or more servings per week.

Source: Fraser GE, Shavlik DJ. Ten years of life: is it a matter of choice? *Arch Int Med* 161:1645–1652, 2001 by permission. Copyright 2001, American Medical Association.

0.5–4.2 and 0.5–1.1 years, respectively (depending on baseline levels of cholesterol) by reducing values to 200 mg/dl and by reducing to ideal weight. Grover et al. (1998) reported similar estimates from the Lipid Research Clinic study.

More recently, an analysis of five large-cohort studies (Stamler et al., 1999) compared hypothetical low-risk individuals with blood cholesterol levels less than 200 mg/dL, systolic and diastolic blood pressures less than or equal to 120/80, and who were not current smokers, with all others who did have one or more of these risk factors. Different studies among this group estimated that the low-risk individuals had 5.8 to 9.5 more years of life expectancy. The greatest advantages were predicted by studies having the youngest baseline ages, as might be expected. One weakness of this analytic approach used by Stamler et al. is that no account is taken of the very different effects of individual risk factors at different ages, which are demonstrated earlier in this chapter. How this may affect the estimates is unclear.

Other studies have noted that greater physical activity, considered alone as a risk factor, is associated with higher life expectancy. A Finnish study found that men with greater physical activity who died during 20 years of follow-up did so at ages that were 2.1 years older, on average, than did others (Pekkanen et al., 1987). The College Alumni Study (Paffenbarger et al., 1986) has also predicted 2.51 extra years of life for a 35–39-year-old man who expends 2000 or more kilocalories per week while walking, climbing stairs, or playing sports, as compared with his expending 500 or fewer calories in these ways. These years were gained before 80 years of age.

There appear to be no similar analyses published, among non-Adventist studies, that jointly include the variety of behavioral risk factors that we have used in the analyses described above. The large-value differences in life expectancy, when comparing high- and low-risk combinations of variables, are broadly similar to those reported by Stamler et al. (1999), even though the variables are different. Behavioral variables, as compared with physiologic risk factors, may affect risk of several disease endpoints, and in theory at least, are amenable to change at little cost or risk.

SUMMARY

1. The poorer health of many older individuals is a consequence of both (*1*) a higher risk of many specific diseases, often resulting from longer exposure to adverse environmental factors, which may interact with one or more specific metabolic abnormalities under genetic control; and (*2*) a

mandatory aging process, also under genetic control, that causes a gradual reduction in metabolic function and efficiency in most, if not all, tissues.

2. Adventists have lower risks of several common causes of mortality, particularly coronary heart disease and several types of cancer. Thus, their increased longevity is at least partly explained by this. Whether the mandatory aging process is also affected by lifestyle is unknown.

3. The Adventist Health Study data clearly indicate that the effects of many risk factors for CHD and for all-cause mortality depend markedly on age. Generally, their effects on CHD risk become weaker with age in a relative sense, but a smaller relative risk may still be associated with a larger difference in the number of CHD deaths if the frequency of the disease is greater, as it generally is, at older ages.

4. These predictions from the whole cohort are confirmed when we restrict analyses to the oldest subjects (over age 84), where many risk factors are still important but have effects of somewhat lower magnitude. Whether the continuing protection occurs because effects at earlier ages have resulted in less pathology at the oldest ages, or whether a change in risk factors at these advanced ages will still change risk of disease, is unknown.

5. The data on black Adventists, even though limited in extent, again show a protective effect of more frequent nut consumption—in this case, on all-cause mortality (data on CHD events were not available). In addition, greater consumption of fruit and green salads appeared to protect against all-cause mortality, while those consuming more cheese may have a modestly higher rate of mortality. Thus, these findings are generally consistent with those for white Adventists, but more information is needed on diet–disease relationships in black study populations.

6. Life table analyses of the white Adventist population indicate that Adventist men and women who choose to eat and exercise in different ways, and who have different histories of smoking and of the use of postmenopausal hormones (women), may experience up to 10 years' difference in life expectancy, probably as a result of these choices.

7. None of the variables studied especially stands out in its effect on life expectancy. Different variables contribute between 1.1 and 2.7 additional years, but combinations may jointly result in large differences.

8. The choice of health habits made by California Adventists may well explain most of their greater life expectancy as compared to other Californians.

8

Vegetarianism and Obesity, Hypertension, Diabetes, and Arthritis

The cohort studies of California Adventists were designed to detect new cases of cancer and coronary heart disease during the follow-up period. Thus, there was no plan for identifying new changes in body weight or new cases of hypertension, diabetes, or arthritis as study endpoints. At the beginning of the studies, however, subjects were required to answer questions about their height and weight and to say whether a doctor had ever diagnosed them as hypertensive, diabetic, or arthritic. This provided a measure of the prevalence of particular values of body mass index (BMI, a measure of obesity) and of the three other listed medical conditions at the beginning of the Adventist Mortality Study (AMS) in 1960, and prior to the Adventist Health Study (AHS) in 1976.

Epidemiologists in recent years, when searching for causal variables, have quite rightly tended not to favor studies reporting associations between disease prevalence and risk factors. The important difference between prevalence and incidence (prospective) studies is that the disease of interest is already present at the beginning of a prevalence study. By contrast, at the beginning of an incidence study the disease of interest is not present and new cases are detected during a follow-up period. The reasons for preferring incidence studies are that (1) prevalence studies tend to include a smaller proportion of subjects with the more severe and perhaps fatal forms of the disease than actually occurs in a population during the follow-up—this is known as length bias (Jekel et al., 1996); and (2) the possible risk factor being investigated (e.g., diet) and the presence of disease are both measured at the same time. Thus, it is possible that the presence of the disease had led subjects to change either their dietary habits or their perception of their previous diet. If so, the reported diet would not correspond to that which may have caused the disease at some time in the past.

As an example of the possible ambiguity in a prevalence study, we found that the more frequent consumers of nuts in our Adventist Health Study population were significantly less obese at the beginning of the study. This can be interpreted in two ways: it could be that nut consumption, or something associated with it, prevents weight gain, or it could be that those who are obese for other reasons tend to avoid nuts, perhaps because they are a relatively fatty food. The causal direction of the association between nut consumption and obesity cannot be determined with prevalence data. It would be better to check whether nut consumption at study baseline was associated with changes in body weight during the follow-up period of a prospective incidence study.

I do not believe that these problems are likely to produce misleading protective associations between vegetarian status and risk of obesity, hypertension, diabetes, or arthritis in Adventists. Rather, the prevalence data on this population can probably produce unambiguous causal insights (Fraser, 1999b). The concern about length bias is not of great relevance to the conditions under investigation, as sudden and severe forms of these disorders, leading rapidly to death, are not common.

Further, it is very unlikely that developing obesity or any of the diseases mentioned above would lead an Adventist to become less of a vegetarian (the reverse causal direction, where the disease causes the risk factor). The Adventist view for many years had indeed been that the vegetarian diet is more healthful. Thus, the onset of a disease will typically prompt an Adventist to reevaluate his or her lifestyle and make changes to conform more closely to the recommended ideal.

Because of this, some Adventists with prevalent diseases will now have become vegetarians, despite having been nonvegetarians during the time that the disease first developed. If protection due to vegetarianism truly occurs, the presence of these subjects in the prevalence data, now as vegetarians, would tend to artifactually reduce any appearance of protection in these data. But if in fact vegetarianism has no true effect it may even appear to increase risk. Thus, if our prevalence data suggest protection, it is probably an underestimate of the true effect. If the data suggest a hazardous effect, this may be either real or artifactual.

Despite the lack of planning for this, we did in fact have the opportunity to also evaluate the incidence of increased body weight, diabetes, and hypertension in vegetarians as compared with nonvegetarians. This was done by using the approximately 8500 subjects who were part of both the Adventist Mortality and the Adventist Health studies (i.e., the overlap population). Only those who told us in 1960 (the Mortality Study) that they did not have a particular disorder were included, and we could then iden-tify those of this group who had developed this medical problem by 1976, when they entered the Adventist Health Study. Thus sometime between 1960 and 1976 their doctors had first told them they had this disorder. It was then possible to relate risk of onset of this disease to vegetarian status in 1960, which had thus been evaluated before the onset of the disease.

The difficulties with these analyses are the relatively small analytic pop-ulation included, the modest numbers of new disease cases, and hence the wider confidence intervals. A difference is that only in these overlap-population analyses are vegetarians defined as those eating meat less than once each week. This is because the 1960 questionnaire did not allow fur-ther discrimination between never eating meat and eating it less than once each week. Nevertheless, these results are especially interesting since other studies that would allow a search for links between vegetarian habits and new-onset obesity, diabetes, and hypertension are uncommon.

RESULTS FROM THE ADVENTIST MORTALITY AND HEALTH STUDIES IN CALIFORNIA

Means and standard errors for BMI, and also the reported prevalence of hypertension, diabetes, and arthritis in both the Adventist Mortality Study (1960) and the Adventist Health Study (1976) populations at study base-lines, are shown in Table 8–1. At the beginning of the Adventist Health Study, about 24% of subjects stated that their doctors had told them they had high blood pressure, about 5% to 6% were diabetic, and about 30% had some form of rheumatism or arthritis. The prevalence is greater for all of these disorders in women, although the possibility that women may visit

Table 8–1. Body Mass Index (BMI) (Mean; Standard Error in Parentheses) and Reported Prevalence (%) of Hypertension, Diabetes, and Arthritis in California Adventists at Baseline of the Cohort Studies[a]

Variable	Adventist Mortality Study (1960)		Adventist Health Study (1976)	
	Men	Women	Men	Women
BMI	25.05 (3.30)	24.75 (4.36)	24.81 (3.55)	24.38 (4.74)
Prevalence of:				
Hypertension	10.4	19.8	20.4	28.4
Diabetes	2.4	2.4	5.1	6.4
Arthritis	17.5	29.0	23.7[b]	42.0[b]

[a]Adjusted for age differences.

[b]Also includes "rheumatism."

doctors more regularly than men, and therefore have a greater opportunity of being given such a diagnosis (a diagnostic bias) should be considered. The corresponding numbers from the earlier Adventist Mortality Study are substantially lower, so there may have been a true increase in the prevalence of these disorders among California Adventists between 1960 and 1976, and it is also possible that some of this secular difference results from the greater diagnostic acumen of doctors. However, the increasing medical sophistication of the California Adventist population, which had become more familiar with the nature of their diagnoses by 1976, is probably a more important factor.

The analyses reported below were rerun, adjusting for education. Because the vegetarians tend to be better educated (see Chapter 1), this could, in principle, create a conservative bias, as the better-educated vegetarians may have received more regular blood pressure checks and their arthritis may have been investigated and diagnosed more completely. However, in fact, the differences due to the adjustment for educational differences were of a small magnitude and of inconsistent direction, so they were not included in the following discussion.

Obesity and Vegetarian Status

We first checked whether the associations between vegetarian status and prevalent obesity, both measured in the 1976 Adventist Health Study, were different at different ages. As this did not appear to be the case, simple age-adjusted regression analyses enabled us to determine whether vegetarian Adventists were more or less likely to be obese than nonvegetarians (see Table 8–2). We found that both vegetarian men and women of average height, at ages 45–64, were approximately 6 kg (13 lb) lighter than their nonvegetarian Adventist counterparts who were the same height. These differences presumably reflect a long-term, often lifelong, exposure to meat intake (and associated factors), or its absence, before enrollment in the study.

The other type of analysis that we used to investigate this question evaluated new changes in body weight, after 1960, among those in the overlap Adventist population who were enrolled in both the AMS and AHS studies. This revealed a complex situation. Those with diabetes, tumors, heart disease, stroke, and cirrhosis in 1960 were removed from the analysis, as it was possible that these chronic disorders would influence body weight, and this is not our present interest. Past smoking was treated as a covariate to avoid confounding. On average, men gained 5.2 lb and women added 5.8 lb during the 16 years. Most subjects in this overlap population were less than 50 years old in 1960.

Table 8-2. Vegetarian Status and Obesity (95% Confidence Interval): The Adventist Health Study[a]

	Index	Vegetarian	Semivegetarian	Nonvegetarian	p
Males	BMI (kg/m^2)	24.26 (24.11–24.42)	25.18 (25.02–25.34)	26.24 (26.11–26.37)	0.0001
Females	BMI (kg/m^2)	23.73 (23.58–23.89)	24.83 (24.66–25.00)	25.88 (25.75–26.02)	0.0001
Males[b]	Weight (kg)	77	80	83	
Females[b]	Weight (kg)	63	66	69	

BMI, body mass index.

[a]For subjects aged 45–64 years. Other ages show similar trends. Vegetarians eat no meat, fish, or poultry; semivegetarians eat one or more of meat, fish, poultry, but in total less than once per week; nonvegetarians eat these foods at least weekly.

[b]At height of 5'10" (1.78 m) for males and 5'4" (1.63 m) for females.

Source: Fraser GE, Associations between diet and cancer, ischemic heart disease, and all-cause mortality in non-Hispanic white California Seventh-day Adventists, *Am J Clin Nutr* 70(Suppl):532s–538s, 1999, by permission. Copyright American Society for Clinical Nutrition.

Nonvegetarians below age 50 in 1960 either gained more weight or lost less weight than vegetarians during the 16 years (1960–1976). However, differences were small and not statistically significant. While female non-vegetarians below age 50 in 1960 gained 1.2 lbs more than vegetarians of similar ages, nonvegetarians aged 50–69 lost 4 lbs less than similar vege-tarians ($p = .02$ for the difference by age) during the 16 years. However, among women over 70 in 1960, the nonvegetarians lost 6 lbs more, on av-erage, than the vegetarians ($p = .16$ for the difference by age). This dif-ferent result in the oldest group, which may be a chance effect, describes the change in weight between ages 70 and 86. Although at first glance, this may not seem to be a favorable response for the vegetarians as they lost less weight, we have previously noted that less weight loss in elderly Ad-ventist women is in fact associated with decreased mortality (Singh, 1999).

In contrast to these rather complicated associations with average weight changes, the relative risks of moving from normal weight (BMI less than 25.0) in 1960 to being overweight (BMI greater than or equal to 25.0) in 1976 were 1.68 (95% confidence interval, 1.13–2.49) for nonvegetarian men and 1.40 (95% confidence interval, 1.11–1.75) for nonvegetarian women, as compared with their vegetarian counterparts (meat less than once per week). These changes occur during a limited period of 16 years during adult life, whereas the apparently much greater influence of vege-tarianism on prevalent obesity, shown in Table 8–2, presumably represents the sum of effects during childhood and the adult life experienced so far.

There is good evidence, from studies of other groups, that vegetarian-ism is associated with lower BMI (Calkins et al., 1984; Famodu et al., 1999; Haddad et al., 1999a; Melby et al., 1993, 1994; Simons et al., 1978; Toohey et al., 1998). Without exception, the vegetarians were thinner, on average. This included black and white Adventists, and populations located in the United States, Nigeria, and Australia. Studies of non-Adventist veg-etarians reach a similar conclusion (see Chapter 12 for more details).

Causal factors for obesity are not completely understood. While there are undoubtedly some genetic influences involved, the focus here is on diet and exercise. Large population-based studies suggest that regular physical activity retards the age-associated increase in weight (Di Pietro, 1999; Jebb and Moore, 1999). As a treatment for established obesity, exercise is ef-fective and may usefully complement dietary changes, although the mag-nitude of its contribution to weight loss is probably quite small (Wing, 1999).

Most dietary research on obesity or weight gain has focused on total energy and total fat intake. Epidemiologic studies of obese subjects are problematic as there is excellent evidence that many subjects, particularly those apparently resistant to dietary interventions, markedly underreport their caloric intake (Heymsfield et al., 1995; Lichtman et al., 1992). There is also the problem of accurately adjusting for exercise or energy expenditure, which is often relatively greater for obese individuals simply due to their greater body size.

Dietary fat is calorie-dense, and its intake is probably poorly regulated by humans (Bray and Popkin, 1998), especially as many prefer the taste of fat to other nutrients. Research has usually indicated that the total intake of calories from fat is related to risk of obesity. However, those eating more fat are usually those with a higher total caloric intake. Is it the fat or the total energy intake that promotes obesity?

A related question—whether dietary fat as a proportion of energy intake, rather than an absolute amount, is associated with obesity—is hotly debated (Bray and Popkin, 1998; Willett, 1998b). As usual, there are the problems of accurate measurement of total energy, fat intakes, and also physical activity, which must be considered at the same time. Many studies have a cross-sectional design and cannot determine whether a high-fat diet, when associated with greater obesity, caused that obesity, or whether obese persons eat more fat for other reasons. Unfortunately, the results of the methodologically stronger prospective studies, which correlate the percentage of baseline dietary calories as fat with a change in BMI, are quite contradictory (Seidell, 1998). Hence the evidence shows that total fat intake, perhaps just reflecting total energy intake, correlates with body weight. Whether fat actually has a greater effect on weight than other equivalent sources of calories is uncertain, but it is unlikely (Fraser et al., 2002).

It may be that the type of fat in the diet is important. For instance, feeding studies of rodents have shown that unsaturated fats, when fed in the same caloric quantities as saturated fats, are less likely to promote obesity (Cha and Jones, 1998; Loh et al., 1998; Shimomura et al., 1990), and may increase the metabolic rate so that more calories are burned (Loh et al., 1998; Shimomura et al., 1990). Cha and Jones (1998) showed that in nonobese rodents, unsaturated, but not saturated, fats increase levels of blood leptin, a protein that causes a sense of satiety. It is also possible that humans can consume more calories from unsaturated than saturated fats, with little gain in weight occurring (Garg, 1998; Kasper et al., 1973), although this idea needs more research support.

Our recent experimental studies of consumption of almonds, a food high in monounsaturated fat, have shown that over a six-month period, adding 320 calories from almonds to the daily diet, without any other nutritional advice, did not cause a significant weight gain. This is despite the fact that estimated reductions in other foods only compensate for about half of the fat calories added by the nuts (Fraser et al., 2002). A further explanation is that nut calories are probably incompletely absorbed when eaten (Haddad and Sabaté, 2000; Levine and Silvis, 1980).

There are at least two possible mechanisms that may underlie the lighter weight of Adventist vegetarians. They are a little more likely to participate in regular vigorous activities than the nonvegetarians (see Chapter 1). Although they take in about as many calories and as much fat as nonvegetarian Adventists (see Table 1–7), the type of fat consumed is quite different. The ratio of polyunsaturated fat to saturated fat is 0.92 in the vegetarians but 0.67 in the nonvegetarians. It is possible that the greater proportion of unsaturated fat may be less likely to result in a weight gain.

In summary, there is strong evidence that vegetarian Adventists are thinner than nonvegetarian Adventists, and that vegetarians are less likely to change from nonobese to obese status during their adult years. However, vegetarian women at the oldest ages may lose less weight as they age. The mechanisms explaining these differences are poorly understood.

Diabetes Mellitus and Vegetarian Status

An interesting observation from the Adventist Mortality Study (Snowdon and Phillips, 1985), regarding its comparison with non-Adventists of the concurrent American Cancer Society (ACS) study, was that the death certificates for Adventists mentioned diabetes mellitus as the underlying cause of death only half as often as those for comparably aged non-Adventists. This result is not likely to be due to chance and suggests that some features of the Adventist lifestyle either reduce risk of diabetes, or reduce its severity to such an extent that it is much less likely to be included as an underlying cause of death.

A multivariate analysis in the AMS adjusted for age, BMI, physical activity (in males), and the intake of a variety of foods, and evaluated associations between vegetarian status and two different diabetic outcome measures. The first of these was the prevalence of self-reported diabetes at the study baseline; the second was an incidence measure—specifically, deceased subjects who did not report diabetes at study baseline but whose death certificates did mention diabetes mellitus. Thus, the latter analysis evaluates the onset of new diabetes that developed after a person's vegetarian status was noted at study baseline. However, the cause of death may have had little to do with the diabetes, as even diabetes as a noncontributing cause on the death certificate would do in this analysis.

Nonvegetarians of both sexes had an increased prevalence of diabetes at study baseline as compared with vegetarians (see Table 8–3). An effect of nonvegetarianism on the second endpoint (new diabetes mentioned on

Table 8–3. Association of Meat Consumption with Endpoints Involving Diabetes: Logistic Regression Analyses in the Adventist Mortality Study

Outcome	Meat Consumption	Multivariate-Adjusted Relative Risk[a] (95% Confidence Interval)	
		Male	Female
Self-reported diabetes prevalence 1960	<1 day/wk (vegetarian)	1.0	1.0
	1+ days/wk (nonvegetarian)	1.7 (1.2–2.4)	1.4 (1.1–1.8)
	<1 day/wk	1.0	1.0
	1–2 days/wk	1.4 (0.9–2.3)	1.1 (0.8–1.6)
	3–5 days/wk	1.5 (0.9–2.5)	1.2 (0.9–1.8)
	6+ days/wk	2.7 (1.6–4.6)	2.3 (1.6–3.3)
Any mention of diabetes on the death certificate (1960–1980)[b]	<1 day/wk (vegetarian)	1.0	1.0
	1+ days/wk (nonvegetarian)	1.9 (1.2–3.1)	1.1 (0.8–1.6)
	<1 day/wk	1.0	1.0
	1–2 days/wk	1.6 (0.9–2.9)	1.3 (0.9–2.0)
	3–5 days/wk	1.6 (0.8–3.0)	1.2 (0.7–1.8)
	6+ days/wk	3.6 (1.9–7.1)	0.6 (0.3–1.2)

[a]For prevalence data, the regression model included age, percentage of desirable weight, physical activity (for males only), and frequency of use of meat, eggs, and milk. For death certificate data, the regression model included these same variables plus frequency of use of fruit, sweet desserts, candy, and soft drinks. The "relative risk" estimates for the prevalence data should be interpreted as prevalence ratios. The reference category for each relative risk is the group of vegetarians.

[b]Among nondiabetics at study baseline.

Source: Snowdon DA, Phillips RI, Does a vegetarian diet reduce the occurrence of diabetes? *Am J Public Health* 1985;75:507–512, by permission. Copyright American Public Health Association.

the death certificate) suggests an increased risk of developing diabetes during the follow-up period, but is seen only in males. An alternative interpretation is that no increase in diabetes occurs among the male nonvegetarians, but that nonvegetarian diabetics are more likely to die, either from other causes or as the result of a complication from diabetes. However, the simplest conclusion is that there is more new diabetes mellitus among the nonvegetarians and that this diabetes, as usual, is an important determinant of mortality. The adjustment for BMI differences in these analyses may have led to an underestimate of the effect as it then amounts to a comparison between vegetarians and nonvegetarians who are at the same BMI levels. However, vegetarians are less obese, and this is an important risk factor for diabetes (Barrett-Connor, 1989).

The prevalence of diabetes mellitus was also measured in the Adventist Health Study at study baseline in 1976. The results of logistic analyses estimating the relative prevalence of diabetes in nonvegetarians, as compared with vegetarians at study baseline, are shown in Table 8–4. This is adjusted for differences in either age alone, or in age as well as BMI. The nonvegetarian Adventists show a near doubling of prevalence as compared with the vegetarians, which is highly statistically significant. Results are consistent for men and women. When an adjustment is made for BMI, the effect of vegetarian status remains important but is of a somewhat reduced magnitude, suggesting that vegetarian status acts partially through effects on obesity. Given the prevalence nature of the data, we did not pursue further analyses to evaluate possible effects of different foods, nutrients, or physical activity on risk.

However, results from the study of the overlap Adventist population, in regard to new-onset diabetes rather than prevalent diabetes (532 new cases between 1960 and 1976), are less clear. As compared with vegetarians (defined here as eating meat less than one time per week), those nondiabetics who ate meat or poultry one to two times per week, or three or more times per week in 1960 had relative risks (95% confidence intervals) for subsequent diabetes of 1.29 (1.04–1.60) and 1.19 (0.96–1.48). Thus this is consistent with the previously mentioned results, given the upper values of the confidence intervals, but is not clearly confirmatory. An adjustment for obesity caused a marked attenuation of these effects.

Overall, it seems that vegetarians experience less diabetes than nonvegetarian Adventists, but that this is at least partly explained by their reduced obesity. It may also be relevant that vegetarians are less insulin-resistant than others (Hua et al., 2001).

Other prospective research on dietary risk factors in new-onset diabetes is not extensive. Associations with dietary fat have not been consistent (Lundgren et al., 1989; Marshall et al., 1991; Salmeron et al., 1995), al-

Table 8–4. Associations between Vegetarian Status, Body Mass Index (BMI), and the Prevalence of Diabetes in Adventists[a]

Exposure Variable	Men				Women			
	Adjusted for Age Only	95% Confidence Interval	Adjusted for Age and BMI	95% Confidence Interval	Adjusted for Age Only	95% Confidence Interval	Adjusted for Age and BMI	95% Confidence Interval
VEGETARIAN STATUS								
Vegetarian	1.00		1.00		1.00		1.00	
Semivegetarian	1.35	1.02–1.78	1.29	0.97–1.71	1.08	0.89–1.32	0.98	0.80–1.20
Nonvegetarian	1.97***	1.56–2.47	1.72***	1.36–2.19	1.93***	1.65–2.25	1.60***	1.36–1.88
BODY MASS INDEX								
First quintile			1.00				1.00	
Second quintile			1.13	0.81–1.59			0.98	0.76–1.27
Third quintile			1.30	0.94–1.81			0.96	0.74–1.23
Fourth quintile			1.13	0.81–1.59			1.19	0.94–1.51
Fifth quintile			2.08***	1.52–2.84			2.94***	2.37–3.64

*** $p < .0001$

[a]Adjusted for age and/or obesity in two separate models.

though it may be important to divide fat into that from animal and from vegetable sources. Vegetable fat appeared to be protective against diabetes in the Nurses' Health Study (Colditz et al., 1992), whereas saturated fat appeared to increase risk, possibly through effects on obesity (Van Dam et al., 2002).

Associations between risk of diabetes and total carbohydrate intake (Lundgren et al., 1989; Marshall et al., 1991), or between risk of diabetes and total dietary fiber (Colditz et al., 1992) are also inconsistent or absent. Cereal fiber, specifically, did appear to protect men in a large prospective study (Salmeron et al., 1995). Intake of one or more of three minerals—potassium, magnesium, or calcium—may reduce risk, but it is not clear which of these is more important (Colditz et al., 1992; Salmeron et al., 1995).

Those who ate more processed meats were at higher risk of diabetes in the Health Professionals Follow-up Study (Van Dam et al., 2002). More frequent consumption of processed meat (7.5 times per week) was associated with a relative risk of 1.46 (95% confidence interval, 1.14–1.86), when compared to consumption of less than once per month. This was not explained by differences in obesity. Other types of meat were not obviously associated with risk, although such effects were not ruled out.

A dietary glycemic index was calculated in the Nurses' Health Study (Salmeron et al., 1997). This is a validated index that accumulates values for all foods in the diet. Foods contributing higher values to the index are those that cause greater blood glucose responses after digestion and greater insulin demand for a given amount of carbohydrate intake. The risk of new diabetes was 37% greater in those individuals in the upper quintiles of this index than in those in the lower quintiles. Foods with a low glycemic index are those particularly favored by many vegetarians and include nonprocessed vegetables, legumes, grains, and nuts.

It is widely known that regular physical activity increases sensitivity to insulin (Horton, 1986; Mayer-Davis et al., 1998), and a number of well-designed prospective studies have now convincingly demonstrated that regular physical activity also reduces the risk of new-onset non-insulin-dependent diabetes mellitus. These studies include the College Alumni Study (Helmrich et al., 1991), the Physicians' Health Study (Manson et al., 1992), the Honolulu Heart Program (Burchfiel et al., 1995; this study may also include a few insulin-dependent diabetics), and the Health Professionals Follow-up Study (Hu et al., 2001).

Physician-Diagnosed Hypertension and Vegetarian Status

The prevalence of hypertension among the nonvegetarian Adventists in the Adventist Health Study was more than double that of the vegetarians ($p <$

.0001), and results were consistent for men and women. However, only 52% of those claiming to be hypertensive were actually taking medication for this condition. It seems probable that these were the more severe hypertensives, on average, and this idea is supported by analyses of the oldest subjects (those over 84), where hypertensives not taking medication had less risk of dying from CHD (Fraser and Shavlik, 1997a) than those who were medicated.

Many supposed "hypertensives" not on medication may not be true hypertensives, and if so, this would dilute the apparent effect of vegetarianism. Thus when hypertension is redefined to mean that antihypertensive medication must be taken, the apparent protective effect of vegetarianism is even greater (Table 8–5), with nearly threefold differences occurring between vegetarians and nonvegetarians. Adjusting for obesity, however, somewhat reduces the magnitude of the effect of vegetarian status, and, as with diabetes, suggests that vegetarianism acts in part through its association with less obesity.

Prediction of the risk of developing new hypertension sufficiently severe to require antihypertensive medication for those in the overlap population—those who were enrolled in both the AMS and the AHS (1008 new cases of hypertension were found between 1960 and 1976)—gave broadly similar results to the prevalence analysis described here. As compared with vegetarians (defined here as eating meat less than one time per week), the relative risks (95% confidence intervals) of subsequent hypertension in those nonhypertensives eating meat or poultry either one to two times per week, or three times per week or more, in 1960 are 1.53 (95% confidence interval, 1.29–1.82) and 1.90 (95% confidence interval, 1.62–2.24). This strong dose–response effect was only modestly reduced by adjusting for differences in obesity, suggesting that the effects of vegetarianism were largely mediated by mechanisms apart from weight reduction. Thus the evidence that vegetarian Adventists, as compared with non-vegetarian Adventists, experience less hypertension is strong and consistent.

Several other studies have compared blood pressure levels of vegetarian and nonvegetarian Adventists. These studies have compared black Adventists in the United States (Melby et al., 1993, 1994) or in Nigeria (Famodu et al., 1998, 1999), and white Adventists in Australia (Rouse et al., 1983a) and in the United States (Melby et al., 1993).

In the Nigerian study, 40 nonvegetarians were compared with 36 vegetarians, but there were no significant differences in blood pressure levels. Melby et al. (1993) compared 27 older black vegetarians with 37 black nonvegetarians (average age, 67.0 years), and 85 white vegetarians with 54 white nonvegetarians (average age, 66.1 years). After an adjustment for age and sex, systolic blood pressure was significantly lower ($p < .05$) for the vegetarians, by 10.2 mm Hg in black subjects and by 1.9 mm Hg in the

Table 8-5. Associations between Vegetarian Status, Body Mass Index (BMI), and the Prevalence of Hypertension in Adventists[a]

Exposure Variable	Men				Women			
	Adjusted for Age Only	95% Confidence Interval	Adjusted for Age and BMI	95% Confidence Interval	Adjusted for Age Only	95% Confidence Interval	Adjusted for Age and BMI	95% Confidence Interval
VEGETARIAN STATUS								
Vegetarian	1.00		1.00		1.00		1.00	
Semivegetarian	1.91	1.54–2.36	1.66	1.34–2.07	1.78	1.55–2.04	1.50	1.30–1.73
Nonvegetarian	2.86	2.83–3.44	2.26	1.87–2.73	2.97	2.86–3.34	2.31	2.04–2.61
BODY MASS INDEX								
First quintile			1.00				1.00	
Second quintile			2.01	1.50–2.70			1.30	1.07–1.51
Third quintile			2.21	1.66–2.96			1.66	1.38–1.99
Fourth quintile			2.96	2.23–3.93			2.52	2.11–3.00
Fifth quintile			5.16	3.91–6.80			5.96	5.00–7.03

[a]Adjusted for age and/or obesity in two separate models. Hypertension is defined as doctor-diagnosed high blood pressure and taking antihypertensive medication. All p values are $<.0001$, except for quintile 2 of BMI in women where $p = .0085$.

white subjects. An adjustment for body mass index attenuated these differences, again suggesting that the vegetarian diet works in part by promoting a lower body mass index. Melby and his coworkers (1994) also reported similar, but nonsignificant, trends in another study of black vegetarian and nonvegetarian Adventists. Further, the comparison of white vegetarian and omnivorous Adventists in Australia (Rouse et al., 1983a) found significantly higher blood pressure among the omnivorous men, but differences among women were not statistically significant.

Other studies, both observational and experimental, have evaluated blood pressure among non-Adventist vegetarians and the effects of an experimental vegetarian diet on blood pressure. Vegetarians typically had moderately lower blood pressure. The details of these studies are discussed further in Chapter 12. Aside from the Adventist studies, there are few, if any, large population studies that have addressed the question of whether meat consumption changes the risk of new hypertension.

It is widely known that more obese persons are at higher risk of hypertension (Mikhail et al., 1999). Physical inactivity also increases the risk of hypertension somewhat, and this cannot be ascribed only to its association with increased obesity (Arroll and Beaglehole, 1993). In addition, there is strong evidence (Appel, 1999; Beilin, 1999; Cappuccio, 1992; McCarron and Reusser, 1999) that dietary sodium and alcohol increase blood pressure levels, and that dietary potassium and possibly calcium tend to decrease blood pressure.

The effects of supplemental dietary calcium on blood pressure have been studied in a meta-analysis of several intervention trials (Bucher et al., 1996). The conclusion was that dietary calcium may lead to a small reduction in systolic, but not diastolic, blood pressure, especially in hypertensive individuals. A similar meta-analysis, of the effects of trials of oral potassium supplementation on blood pressure (Whelton et al., 1997), concluded that potassium supplementation was associated with lower systolic and diastolic blood pressure by approximately 3 mm Hg and 2 mm Hg, respectively. The effect appeared to be strongest where sodium intake was higher.

The effect of salt consumption in elevating blood pressure has been confirmed by two large population studies (Stamler, 1997; Stamler et al., 1996). Although the analyses were cross-sectional in nature, it seems unlikely that hypertensives would choose to take in more salt and so distort the association. This confirms work from many smaller randomized trials on the effect of dietary salt.

Dietary cholesterol, saturated fatty acids, starch, and alcohol have been positively related to blood pressure in a large population study (Stamler et al., 1996), whereas more dietary protein and polyunsaturated acids were associated with lower blood pressure. Fruit fiber intake (undoubtedly also correlated with potassium and magnesium) was associated with lower blood pressure in a multivariate analysis from a large prospective study (Ascherio et al., 1992). A similar pattern was found when these variables were related to changes in reported blood pressure values between 1986 and 1990. More work is necessary to confirm the causal nature of these associations.

Finally, the recently published Dietary Approaches to Stop Hypertension (DASH) Trial (Harsha et al., 1999; Moore et al., 1999) is of interest as an attempt to put many of these dietary factors together in an experimental study of three different diets and their effects on blood pressure. The control diet was a typical American diet. A second diet emphasized fruit and vegetables, but was similar to the control diet in macronutrient content. Potassium and magnesium were markedly higher in the fruit-and-vegetables diet, but sodium intakes did not differ. The third diet was also high in fruit and vegetables, but included only low-fat dairy products. The third diet also had markedly more potassium, magnesium, and calcium than the control diet, but less total and saturated fat, cholesterol and meat, and, again, there was no difference in sodium intake.

The effects of these diets were quite dramatic over the eight-week period of the study. The third diet showed the greatest effect with drops of 5.5 mm Hg and 3.0 mm Hg, respectively, in systolic and diastolic pressures, as compared with corresponding changes in the control group. The differences were highly statistically significant, quite consistent for men and women, and much greater among hypertensives (relative drops of 11.4 mm Hg in systolic pressure and 5.5 mm Hg in diastolic).

Thus, vegetarians have lower blood pressure and less hypertension. However, it is not clear that lack of meat is the important factor. Evidence suggests that lower salt intake, higher potassium, less alcohol, and more fruit, all of which characterize many vegetarian diets, will lower blood pressure (see Chapter 12 for further comments).

Rheumatoid Arthritis, Other Forms of Arthritis and Rheumatism, and Vegetarian Status

Male and female nonvegetarian Adventists in the Adventist Health Study reported about a 50% greater prevalence of both rheumatoid arthritis and other forms of arthritis/rheumatism than vegetarian Adventists (see Table 8–6). There was little evidence that obesity is associated with the prevalence of rheumatoid arthritis, although the analysis shown does adjust for BMI. However, for "other arthritis/rheumatism," probably largely osteoarthritis, obesity is associated with increased risk, especially in women. When adjusting for obesity, the effect of vegetarianism remains important

Table 8-6. Associations between Vegetarian Status, Body Mass Index (BMI), and the Prevalence of Arthritis in Adventists[a]

	Men				Women			
Exposure Variable	Adjusted for Age Only	95% Confidence Interval	Adjusted for Age and BMI	95% Confidence Interval	Adjusted for Age Only	95% Confidence Interval	Adjusted for Age and BMI	95% Confidence Interval
RHEUMATOID ARTHRITIS								
Vegetarian status								
Vegetarian			1.00				1.00	
Semivegetarian			1.16	0.84–1.61			1.16	0.97–1.40
Nonvegetarian			1.56***	1.19–2.05			1.54***	1.31–1.80
OTHER ARTHRITIS AND RHEUMATISM								
Vegetarian status								
Vegetarian	1.00		1.00		1.00		1.00	
Semivegetarian	1.20	1.03–1.39	1.15	0.98–1.34	1.28	1.16–1.41	1.21	1.01–1.45
Nonvegetarian	1.48***	1.31–1.68	1.37***	1.20–1.55	1.61***	1.49–1.75	1.44***	1.32–1.57
BODY MASS INDEX								
First quintile			1.00				1.00	
Second quintile			0.96	0.80–1.16			1.17	1.04–1.33
Third quintile			0.96	0.80–1.15			1.40***	1.24–1.59
Fourth quintile			1.15	0.96–1.37			1.62***	1.44–1.83
Fifth quintile			1.46***	1.22–1.75			2.16***	1.91–2.43

*** $p < .0001$

[a]Adjusted for age and/or obesity in two separate models.

for both arthritic endpoints but has a slightly diminished magnitude in the second case, suggesting that the beneficial effect of vegetarianism here may be partly mediated by the lower body weights for vegetarians of any particular height.

There is little other prospective work associating lifestyle with new osteoarthritis. However, obesity is clearly a risk factor (Cooper et al., 1998), as is occupational heavy lifting among men (Coggon et al., 1998). There is limited evidence of a vascular component to spondylosis, a common form of arthritis of the spine. Finnish investigators performed postmortem angiographic examinations and found significant correlations between the number of missing (or stenosed) lumbar arteries and the severity of antemortem back-related symptoms (Kauppila and Tallroth, 1993). Moreover, there was a significant correlation between the severity of aortic atherosclerosis and vertebral disk degeneration (Kauppila et al., 1993). Smoking, a widely established risk factor for vascular disease, may be more common among those with spondylosis (Battie et al., 1991).

There is little support in the literature for the idea that nonspinal osteoarthritis has a vascular component, although one study has found that patients with generalized osteoarthritis were more likely to be hyperlipidemic than those who have only one hip or one knee joint affected (Sturmer et al., 1998). Thus, if vegetarianism does indeed protect against osteoarthritis (including spondylosis), it is possible that this is partly mediated through vascular effects. However, the etiology of osteoarthritis is at present poorly understood, as are the possible roles played by dietary factors.

Folklore has long held that diet is related to rheumatoid arthritis and other types of arthritis. In fact, only preliminary and inconclusive evidence is available. In Italy, LaVecchia et al. (1998) found a 16% reduction in prevalence of rheumatoid arthritis among those in the highest category of vegetable intake as compared with those in the lowest. Another Italian case-control study found a protective association with higher consumption both olive oil and cooked vegetables (Linos et al., 1999). A vegetarian diet may improve symptoms in some patients, according to two experimental studies conducted among rheumatoid arthritics (Kjeldsen-Kragh, 1999; Kjeldsen-Kragh et al., 1991, 1995; Peltonen et al., 1997). Both supplements of dietary omega-3 polyunsaturated fatty acids (Cleland and James, 1997; Nielsen et al., 1992) and fasting (Mangge et al., 1999) have also been reported to improve the clinical status of some patients. However, the latter studies all have design flaws and there is the possibility of different interpretations (Mangge et al., 1999; Nenonen, 1998). Thus, more evidence is necessary before concluding that such dietary manipulations are clinically effective.

Grant (2000) has summarized ecologic evidence for an association between meat consumption and the risk of rheumatoid arthritis, but such evidence cannot strongly support causality. He and others have also described some possible mechanisms by which a vegetarian diet may improve the clinical status of those with rheumatoid arthritis. Omega-6 polyunsaturated fatty acids, mainly linoleic acid, are increased in many vegetarian diets but are not clearly helpful in treating rheumatoid arthritis (Haugen et al., 1994) and do not seem to suppress cell-mediated inflammatory responses (Rosetti et al., 1997).

Omega-3 fatty acids (Henderson and Panush, 1999; Shapiro et al., 1996), in contrast, can act by inhibiting cellular immune and inflammatory responses (Rosetti et al., 1997). They promote the formation of a family of prostaglandins—thromboxanes and leukotrienes. These eicosanoids are important mediators of platelet function, vascular homeostasis, and inflammation, and those that incorporate omega-3, rather than omega-6, fatty acids may protect against some inflammatory diseases (Cleland and James, 1997). A small, but carefully conducted, double-blind randomized trial for an omega-3 fatty acid, gamma linolenic acid (Zurier et al., 1996), did show quite impressive differences in favor of this treatment, although minor differences in the baseline characteristics of the subjects suggest the need for confirmation in a larger trial. Aside from their presence in fatty deepwater fish, omega-3 fatty acids are also found in certain vegetables, mainly as linolenic acid. Good sources are flaxseeds, primrose oil, and walnuts (Callegari et al., 1991; DeLuca et al., 1995).

Finally, it has been suggested that antibodies to the colonic bacterium *Proteus mirabilis* may be involved in the etiology of rheumatoid arthritis (Deighton et al., 1992; Ebringer et al., 1985; Rogers et al., 1988). In the experimental study by Kjeldsen-Kragh (1999), the vegetarian diet caused a decrease in IgG antibody production against this bacterium, and it was these changes, rather than changes in fatty acid constituents of the blood (Kjeldsen-Kragh et al., 1995), that correlated significantly with the reported improvement in clinical status (Kjeldsen-Kragh et al., 1991).

SUMMARY

1. Vegetarian Adventists have a much lower weight for a given height than do nonvegetarian Adventists. This result is supported by other studies of vegetarians. Vegetarians probably gain less weight during their adult years, but vegetarian women, at least, lose less weight at the oldest ages—both probably being beneficial effects.

2. Vegetarian Adventists are less likely to develop diabetes. The existing studies were not specifically designed to test this hypothesis but nevertheless suggest a moderate protective effect. Much of this "vegetarian" effect is probably due to the lower prevalence of obesity in the vegetarians.

3. Adventist vegetarians are much less likely to develop new hypertension than are nonvegetarians. This is supported by other studies of the vegetarian diet. It is not clear that meat is the hazardous agent, and the intake of less salt and more potassium and fruit probably accounts for at least part of this difference. Adjustment for obesity modestly attenuated the vegetarian effect, suggesting that some, but not all, of this is mediated by the lower weight of vegetarians.

4. Self-reported (ostensibly, doctor-diagnosed) rheumatoid arthritis was substantially less prevalent in vegetarian than in nonvegetarian Adventists. Adjustment for obesity changed the results very little, suggesting that effects of vegetarianism on this form of arthritis are mediated in ways aside from differences in body weight. Limited evidence suggests that a vegetarian diet, and a diet with increased omega-3 fatty acids, may improve the clinical status of those with diagnosed rheumatoid arthritis, and some mechanisms have been suggested.

5. Vegetarians also have a decreased risk of other forms of arthritis/rheumatism, probably most of which is osteoarthritis. Although obesity was clearly a risk factor for these other types of arthritis, the lower weight of the vegetarians could only partly explain the protective effect. Some evidence suggests that there is a vascular component to spondylosis, and one idea is that diet may act here by improving vascular function, but more evidence is necessary.

9

Social Support, Religiosity, Other Psychological Factors, and Health

JERRY LEE, GRAHAM STACEY, AND GARY FRASER

Rather than providing a comprehensive analysis of psychosocial and religious commitment variables and their effects on mortality rates, we will focus here on the roles that some of these factors might play in distorting our dietary analyses. For instance, vegetarian Adventists may have better social support or attend church more regularly. If social support or church attendance are independent predictors of mortality, the apparent influence of vegetarianism would involve a mixture of effects of the related psychosocial variables and of any true effect of vegetarianism. In other words, the dietary and psychosocial variables would then be confounded and both would need to be included in the statistical models if their independent effects were to be estimated. Some possible interrelations between different kinds of variables are shown in Figure 9–1.

A confounding variable needs to be related to both the variable of interest (say, meat consumption) and the endpoint it affects (say, CHD mortality). Hence, in the sections that follow, we provide definitions of some of the psychosocial and religious variables of interest and describe mechanisms by which they may influence mortality. To the extent that the Adventist data allow, associations between psychosocial variables and dietary factors, and between psychosocial factors and mortality, are explored separately to decide if confounding is likely. Finally, analyses that include both dietary variables and the psychosocial variables suspected to be confounders, are used to estimate the independent effects of both kinds of factors.

SOCIAL SUPPORT AND HEALTH

Social isolation can be considered a chronically stressful condition that may have harmful physiologic and psychologic consequences. Social support

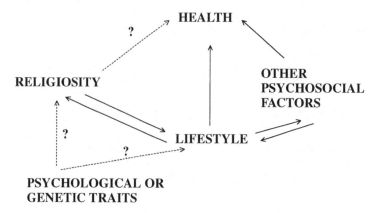

Figure 9–1 Possible pathways between religiosity, other causal factors, and health status. Question marks and dotted lines indicate the more speculative links. Although arrows directed from "health" to other factors are likely, these are not relevant to this discussion.

will help counteract these problems. The broad concept of social support is understood to comprise several components. First, there is a structural aspect—how large and complex is the social network? This is usually measured as the number of friends and close family members that a person can count on, marital status, and participation in social groups and religious organizations.

Second, this network can potentially act in several different ways to influence health. It may provide personal support, social influence, social engagement, and better access to and information about supportive community resources (Berkman and Glass, 2000). Thus, simply knowing the size and structure of a network identifies only potential benefits. Whether the supportive mechanisms actually operate is more important, and depends on other characteristics of the network and the person.

Personal support has an emotional "loving and caring" component but also includes what has been labeled instrumental support, where others provide tangible assistance, when necessary, for cooking, shopping, or even providing money. Social influence refers to the way that social interactions may influence a person's opinions and behaviors. In some instances, these influences can be powerful determinants of dietary, exercise, and smoking habits that have important health consequences. Social engagement is especially important for elderly subjects. The emphasis here is that social participation in clubs or church activities, for instance, will often enhance a sense of well-being and self-worth. Finally, social involvement and participation in networks can often provide better information about and access to job opportunities and health care—which also have health consequences.

Psychological and biological mechanisms have been proposed to explain how these social factors may cause or prevent physical disease. First, as mentioned, greater social support may allow better access to medical care. Second, there is some evidence that increasing social disconnection is associated with a greater prevalence of health-damaging behaviors, such as cigarette smoking and physical inactivity (Hanson et al., 1987; Murray et al., 1995; Trieber et al., 1991). Third, better social support improves perceived self-efficacy and reduces the risk of depression. Socially isolated individuals, particularly when elderly, are more prone to depression (Murphy, 1982). Oxman and colleagues (1992) found that the previous loss of one's spouse, inadequate emotional support, inadequate tangible support, recent loss of a confidant, and the numbers of children visiting weekly were all predictive of depression. As depression itself is associated with poorer physical health, social isolation may partly act, through depression, to affect physical health.

Finally, there is an extensive literature describing research among animals that have been deprived of social contacts, either at critical stages of development or permanently. As compared with other animals, they often have higher resting pulse rates and blood pressure (Watson et al., 1998), along with exaggerated hormonal responses to stress. Cortisone and epinephrine levels are more responsive to stress in these than in nondeprived animals and are often slower to recover after the stress ends (Suomi, 1997). Other work indicates that the endothelial function of arteries and vasomotor responses to acetylcholine are markedly impaired in socially deprived monkeys (Williams et al., 1991). There is some suggestion of similar hormonal and cardiovascular responses in socially deprived humans subjected to stress, although much less information is available (Knox and Uvnas-Moberg, 1998). Uchino et al. (1996, 1999) have reviewed this literature in more detail.

That these physiologic changes can result in arterial pathology has been shown in socially disrupted cynomolgus monkeys (Kaplan et al., 1991). Such monkeys develop significantly more arterial atherosclerosis. In a large population study of Finnish men, those with more exaggerated blood pressure responses to mental stress had evidence of significantly greater carotid atherosclerosis than others (Kamarck et al., 1997).

Cellular immunocompetence in humans may also respond to social support (Adler and Hillhouse, 1996; Kiecolt-Glasser et al., 1994; Thomas et al., 1985). For example, a recent experimental study showed that, when intentionally exposed to the common cold virus, those subjects with more types of social contacts were less susceptible to infection (Cohen et al., 1997). Further details of such possible mechanisms can be found in Berkman and Glass (2000).

That lack of social support is associated with increased mortality in humans has been shown many times. Many of these studies measured social support in terms of the structure of the social network. This was simply scored as combinations of factors such as marital status, contacts with friends and relatives, church membership, and membership in other groups. This total social network index was an important predictor of both all-cause and CHD mortality (Berkman and Breslow, 1983; Berkman and Syme, 1979; Reed et al., 1983). There were twofold to fourfold differences in all-cause mortality in different age and sex groups when those with the fewest connections and those with the most connections were compared. Those who were least connected were at an increased risk of dying from cerebrovascular and circulatory disease and from cancer. While these structural and functional measures of support are related to health outcomes, it is interesting that, on reviewing the existing literature, Penninx et al. (1996) conclude that perceived social support is probably even more important.

Thirteen prospective studies that evaluated the health effects of social support were reviewed by Berkman and Glass (2000); by their design, these studies had the ability to determine that any inferred causality must run in the direction that poor social support causes disease, rather than the converse occurring. In general, the effects on mortality in these studies have been stronger than effects on incidence. This suggests that social support may affect survival after a diagnosis more strongly than it affects the risk of disease in the first place. Although significant effects in women were sometimes demonstrated, they were often stronger in men.

Social Support in California Adventists

The California Adventist cohort studies collected relatively little information on social support. They included questions on whether subjects were presently married, whether they considered their mother and father to have been "warm and understanding," and "how satisfied" they were with their "present family life." Thus these questions provided quite limited information about emotional support both during childhood and at study baseline.

Briefly, these social support variables were often modestly but still significantly related to all-cause mortality for the California Adventists. When adjusted for age, married men and women had mortality ratios of 0.82 and 0.90, respectively, when compared with single subjects (both $p = .004$). Those men and women who reported that their mother was "warm and understanding" had mortality ratios of 0.86 ($p = .03$) and 0.88 ($p = .009$), respectively, as compared with those not checking this box in the questionnaire. A similar question regarding feelings toward their fathers was not a significant predictor of mortality in either sex. Those men who claimed to be satisfied with their family life had the same mortality ratio as others (1.01), but women with a similar claim had a ratio of 0.90 ($p = .03$) as compared with those who were not satisfied with their family life. These same variables also showed a low order of protection for CHD mortality but without statistical significance. Thus, the effects are small, although often statistically significant, and it seems unlikely that these variables would significantly confound dietary associations with CHD or all-cause mortality. However, it is worth emphasizing again that our ability to measure social support in this cohort was quite limited.

There is a link between social support and religiosity. Religiosity is a complex concept, and greater participation in religion may affect health through several mechanisms. One of these involves increased social support. Greater religious involvement will often provide more personal emotional support, social influence, and social engagement. We will adjust for measured aspects of social support when examining any effects of religiosity on health.

RELIGIOSITY AND HEALTH

The idea that religion and health are related is not new. For example, Proverbs 3:7–8 (Revised Standard Version of the Bible) states: "Be not wise in your own eyes; fear the LORD, and turn away from evil. It will be healing to your flesh and refreshment to your bones." In 1890, Ellen White, one of the founders of the Seventh-day Adventist Church, also emphasized the connection between religion and health: "True religion brings man into harmony with the laws of God, physical, mental, and moral. It teaches self-control, serenity, temperance. Religion ennobles the mind, refines the taste, and sanctifies the judgment. . . . Faith in God's love and overruling providence lightens the burdens of anxiety and care. . . . Religion tends directly to promote health, to lengthen life, and to heighten our enjoyment of all its blessings" (White, 1890, p. 600).

However, there had been relatively little interest in this subject among mainline health researchers and professionals until the late 1980s. Much of the earlier research had emphasized membership, particularly in denominations such as the Seventh-day Adventists and the Mormons, whose religion advocated certain lifestyle practices that may promote better health (Jarvis and Northcott, 1987). However, denominational affiliation is severely limited as a causal variable—between-group differences may be severely confounded by even greater within-group differences.

Research on religiosity (Comstock and Partridge [1972] reported one of the first studies) then shifted toward an examination of the association between church attendance and health (Levin and Vanderpool, 1987). However, if the effect of poor health in decreasing church attendance is not accounted for, conclusions from this research can be problematic. More recently, a greater emphasis has been placed on the study of how personal religious experience and motivation relate to health. Initially, Allport and Ross (1967) defined intrinsic and extrinsic religiosity. Those with intrinsic religious motivation believe and participate because of the value they see in the beliefs themselves. An extrinsic religious motivation, however, reflects more sensitivity to the possible gains that will result from religion or religious activity, whether they will be social gains from church attendance or comfort from prayer. Some (e.g., Genia, 1996; Koenig et al., 1992) have found associations of these two types of religiosity with mental and physical health.

Since 1985 there have been at least 16 reviews of this literature—8 dealing with possible effects of religiosity on physical health (Ellison and Levin, 1998; Hill and Butter, 1995; Jarvis and Northcott, 1987; Levin, 1994; Levin and Schiller, 1987; Levin and Vanderpool, 1987, 1991; Matthews et al., 1998), and 8 covering effects on mental health (Gartner et al., 1991; Larson et al., 1992; Levin and Chatters, 1998b; McCullough and Larson, 1999; Mickley et al., 1995; Payne et al., 1991; Weaver et al., 1998, 2000). There is room for concern about the methodologic adequacy of many of the studies reviewed (see Levin, 1994; Sloan et al., 1999), but most reviewers have concluded that the consistency in finding a salutatory association between religion and health is impressive.

In adolescence, religious attendance, importance of religious belief, and adherence to religious beliefs have been associated with less injury-related behavior (e.g., violent actions, riding with a drinking driver, or not wearing seat belts) (Wallace and Forman, 1998); less drug use, including use of alcohol and tobacco, among both Adventist and general samples of American youth (Dudley et al., 1987; Wallace and Forman, 1998; Weaver et al., 2000); less, or delayed, sexual activity (Weaver et al., 2000); and less "delinquency" among Mormons (Chadwick and Top, 1993).

Among adults, religion—most commonly religious attendance—has been associated with lowered mortality and morbidity (Jarvis and Northcott, 1987), a reduction in cancer (Troyer, 1988), lowered blood pressure (Levin and Vanderpool, 1989), lower levels of stress (Anson et al., 1990b; Maton, 1989), increased subjective well-being (Ellison, 1991; Ellison and Gay, 1990; Maltby et al., 1999; Pollner, 1989; Poloma and Pendleton, 1991), and better immune function in HIV-seropositive gay men (Woods et al., 1999). In elderly participants, religious behaviors and beliefs have been associated with better subjective health among those with important physical problems (Musick, 1996), faster remission of depression for intrinsically religious individuals (Koenig et al., 1998a), and a greater sense of psychological well-being (Levin and Chatters, 1998a).

However, some of these associations are complex and puzzling. For example, Strawbridge et al. (1998) report that both organizational religiosity (church attendance and involvement in church activities) and personal religiosity (prayer and the importance of religious and spiritual beliefs) reduced the effect of nonfamily stressors on depression. However, both types of religiosity also increased the influence of certain family stressors on depression.

The literature is not entirely uniform in citing beneficial associations, and a few studies have shown either no association or negative associations of religion with various aspects of health. For example, rehabilitation patients who were more religious than others did not recover sooner (Fitchett et al., 1999) and patients who "professed some form of spiritual belief, whether or not they engaged in a religious activity" were more likely to "remain the same or deteriorate clinically nine months later" (King et al., 1999, p. 1291).

So far this discussion has mentioned only statistical associations. It is much more difficult to establish whether or not religious participation or beliefs are causally related to better health. Only fairly recently have a few reports been published that incorporate a longitudinal study design and the appropriate controls necessary to tease out causality. These often continue to support a positive religion–health relationship. In one series of studies, Idler and Kasl found that improvements in functionality and depression were associated with greater religious participation and that the religious elderly were apparently able to delay death until, or after, religious holidays (Idler and Kasl, 1992, 1997). Oxman et al. (1995) showed that, among the elderly, following elective open-heart surgery, mortality rates were higher for individuals with lower rates of participation in social or community groups and those who felt that they had no strength or comfort from religion.

Lower mortality among subjects with more frequent religious attendance (prior to the research) has been noted in four prospective studies (Bryant and Rakowski, 1992; Hummer et al., 1999; Oman and Reed, 1998; Strawbridge et al., 1997). These associations persisted despite controls for initial health and social support, though with reduced strength. Other prospective research, however, has failed to find relationships between religion and later health experience (Anson et al., 1990a; Fitchett et al., 1999; Levin and Taylor, 1998c), although the study by Fitchett et al. had a small sample size of only 96.

Thus, although the prospective studies have a stronger design, they have used a confusing variety of measures of "religiosity," and the control for other possibly causal confounding variables has often been inadequate. The strongest evidence of the benefits of religiosity is for religious attendance and participation variables, but it is unclear whether there is some intrinsic benefit to this, or whether it is a mark of more personal religiosity or of other nonreligious behavioral variables and risk factors. More prospective research that incorporates measures of personal religiosity and better control of confounding variables is necessary before conclusions can be drawn.

Possible Mechanisms for a Religiosity–Health Connection

As usual, it is difficult to conclude that associations are causal ones in the absence of biological mechanisms. If religious practice and belief are connected to health, then it is important to understand where such connections might come from. One early suggestion of possible mechanisms was made by Vaux (1976) and was briefly mentioned in Chapter 1. A more recent and comprehensive search (Ellison and Levin, 1998) has suggested seven possible mechanisms.

Regulation of health behaviors and personal lifestyles

Religious beliefs may cause a reduction in harmful behaviors or an increase in healthful behaviors. This idea is not new. Maimonides, the twelfth-century rabbi and physician, argued that people had a positive duty to "avoid whatever is injurious to the body, and cultivate habits conducive to health and vigor" in order to clearly understand how to "walk in the ways of God" (*Mishneh Torah*, quoted in Tomlinson, 1991, p. 114). Matthew Henry, who published a commentary on the Bible in 1607, made a more explicit connection between religion and improved health behaviors: "The prudence and sobriety which religion teaches, tend not only to the health of the soul, but to the health of the body" (Henry, 1983, p. 462).

Social integration and social support

As was pointed out earlier, there is considerable evidence that support from others is related to decreased mortality and morbidity. Religious participation is one source of such support. Ellison and Levin (1998) cite studies showing that more frequent church attenders have larger and denser social networks and exchange information, goods, and services more often than less frequent attenders. Religious organizations bring together individuals of similar beliefs and values. Friendships are more likely to arise between church participants and similar others (Berscheid and Reis, 1998).

Several have also argued that the perceived support that the religious person has from God may be health-enhancing, and they have provided some supporting data (Maton, 1989; Pollner, 1989).

Self-esteem and personal efficacy

Religion may help people maintain their self-esteem, sense of self-worth, and sense of personal efficacy (Bergin et al., 1987; Gartner et al., 1991; Payne et al., 1991), and this may promote better health (Ellison and Levin, 1998). However, these relationships are complex. Watson et al. (1988) found that an intrinsic orientation to religion, along with a belief in grace, predicted less self-consciousness, depression, hopelessness, and self-efficacy among undergraduates; however, an "extrinsic orientation to religion" and "orthodox religious beliefs dealing with guilt, tended to predict maladjustment" (p. 270). These matters are still far from settled and the answers will probably not be simple.

Coping resources and behaviors

Isaiah said, "Thou wilt keep him in perfect peace, whose mind is stayed on thee" (Isaiah 26:3) and suggested that religious belief may reduce mental stress. Hindus have a similar concept: "He who knows the joy of Brahman . . . is free from fear" (*Taittiriya Upanishad* 2.7–9). Lazarus and his colleagues (Folkman, 1984; Lazarus and Folkman, 1984; Lazarus and Launier, 1978) have argued that the experience of stress depends on how one appraises an event and the resources one has to cope with it. To the extent that religion increases such resources and changes the way that events are appraised, it may reduce the influence of stress on health.

Ellison and Levin (1998) suggest that meditation and prayer may help a believer cope with stress by increasing the sense of personal control (see also, McCullough [1995], for a review of some of these issues). Prayer may be a religious person's coping mechanism that improves the health of both the person praying and the person who knows he or she is being prayed for (Harmon and Myers, 1999; Levin and Taylor, 1998; McCullough, 1995; Poloma and Pendleton, 1991). It has been shown that another type of coping—confession, a practice encouraged among Christians (James 5:16; 1 John 1:9)—may reduce physician visits and perhaps improve immune system function (Pennebaker, 1989, 1995). Finally, some (Goldberg, 1986, 1987; Golner, 1982) believe that Sabbath-keeping can promote better mental health, but there seems to be little research on this as a form of religious coping behavior or on its effect on health.

As McCullough (1995) points out, however, some other forms of "religious coping" can actually lead to increased problems in dealing with stress. The extensive research done by Pargament and his colleagues

(Pargament, 1990; Pargament and Brant, 1998; Pargament et al., 1988, 1992, 1998a, 1998b) has shown both advantages and disadvantages to using "religious coping" to deal with stress. By "religious coping," Pargament means attempting to deal with stressful events by using religious imagery or explanations. Framing a negative event as somehow being the will of God or the result of loving God's actions was associated with positive outcomes. Attributing the negative event to God's act of punishment was associated with negative outcomes.

Positive emotions

Salovey and colleagues (2000) review literature suggesting that positive emotional states may promote better physical health. Other researchers have documented an adverse impact of at least some negative emotions on health and mortality (Cohen and Herbert, 1996; King, 1997; Miller et al., 1996; Musselman et al., 1998; Penninx et al., 1999; Wulsin et al., 1999). Religion, however, may induce positive emotional states such as "forgiveness, contentment, and love" (Ellison and Levin, 1998).

Specific research in this area of the connection between religion and health is limited. Levin and Chatters (1998a), in a cross-sectional study of three national probability samples, present evidence that religious beliefs promote a sense of positive well-being and health; Myers (2000) concludes, after a review of evidence, that religious people tend to be happier than the nonreligious. However, there is also the potential for certain religious experiences to produce "negative emotions such as guilt and fear" (Ellison and Levin, 1998, p. 708), as was pointed out by Freud (1927).

Healthy beliefs

Research on placebo (Fisher and Greenberg, 1997) and nocebo effects (Hahn, 1999) suggests that expectations that one will become healthy or ill can affect health. Ellison and Levin (1998) suggest that religion may encourage positive expectations and that these expectations can improve health. There is evidence that feelings of hope or optimism (Peterson, 1995, 2000; Scheier and Carver, 1992), various forms of positive illusions (Taylor et al., 2000), and a sense of coherence (a belief that life is meaningful, manageable, and comprehensible) (Antonovsky, 1992; Coe et al., 1998) are associated with improved physical health. However, while it is reasonable to suggest that religion may promote such beliefs, the direct evidence is limited.

Additional mechanisms

Byrd (1988) found positive effects of intercessory prayer on the health of hospitalized patients in a double-blind randomized clinical trial. Individuals who did not know or meet the patients were asked to pray for a randomly selected group of patients, who also did not know whether they would receive this intercessory prayer. As compared with the group not receiving these additional prayers, the experimental group seemed to have better outcomes. Since then, at least two other randomized, double-blind clinical trials (Harris et al., 1999; O'Laoire, 1997) have apparently demonstrated some effectiveness of intercessory prayer. But Walker et al. (1997) failed to find any effect of intercessory prayer on individuals in an alcohol treatment program.

Targ (1997) has provided a review on the effectiveness of such "distant healing," and Levin (1996) has discussed possible theoretical models to explain its claimed effectiveness. None of the six primary mechanisms that Ellison and Levin (1998) have described can account for such effects, and, indeed, a variety of "unusual hypotheses" have been offered to account for them. These include "the operation of subtle bioenergies, morphogenetic fields, psi effects, non-local consciousness, and 'divine' or supernatural influences" (p. 709).

In summary, there is no shortage of possible ideas as to how religiosity may affect physical and mental health, but the existing data are quite limited, and the results often require complicated explanations. Further, religion is a multidimensional phenomenon, and any one measure fails to capture its entire meaning. Examining the religion-and-health relationship with clear, unambiguous, and agreed-upon operational definitions is a serious methodological challenge.

Research on the Religiosity–Health Connection among Adventists

Traditional Adventism belongs to the fundamentalist branch of Christianity, and emphasizes a fairly literal understanding of the scriptures. Although not always acknowledged, historically, there has often been a substantial emphasis on works and performance as indicators of piety. However, church members today span a spectrum of practice and may differ in many of the details of belief, motivation, and practice. Nearly all Adventists support a "whole-person" model of health and well-being, which includes physical, mental, and spiritual dimensions. This justifies the church's emphasis on personal health and its commitment to medical institutions.

There has been little previous peer-reviewed research on the association between religion and health among Seventh-day Adventists. Dudley et al. (1987) found an association between religious belief and lowered drug use in adolescent Adventists. Lee et al. (1997) found that the experience of regular family worship that rotated among family members was associated with lower drug use among adolescent Adventists. These associations raise the possibility of causal connections but do not prove them.

The religiosity data gathered from participants in the 1976 Adventist Health Study in California are confined to attendance and participation variables. There is no information about personal beliefs and motivations. However, as others have often found attendance and participation to be predictive of mortality, analysis of the Adventist data is of interest.

The distribution of these participation variables among the Adventists is shown in Table 9–1. The main variable, "frequency of church attendance," refers to attendance at the worship hour of a Saturday morning. In addition, most Adventist churches have an optional midweek evening prayer meeting that is attended by some members. Lay members hold important church offices—for example, church elders, Sabbath school (similar to Sunday school) leaders, treasurer, musicians, and many others that enable the church to function.

The Adventist participants in this study group were overwhelmingly frequent church attenders, which is quite typical of Adventists in general (see Chapter 1). However, much more diversity is found in the frequency of holding church office and in attendance at midweek prayer meetings. Participation appears to be very similar among men and women.

Further, these participation variables, measured in 1976, are related to subsequent risk of incident CHD and also to all-cause mortality (see Table 9–2). Strong associations are found between church attendance and both coronary and all-cause mortality, suggesting that those Adventist men who attend infrequently have a 60–70% increase in the risk of incident CHD mortality and a 20–50% increase in all-cause mortality.

Table 9–1. Frequency of Attendance or Participation in Religious Activities: The California Adventist Health Study[a]

Variable	Level	Men	Women
		Percentages	
Church attendance	<1/mo	4.5	4.6
	1–2/mo	5.3	6.8
	3–4/mo	90.2	88.6
Holds church office	Never	14.0	18.7
	Occasionally	20.9	26.7
	Often	27.4	26.3
	Nearly always	37.7	28.3
Attendance at midweek prayer meeting	Never	31.6	26.9
	Occasionally	36.5	38.4
	Frequently or nearly always	31.8	34.8

[a]This excludes those in low-participation categories with known heart disease, cancer, stroke, or arthritis or rheumatism that might have caused their diminished participation and may also effect subsequent mortality.

Table 9-2. Attendance at Religious Services and Other Religious Participation among Adventists in Relation to Incident Coronary Heart Disease (CHD) and All-Cause Mortality[a]

		CHD Mortality		All-Cause Mortality	
Variable	Level	Men	Women	Men	Women
Church attendance	3–4/mo	1.00	1.00	1.00	1.00
	1–2/mo	1.37 (.39–2.08)	2.03 (1.11–3.71)	1.05 (.74–1.48)	1.30 (1.00–1.68)
	<1/mo	1.73 (1.01–2.98)	1.63 (1.00–2.66)	1.44 (1.09–1.89)	1.23 (.98–1.53)
Holds church office	Never	1.00	1.00	1.00	1.00
	Occasionally	0.52 (.32–.83)	0.99 (.66–1.48)	0.70 (.56–.87)	0.88 (.74–1.04)
	Often	0.56 (.36–.88)	0.74 (.48–1.14)	0.78 (.63–.96)	0.89 (.75–1.06)
	Nearly Always	0.42 (.27–.66)	0.93 (.61–1.40)	0.74 (.60–.90)	0.89 (.75–1.06)
Attendance at midweek prayer meeting	Never	1.00	1.00	1.00	1.00
	Occasionally	1.12 (.74–1.69)	0.86 (.54–1.35)	0.91 (.76–1.10)	0.87 (.74–1.03)
	Frequently or nearly always	1.08 (.69–1.69)	1.22 (.79–1.89)	0.94 (.77–1.13)	0.88 (.74–1.05)

[a]Subjects who had known chronic diseases (prevalent CHD, stroke, cancer, arthritis/rheumatism) that may interfere with attendance and participation were excluded from this analysis. Each variable in these analyses is adjusted for age, each other, and the other social support variables that we had available, specifically "a warm and understanding mother," "marital status," "satisfaction with family life," "participation in church social activities."

Table 9–3. Association (%) between Church Attendance and Other Behavioral Risk Factors[a]

Church Attendance	High Exercise	Meat <1/mo	Nuts ≥5/wk	Past Smoking	High Quartile Depression
MEN					
3–4/mo	47.1	35.5	26.2	30.9	16.9
1–2/mo	40.0	12.0	15.5	29.2	26.5
<1/mo	41.2	8.9	13.9	41.3	24.9
WOMEN					
3–4/mo	37.3	35.4	24.6	12.8	23.9
1–2/mo	33.5	13.6	15.1	15.8	33.7
<1/mo	29.1	12.1	12.5	17.9	35.0

[a]Age-adjusted test of no association $p < .0001$ for both sexes for all variables.

These relationships are strong and statistically significant for men, and, although a little weaker, are almost statistically significant for women. Holding church office also appears to be protective for men, but is much less clearly predictive for women. These statistical effects of church attendance and of holding church offices are independent of each other, as both sets of variables are placed together in the statistical model. Note that the analyses also adjust for the social support variables that are available (see the data discussed above). In fact, this adjustment hardly changed the estimates at all, suggesting that effects of religious participation on mortality are acting through mechanisms that are separate from the few social support variables that we measured.

Those Adventists who attend church more regularly generally have a more healthful lifestyle (see Table 9–3). Those who attend three to four times per month also exercise more, eat nuts more frequently, are much more likely to be vegetarians, and are less likely to be past smokers or depressed, when compared with less frequent attenders. Hence, religious participation may in part be a marker for lower risk values for these variables rather than a risk factor in its own right. Even then religiosity would still be a potent force for risk reduction if it were a cause of these lower risk values among this population. This point is considered further in the final section of this chapter.

SELECTED PSYCHOLOGICAL VARIABLES, FATAL CHD, AND ALL-CAUSE MORTALITY

A large number of psychological factors have been studied in relation to mortality (Shepherd and Weiss, 1987), but here we will briefly focus on three variables for which the Adventist Health Study provides some data: a sense of "time urgency," depressive feelings, and frequent feelings of hostility. Prospective studies are emphasized in the brief review of related work by others that follows; in retrospective studies the presence of disease may bias subjects' perceptions of psychological factors.

The type A behavior pattern was originally described by Friedman and Rosenman (1959), and a sense of increased "time urgency" was one of the components of this behavior pattern. In their data, type A behavior was associated with an elevated risk of CHD (Rosenman et al., 1975). However, some later studies did not confirm this association (Leon et al., 1988; Shekelle et al., 1985) or even found that it was associated with fewer events (Ragland and Brand, 1988). The evidence for type A behavior as a risk factor was perhaps strongest in predicting recurrent events for those with existing heart disease, but even here the results are mixed (Ahern et al., 1990; Case et al., 1985; Friedman et al., 1984; Jenkins, 1976; Williams, 1987a). One result from the analysis of a large Duke University data set suggested that type A behavior was hazardous for younger patients but may even be protective for older patients (Williams et al., 1988). Different investigators measured what they call type A behavior either using the original structured interview or by a questionnaire, and these measures are probably not equivalent. Moreover, the several different components of type A behavior, as originally described, almost certainly have quite different effects on CHD risk (Williams, 1987a).

In a more detailed analysis, a component that seemed to be more strongly related to risk than others was labeled hostility. A number of prospective studies have subsequently examined this attribute in relation to all-cause mortality and risk of CHD events (Barefoot et al., 1983, 1995; Everson et al., 1997; Leon et al., 1988; McCranie et al., 1986; Shekelle et al., 1983). Most of these studies used the Ho Personality scale of the Minnesota Multiphasic Personality Inventory (MMPI), which has been described as measuring a tendency toward hostility, cynicism, and anger (Williams, 1987b). Several showed relative risks for CHD that were 1.5- to 2 times higher among those with higher hostility scores as compared with those with lower scores. However, a few studies did not find a significant effect (Leon et al., 1988; McCranie et al., 1986), and one found that an adjustment for other behavioral risk factors (smoking, alcohol consumption, physical activity, and body size) eliminated the hostility association, suggesting that hostility may operate through these factors (Everson et al., 1997).

There is a good deal of evidence from prospective studies that depression creates an increased risk of heart attack (Musselman and Nemeroff, 1998). This is true when we are predicting incident or new coronary events (Anda et al., 1993; Barefoot and Schroll, 1996; Ford et al., 1998; Pratt et al., 1996), and also recurrent events (Ahern et al., 1990; Frasure-Smith et al., 1993, 2000; Ladwig et al., 1991). The Frasure-Smith et al. study suggested that greater social support may improve depression scores and thus decrease CHD mortality in this way. Different studies found significant relative risks for CHD of between 1.5 and 4.5 for depression even after an adjustment was made for other risk factors or, when appropriate, for the severity of existing coronary disease. More generally, a 35-year longitudinal study of Harvard University alumni found that a "pessimistic explanatory style" in the early adult years did predict poor health at ages 45 to 60 when this was evaluated at a subsequent physician examination (Peterson et al., 1988).

Possible mechanisms by which depression may affect risk include sympathoadrenal hyperactivity, ventricular arrhythmias, and increased platelet reactivity (Musselman and Nemeroff, 1998; Nair et al., 1999). Depressed individuals have higher blood levels of catecholamines and higher cerebrospinal fluid levels of the corticotrophin-releasing factor than others, perhaps indicating chronic stimulation of the sympathoadrenal system. Among patients with existing heart disease and depression, the presence of frequent premature ventricular beats seems to be unusually predictive of subsequent mortality.

Selected Psychological Factors, Fatal CHD, and All-Cause Mortality in California Adventists

Now we turn to the Adventist data. In order to find a smaller number of variables to work with, we first applied factor analysis to the 15-odd psychological variables that were available from the Adventist Health Study questionnaire. Some of these variables had somewhat similar meanings, and the factoring technique allowed us to detect groups of similar variables, or factors, and then identify subjects who had higher or lower values for these factors. The idea is that variables contributing heavily to the value for a particular factor may all be measuring some common underlying trait. By studying the content of the questions and answers that contributed strongly to a particular factor, we could provide a label for these common themes. For instance, one group of questions elicited answers that showed that higher scores on certain questions tended to occur in the same individuals. The answers were as follows: "I often feel that I face so many difficulties that I cannot overcome them," "I wish that I could be as happy as others," "I am not satisfied with my present family life." The trait indicated by these answers was labeled a "depressive tendency."

We then formed an index by summing quantile values for each component question. If age-specific quantiles are used for the component questions, the resulting indices allow age-adjusted comparisons between men and women for the depression, authoritarian, and hostility indices. Thus, age- and sex-specific quantiles for the component questions were used when calculating these indices.

Summing quantiles in this way allows each component question to be placed on an equivalent scale (0 to 100%, or lowest to highest) that reflects the ranking of responses among the Adventist study population. Then two questions that have the same rankings, for instance, will contribute the same weights to the index. Indices were formed based on "factors" from the factor analysis that we labeled "time urgency," "depression," "authoritarianism," and "hostility." (The component questions for these factors are given in the note.[1]) Nevertheless, it must be pointed out that these indices have not been independently validated as measures of the corresponding clinical diagnoses. Although they have good face validity, this reservation should be borne in mind when interpreting the results. The time-urgency index was based on items taken from the Bortner pattern A short rating scale (Bortner, 1969). Items for the authoritarianism index were taken from the Adorno scale (Adorno, 1950).

Men were found to be less hostile, but more authoritarian, and they had a greater sense of time urgency. The women were found to be more depressed (hopefully, these gender differences are not causally related!). A standardized score of zero represents the score for the average person if we combine men and women. The separate mean standardized scores for men and women were 0.067 and −0.042 for time urgency ($p < .0001$); −0.135 and 0.073 for depression ($p < .0001$); 0.024 and −0.015 for authoritarianism ($p < .002$); and −0.024 and 0.015 for hostility ($p < .002$). Although statistically significant due to the large numbers, probably only those gender differences found for time urgency and depression are of a sufficient magnitude to be, practically speaking, important.

A greater sense of time urgency is associated with a substantially and significantly lower risk of both CHD and all-cause mortality among both men and women (see Table 9–4). This is a superficially unexpected result, especially given the earlier associations between type A behavior, with its increased sense of time urgency, and higher risk of CHD. Clearly, type A behavior has many components, with effects that may not all be in the same direction. It is possible to think that a sense of increased time pressure may reflect a person's optimism, enthusiasm, and desire to achieve— which may be a psychologically and physiologically beneficial situation. Recall that those in the Adventist cohort were relatively well educated, and they may often have a degree of flexibility in their job performance. In that case, the sense of time urgency is more likely to be a choice, rather than an imposition.

Another finding is that higher scores on the depression scale for women predicted a modestly greater all-cause mortality and a 33% greater mor-

Table 9-4. Relative Risks (95% Confidence Intervals) Comparing the Highest and the Lowest (Reference) Quintiles of Selected Psychological Variables in Relation to Fatal Coronary Heart-Disease (CHD) and All-Cause Mortality

Variable	Age-Adjusted			Psychosocial Multivariate[a]		
	Men	Women	Combined	Men	Women	Combined
ALL-CAUSE MORTALITY						
Time urgency	0.73 (0.64–0.84)	0.68 (0.61–0.76)	0.70 (0.64–0.76)	0.75 (0.66–0.86)	0.70 (0.63–0.78)	0.72 (0.66–0.78)
Depression	1.23 (1.09–1.37)	1.24 (1.14–1.35)	1.26 (1.17–1.36)	1.10 (0.98–1.25)	1.17 (1.07–1.27)	1.16 (1.07–1.25)
Authoritarian	1.29 (1.13–1.48)	1.27 (1.14–1.41)	1.28 (1.18–1.39)	1.22 (1.06–1.40)	1.14 (1.02–1.28)	1.17 (1.07–1.28)
Restricted feelings	1.01 (0.87–1.16)	1.05 (0.93–1.19)	1.03 (0.94–1.12)	—[b]		—
Hostility	1.08 (0.94–1.25)	1.03 (0.91–1.17)	1.06 (0.96–1.16)			
FATAL CHD						
Time urgency	0.64 (0.47–0.89)	0.67 (0.51–0.88)	0.66 (0.54–0.81)	0.80 (0.65–0.98)	0.67 (0.51–0.89)	0.69 (0.56–0.85)
Depression	0.98 (0.73–1.31)	1.42 (1.15–1.76)	1.25 (1.04–1.51)	0.87 (0.64–1.18)	1.33 (1.07–1.67)	1.13 (0.93–1.37)
Authoritarian	1.24 (0.91–1.70)	1.71 (1.30–2.26)	1.51 (1.23–1.86)	1.18 (0.85–1.64)	1.52 (1.14–2.03)	1.39 (1.12–1.72)
Hostility	0.97 (0.68–1.38)	0.97 (0.69–1.36)	0.98 (0.77–1.24)	—		—

[a]Adjusted for other psychosocial variables that showed significant associations with these two endpoints. Social support: marital status, "mother warm and understanding"; church participation: frequency of church attendance, frequency of holding church office. Combined analyses also adjusted for sex.

[b]Not included in the multivariate model due to lack of important effects in either gender on univariate analysis.

tality from CHD in the multivariate analyses. This result was not found for men, which is consistent with the findings from the Established Populations for Epidemiologic Studies of the Elderly Project (Mendes de Leon et al., 1998). The reason for such a sex difference is not well understood. An authoritarian attitude also predicted a modestly higher all-cause mortality rate for men and women, and a 52% higher CHD mortality rate for women alone. Higher scores for the questions in the hostility scale were not associated with increased CHD or all-cause mortality for this population, although the confidence interval still admitted the possibility of a modest-size association.

Thus, our findings relating depression to mortality among women are in line with the findings of others, but the relatively strong associations that we find with an increased sense of time urgency and authoritarianism are new. This work therefore needs to be duplicated by others before we can generalize the findings to other populations.

ARE EFFECTS OF RELIGIOUS PARTICIPATION AND PSYCHOLOGICAL FACTORS INDEPENDENT OF TRADITIONAL RISK FACTORS?

An obvious concern with the preceding results, regarding religious participation (see Table 9–2) is that it is the vegetarians, and those who have a healthier lifestyle in other ways, who are more likely to attend church regularly. This is not unexpected since the avoidance of meat at least, and, to a lesser extent, obtaining regular exercise, are characteristics of traditional Adventism. So, is there an independent effect of religious participation on mortality, or does this just reflect a healthier lifestyle among those who attend church more often?

Effects of both vegetarian status and nut consumption on CHD mortality in the analyses reported below are apparently somewhat smaller than those noted in Chapter 5. This is probably because the focus here on fatal events allowed a longer follow-up period of 12 years (1976–1988), whereas the major analyses in Chapter 5 included only a 6-year follow-up (1976–1982). This longer follow-up period has the advantage of increasing the number of events for the relatively few infrequent church attenders, thus improving statistical power. However, a disadvantage is that the assessment period for diet and exercise is now up to 12 years before some of the deaths. Any changes in these variables during the follow-up period will add to measurement errors, and this probably accounts for the smaller effect estimates. Analyses incorporating vegetarianism, other traditional lifestyle factors that predict mortality in Adventists, and church attendance and other important psychological variables, are included in Tables 9–5

Table 9–5. The Independent Effects of Traditional Lifestyle Risk Factors and Psychosocial and Religious Participation Variables on All-Cause Mortality in California Adventists

| | | Relative Risks | | | | | | | | |
| | | Traditional Lifestyle Factors Alone | | | Lifestyle Variables and Church Attendance | | | All Variables[a] | | |
Variable	Level	Men	Women	Combined	Men	Women	Combined	Men	Women	Combined
Sex	Women			1.00			1.00			1.00
	Men			1.43***			1.49***			1.50***
Meat	Vegetarian	1.00	1.00	1.00	1.00	1.00	1.00	1.00	1.00	1.00
	<1/wk	1.01	1.03	1.02	1.01	1.02	1.02	0.99	1.02	1.01
	≥1/wk	1.15*	1.15**	1.15*	1.12*	1.11*	1.12**	1.09	1.08	1.09*
Exercise	Low	1.00	1.00	1.00	1.00	1.00	1.00	1.00	1.00	1.00
	Medium	0.76***	0.78***	0.78***	0.78***	0.79***	0.79***	0.80***	0.81***	0.81***
	High	0.71***	0.78***	0.75***	0.73***	0.80***	0.77***	0.75***	0.81***	0.79***
Nuts	<1/wk	1.00	1.00	1.00	1.00	1.00	1.00	1.00	1.00	1.00
	1–4/wk	0.84**	0.86***	0.85***	0.85**	0.87**	0.86***	0.87*	0.89**	0.89***
	≥5/wk	0.74***	0.85***	0.80***	0.76***	0.86**	0.82***	0.78***	0.88**	0.84***
Smoking	Never	1.00	1.00	1.00	1.00	1.00	1.00	1.00	1.00	1.00
	Past	1.16***	1.18**	1.18***	1.13**	1.17**	1.16***	1.09*	1.15*	1.13**

		(1)	(2)	(3)	(4)	(5)	(6)
Church attendance[b]	3–4/mo	1.00	1.00	1.00	1.00	1.00	1.00
	1–2/mo	1.01	1.18	1.13	0.99	1.20	1.12
	<1/mo	1.43**	1.18	1.29**	1.32*	1.17	1.25**
Time urgency[c]	Low				1.00	1.00	1.00
	High				0.72***	0.66***	0.72***
Depression[c]	Low				1.00	1.00	1.00
	High				1.23**	1.36***	1.34***
Authoritarian[c]	Low				1.00	1.00	1.00
	High				1.15*	1.16**	1.17***

*$p \leq .05$, **$p \leq .01$, ***$p \leq .001$.

[a]The model excludes psychosocial variables that in multivariate analysis showed neither statistical significance nor important effects. It includes all variables listed in this table plus frequency of holding church office, BMI and BMI^2.

[b]The effect of church attendance is that estimated for those who are not potentially disabled by previous CHD, stroke, cancer, or arthritis/rheumatism.

[c]Comparing mid-points of extreme quintiles of these indices. Lowest quintile is the reference.

Table 9–6. The Independent Effects of Traditional Lifestyle Risk Factors and Psychosocial and Religious Participation Variables on Coronary Heart Disease (CHD) Mortality in California Adventists

Variable	Level	Relative Risks								
		Traditional Lifestyle Factors Alone			Lifestyle Variables and Church Attendance			All Variables[a]		
		Men	Women	Combined	Men	Women	Combined	Men	Women	Combined
Sex	Women			1.00			1.00			1.00
	Men			1.61***			1.62***			1.63***
Meat	Vegetarian	1.00	1.00	1.00	1.00	1.00	1.00	1.00	1.00	1.00
	<1/wk	1.63**	1.20	1.34***	1.63**	1.20	1.34**	1.56**	1.18	1.31**
	≥1/wk	1.70***	1.04	1.27***	1.68***	1.04	1.26**	1.59**	1.03	1.21*
Exercise	Low	1.00	1.00	1.00	1.00	1.00	1.00	1.00	1.00	1.00
	Medium	0.83	0.82	0.81*	0.85	0.82	0.82*	0.86	0.84	0.85
	High	0.67**	0.73**	0.69***	0.68**	0.73**	0.69***	0.70**	0.73**	0.71***
Nuts	<1/wk	1.00	1.00	1.00	1.00	1.00	1.00	1.00	1.00	1.00
	1–4/wk	0.97	0.75**	0.82*	0.98	0.74**	0.83*	1.04	0.77*	0.87
	≥5/wk	0.78	0.66***	0.70***	0.80	0.66***	0.71***	0.85	0.68**	0.73**
Smoking	Never	1.00	1.00	1.00	1.00	1.00	1.00	1.00	1.00	1.00
	Past	1.12	1.08	1.09	1.11	1.07	1.08	1.04	1.09	1.04

Church attendance[b]	3–4/mo	1.00	1.00	1.00	1.00	1.00	1.00
	1–2/mo	0.81	1.59	1.22	0.76	1.70	1.23
	<1/mo	1.93**	1.35	1.65**	1.55	1.38	1.58**
Time urgency[c]	Low				1.00	1.00	1.00
	High				0.67	0.65**	0.69**
Depression[c]	Low				1.00	1.00	1.00
	High				1.33	2.23***	1.88***
Authoritarian[c]	Low				1.00	1.00	1.00
	High				1.08	1.47**	1.32**

$^{*}p \leq .05,\ ^{**}p \leq .01,\ ^{***}p \leq .001.$

[a]The model excludes psychosocial variables that in multivariate analysis showed neither statistical significance nor important effects. It includes all variables listed in this table plus frequency of holding church office, BMI and BMI^2.

[b]The effect of church attendance is that estimated for those who are not potentially disabled by previous CHD, stroke, cancer, or arthritis/rheumatism.

[c]Comparing mid-points of extreme quintiles. Lowest quintile is the reference.

and 9–6. Adding the few social support variables that we have available as covariates did not change these results.

By comparing Table 9–5 with Table 9–2, we can see that the protective effect of regular church attendance on all-cause mortality is hardly affected when adjustment is made for the nonpsychological lifestyle factors. For instance, in Table 9–2, the apparent effect of church attendance of less than once per month for men was a relative risk of 1.44 for all-cause mortality, but the corresponding quantity in Table 9–5, when lifestyle variables are added, is 1.43. This suggests that in Table 9–2, the effect was not due to the poorer lifestyle profile for infrequent church attenders. Adding the available psychological variables to the model (see the right-hand columns of Table 9–5) does reduce the effect of infrequent attendance a little. Despite this, there is a suggestion that some independent effect of attendance remains for both sexes, especially men.

Turning to CHD mortality, the adjustment for other lifestyle and psychological factors substantially reduces the initially stronger effect of church attendance on this endpoint for both men and women (if we now compare Tables 9–2 and 9–6). When data for both sexes are combined, however (see Table 9–6), there remains a 58% increase in CHD mortality ($p < 0.01$), when we compare infrequent with frequent attenders. This occurs when other lifestyle differences between the attendance groups have been controlled. By contrast, when Table 9–4 is compared with Tables 9–5 and 9–6, the effects of time urgency and authoritarian attitudes on either all-cause or CHD mortality are hardly changed by the additional adjustment for traditional risk factors and church attendance. However the independent effects of depression are strengthened, and although not shown, were not modified by the presence or absence of pre-existing chronic diseases (CHD, stroke, arthritis or cancer).

How should we interpret the apparent reduction in the effect of religious participation on CHD mortality once traditional risk factors are controlled? One reasonable explanation is in line with the first of the mechanisms proposed by Ellison and Levin (1998) and with the suggestions of Vaux (1976), described above to explain a connection between religiosity and health. That is, greater religiosity causes a reassessment of health values and health habits, and then prompts changes to correct suboptimal behaviors. If this is the case, these traditional risk factors are intervening variables between religious participation and health experience. Then the diminution in the apparent effect of religious participation, after controlling for traditional risk factors, should not be interpreted as evidence of a small effect but, rather, as evidence that religiosity has an important effect on health and that this is partially mediated by its positive influence on health behavior and traditional risk factors.

Another possibility, however, is that people who become regular church participants are also those who are predisposed to being health conscious. This predisposition could be due to some psychological, or even genetic, mechanism (see Fig. 9–1) that encourages both religious participation and special attention to healthful behaviors. However, there is no evidence in support of this.

If religiosity can promote adherence to more healthy behaviors, this may explain why Adventists have been able to adopt somewhat of a countercultural lifestyle for more than 100 years. While there are few religions that formally incorporate a healthy lifestyle into their belief structure, Adventists do so, and this is a natural fit for at least Christianity, Judaism, and Islam. There is a need to better understand religion's role in health promotion. Could other religious groups, like Adventists, benefit from incorporating health as a core belief and by providing learning opportunities and social support for their members (Fraser, 1999c)? These matters are discussed in more detail in Chapter 14.

ARE THE EFFECTS OF VEGETARIANISM AND TRADITIONAL RISK FACTORS INDEPENDENT OF RELIGIOUS PARTICIPATION AND PSYCHOLOGICAL VARIABLES?

Another natural question is whether the inclusion of psychological variables and church attendance together in the statistical model has influenced the estimated effects of vegetarianism and other traditional risk factors on all-cause and CHD mortality. This is particularly relevant as strong associations were found between vegetarian status and religious participation (see Table 9–3), showing that vegetarians usually participated more frequently in formal religious activities. Associations between vegetarian status and psychological variables, however, were of a small magnitude (see Table 9–7), though usually statistically significant, given the large number of subjects. They suggested that vegetarian men and women had a lesser sense of time urgency, were less likely to be depressed, and were less au-

Table 9–7. Associations with Vegetarian Status: Age-adjusted Spearman's Rho Correlation with Religious Participation and Psychosocial Variables

Variable	Men		Women	
	Rho	p	Rho	p
Time urgency	−0.06	<.0001	0.005	.50
Depression	−0.07	<.0001	−0.10	<.0001
Authoritarian	−0.06	<.0001	−0.04	<.0001
Hostility	0.07	<.0001	0.02	<.006

thoritarian but more likely to be hostile! Associations with social support variables (not shown here) were few, but again suggested that vegetarians had a little more social support. Then it is possible that vegetarianism is just an indicator of certain religiosity and psychological risk factors, rather than being a risk factor itself. Again, this can be resolved by putting all variables in the model together.

The effect of vegetarianism on all-cause and CHD mortality was previously seen largely among men and among younger and middle-aged women (see Tables 9–5 and 9–6). The effect on CHD mortality is only slightly reduced when the psychological and religious participation variables are added. However, the moderate effect of vegetarianism on all-cause mortality is attenuated, but not nullified, by adding the new variables. It is also interesting that there was virtually no influence on the estimated effects of other traditional risk factors when church attendance was added to the model, and only very slight attenuation toward the null result when the psychological variables were also added. Thus in the context of this book, an important result is that the effects of vegetarianism (and other traditional risk factors) cannot be explained by their associations with the available measures of religiosity or psychological factors.

SUMMARY

1. Although our ability to measure social support among Adventists was quite limited, modest but statistically significant protective effects for all-cause mortality were found for men and women who were married as compared with those who were single, and also for those who had had a warm and understanding mother, and for women who were satisfied with their family life. These factors had less of an effect on CHD mortality.

2. Participation in religious life, as well as personal religious experience, is hypothesized to be protective through several different mechanisms.

3. Several epidemiologic studies, some being prospective, have found evidence that frequent attendance at religious services is associated with decreased mortality. This raises the question of how such frequent attenders may be different from less frequent attenders in more traditional behavioral and other risk factors. The Adventist Health Study is unusual in having a wealth of lifestyle information, as well as some religious participation variables. Hence independent effects can be sought.

4. Adventist men and women who attend church less frequently have a higher all-cause mortality rate and a much higher CHD mortality rate than frequent attenders have. The effect of church attendance on CHD mortality is somewhat attenuated by an adjustment for other factors, but confidence intervals are quite wide. Thus our data suggest that there are probably important effects of church attendance on all-cause and CHD

mortality that are independent of traditional risk factors, although larger studies, with repeated assessments of dietary and exercise habits, would give more credibility to this conclusion.

5. It is also possible that the attenuation of the church attendance effect on CHD risk, when it is adjusted for other factors, indicates that religiosity is not just a marker for lifestyle variables but may act in part by improving values for these other factors. Indeed, frequent attenders do appear to have a better lifestyle, which may have been caused in part by their religious participation, although our data cannot prove this. If this is correct, the true effects of religiosity would be greater and closer to those shown in Table 9–2, when data are unadjusted for traditional risk factors. Future studies should measure more specific aspects of religiosity.

6. A strong protective effect of a greater sense of time urgency is seen for both all-cause and CHD mortality among both sexes. This is not significantly attenuated by an adjustment for other factors.

7. For women, feelings of depression are associated with an important increase in risk of both all-cause and CHD mortality. However, this effect appears to be less for men. For both sexes there is a modest tendency for those scoring higher on the authoritarian scale to have a greater risk of all-cause mortality, and for women there is a 47% increase in risk of CHD mortality.

8. The most important result, in the context of this book, is that an adjustment for church attendance and the other psychosocial factors that we have available had little influence on the estimated effects of vegetarianism on risk of CHD mortality and on effects of traditional risk factors for all-cause or CHD mortality. Thus these effects cannot be accounted for by confounding with the religiosity or psychological variables that we measured.

NOTES

1. The following is a list of the psychological factors and their component questions. The questions for the time urgency factor allowed subjects to mark one of 10 positions between the two named extremes. The questions for all other factors were scored as "Yes/No" and (−) after the question means that a "Yes" response is given a negative score. (a) Time urgency: "Always feel rushed—Never rushed even under pressure," "Fast eating, walking etc—Slow doing things," "Very competitive—Not competitive," "Try to do many things at once—Take things one at a time"; (b) Depression: "I often feel that I face so many difficulties that I cannot overcome them," "I wish I could be as happy as others," "Are you satisfied with your present family life?" (−); (c) Authoritarianism: "Obedience and respect for authority are the most important virtues a child should learn," "These days a person does not really know whom he can count on," "It is best never to show your feelings to others;" (d) Hostility: "I sometimes try to get even, rather than forgive and forget," "I have never intensely disliked someone" (−).

10

Coronary Heart Disease Mortality among British, German, and Indian Vegetarians

Researchers have reported the results of three prospective studies and one retrospective study of non-Adventist vegetarians' dietary habits and the risk of CHD. The studies are smaller than the California Adventist studies, and the prospective studies included only cases of CHD that resulted in death. Nevertheless, they add substantially to the total amount of information that is available.

These studies bring a greater diversity of experience to bear on the research questions, in part because they were done in other countries: the United Kingdom, Germany, and India. Also, while Adventists are vegetarians for reasons of health and, in some cases, for "moral purity," the non-Adventist vegetarians are much more likely to be motivated by concerns about animal rights or the environment. This is not to deny that many non-Adventists expect some health benefits or that many Adventists feel satisfied that their choices spare animal lives and reduce the exploitation of scarce environmental resources (Gussow, 1994; Lewis, 1994). Another difference is that although most of the non-Adventist subjects are lacto-ovo vegetarians, as were the Adventists, there is a higher percentage of vegans among the non-Adventist vegetarians.

The four studies of non-Adventist vegetarians are the Health Food Shoppers and the Oxford Vegetarian Studies, both done in the United Kingdom; the Heidelberg Vegetarian Study, in Germany; and a case-control study of acute myocardial infarction, in Bangalore, India. Another cohort of approximately 25,000 British vegetarians has been established at Oxford University as part of the European Prospective Investigation into Cancer and Nutrition (EPIC), but the investigators have not yet reported findings on new disease events.

THE HEALTH FOOD SHOPPERS STUDY

Subjects for this study were recruited by distributing a short questionnaire to customers at health food shops and clinics, subscribers to health food magazines, members of vegetarian and health food societies, and also to subscribers to a Seventh-day Adventist publication (but in the end, only a very small percentage of subjects in this cohort were Adventists). Between 1973 and 1979, some 10,977 subjects were recruited (Burr and Sweetnam, 1982; Key et al., 1996).

The dietary portion of the questionnaire was very simple. It asked whether the subject was a vegetarian or not (with no further definition) and asked about the frequency of consumption of whole-meal bread, bran cereals, nuts and dried fruits, fresh fruit, and raw vegetable salads. Each question had three frequency categories: at least daily; less than daily, but more than once per week; and less than once per week.

To assess the stability of dietary habits, the researchers interviewed 289 of these subjects initially and then between 18 months and six years later (Burr and Sweetnam, 1982). Of those initially stating that they were vegetarians, 66% still ate meat or fish less than once per month at the later time. Of those initially stating they ate whole-meal bread, 67% still did so. Other substudies demonstrated that the subjects were quite accurate in their reports of whole-meal bread consumption (Westlake et al., 1980), and that vegetarian males and females consumed substantially more fiber than nonvegetarians (Burr et al., 1981).

The follow-up period to find fatal events continued until March 1995, using computerized national vital status data. By December 1980 (Burr and Sweetnam, 1982), 585 deaths had been recorded, and by March 1995, there were 2562 fatalities (Key et al., 1996). Death certificates were obtained and coded according to ICD8 or ICD9 criteria. In the calculations of standardized mortality ratios, numbers of expected deaths were based on mortality rates for England and Wales. The first year of the follow-up period was excluded in the researchers' first report (Burr and Sweetnam, 1982) as an attempt to eliminate the effect of any healthy-volunteer bias. Some idea of the dietary and other characteristics of this cohort is shown in Table 10–1. About 43% were self-reported vegetarians, and relatively high percentages of these ate nuts or dried fruit, fresh fruit, or raw salads at least daily.

The mortality results by 1980 showed that the whole study group had only about 43% of the deaths expected for such a group in England and Wales. They were "health conscious," by definition, and as a group did have a much lower CHD mortality. At that point in the study, age- and sex-standardized mortality ratios, as compared with the average British res-

Table 10–1. Characteristics of Subjects and Intake of Certain Foods in Men and Women of the Health Food Shoppers Study: Values Are Numbers of Subjects (Percentages) unless Stated Otherwise

	Men ($n = 4336$)	Women ($n = 6435$)
Mean (SD) age (years)	45.7 (17.7)	45.9 (18.3)
Current smokers	1100 (25.4)	964 (15.0)
Pipe or cigars, or both	375 (8.6)	33 (0.5)
1–14 cigarettes[a]	373 (8.6)	579 (9.0)
≥15 cigarettes	352 (8.1)	352 (5.5)
Mean (SD) weight (kg)	70.3 (9.9)[b]	58.3 (8.7)[c]
Vegetarian	1851 (42.7)	2776 (43.1)
Wholemeal bread daily	2732 (63.0)	3967 (61.6)
Bran cereals daily	1279 (29.5)	1669 (25.9)
Nuts or dried fruit daily	1660 (38.3)	2431 (37.8)
Fresh fruit daily	3103 (71.6)	5201 (80.8)
Raw salad daily	1486 (34.3)	2619 (40.7)

SD, standard deviation.

[a]Includes 21 cigarette smokers (8 men and 13 women) with unknown amount smoked.

[b]$n = 4111$.

[c]$n = 6112$.

Source: Reprinted by permission from Key TJA, Thorogood M, Appleby PN, Burr ML, Dietary habits and mortality in 11,000 vegetarians and health-conscious people: result of a 17-year follow up, *Br Med J* 3113:775–779, 1996. Published by BMJ Publishing Group.

ident were 0.36 for vegetarians and 0.50 for nonvegetarians, and the difference between vegetarians and nonvegetarians within the study was nearly statistically significant at the traditional level ($\alpha = 0.05$). Interestingly, the difference between vegetarians and nonvegetarians was found only for males (SMRs of 0.33 and 0.58, respectively), whereas for females the SMR values were 0.39 and 0.37. Although the number of CHD deaths was relatively small by 1980, and there was little adjustment made for other risk factors, it was shown that these results for men or women were not due to differences in cigarette smoking habits between the vegetarians and nonvegetarians.

A longer, 10- to 12-year, follow-up study of this cohort (Burr and Butland, 1988) again showed that the vegetarians had significantly lower CHD mortality rates ($p < .01$) when compared to nonvegetarians, and that this was still more pronounced for the men. However, the cerebrovascular disease death rates for the vegetarians were not significantly lower. A yet later report (Key et al., 1996) contained a somewhat more robust analysis because of the many more deaths that occurred during this much longer follow-up period. The frequency of consumption of foods was categorized by daily and less-than-daily use. Only deaths that occurred between ages 16 and 79 were included, as documentation of the cause of death for the more elderly was considered less reliable. The follow-up period was quite

Table 10–2. Relative Risks for Fatal CHD Associated with Nonvegetarian Status, or at Least Daily Consumption of Selected Foods, as Compared to Alternative Habits: The Health Food Shoppers' Study[a]

Food	Relative Risk	95% Confidence Interval
Nonvegetarian	1.18	0.94–1.47
Whole meal bread at least daily	0.85	0.68–1.06
Bran cereals at least daily	0.99	0.79–1.25
Nuts or dried fruits at least daily	0.89	0.72–1.11
Fresh fruit at least daily	0.76	0.60–0.97
Raw salads at least daily	0.74	0.59–0.92

[a]Adjusted for age, sex, and cigarette smoking.

Source: Key TJA, Thorogood M, Appleby PN, Burr ML, Dietary habits and mortality in 11,000 vegetarians and health-conscious people: result of a 17-year follow up, Br Med J 313:775–779, 1996. Published by BMJ Publishing group. Adapted and printed by permission.

long (up to 21 years, with a mean of 16.8 years), so the expected death calculation used the national mortality rates for the five-year period corresponding to the individual deaths.

As in the earlier analyses, the whole cohort experienced a much lower mortality rate from CHD (about 50%) than that predicted from national data. Analyses within the cohort again compared the CHD mortality experience of vegetarians and nonvegetarians, and of those who ate whole meal bread, bran cereals, nuts or dried fruits, fresh fruit, raw salads, daily as compared to those consuming these foods less frequently. The results are shown in Table 10–2, after adjusting for age, sex, and cigarette smoking habits. The nonvegetarians had a nonsignificant 18% higher risk than the vegetarians, although the 95% confidence interval was wide, ranging from a 6% decrease in risk to a 47% increase in risk. The implication is that the CHD mortality reduction seen in the whole study group can only partly be ascribed to lower meat consumption. Unfortunately, these data were not reported separately for men and women, which would have been interesting given the differences by gender that were found in the earlier analyses.

Consumption of fruit and/or salads at least daily, as compared with less than daily, was associated with a 25% reduction in CHD risk. When fruit and salads are adjusted for each other, both remained significant, or nearly so, but the effect of fruit was somewhat attenuated. For cerebrovascular disease mortality, daily fruit consumption was also associated with a protective relative risk of 0.68 (95% confidence interval, 0.47–0.98). Vegetarianism was not clearly associated with cerebrovascular disease, although the confidence interval was wide.

As pointed out by the authors, a very long follow-up period such as this, after a single simple assessment of diet, almost certainly leads to some attenuation of the calculated effects due to undocumented changes in dietary habits during the follow-up period. None of the analyses cited here excluded cases of CHD present at the study baseline. Nevertheless, the estimated effects of diet, although relatively weak, are consistent with a benefit gained from more fruits and salads, and possibly from less meat and more whole-meat bread—all characteristics of a vegetarian diet. Most of the health-conscious subjects in this study had dietary habits that at least trended in this direction and, on average, had a greatly reduced CHD mortality rate as compared with the general population.

THE OXFORD VEGETARIAN STUDY

The Oxford Vegetarian Study is also a cohort study and included 11,130 subjects. These were 6115 vegetarians defined as subjects who ate meat less than once each week, and 5015 nonvegetarians (Thorogood et al., 1994). The vegetarians were recruited through the Vegetarian Society of the United Kingdom, by publicity in the national and local media, and by word of mouth. The nonvegetarian "controls" were found by the vegetarians and were typically friends and relatives who had a similar lifestyle and were from the same social class, but who ate more meat. This design was an attempt to keep the consumption of meat as the major difference between the vegetarians and the nonvegetarians. On average, the nonvegetarians consumed 22.6 oz of meat per week. However, fewer than half ate meat daily, so these controls were not actually typical British omnivores. Recruitment was done from September 1980 through January 1984. Only 24 of these subjects were Adventist.

Subjects completed a questionnaire concerning their diet and their demographic, medical history, and lifestyle data at study baseline. The dietary questionnaire was a food-frequency instrument that included 28 foods, each with five possible frequency categories for response. In addition, there were questions about the consumption of fats and alcohol.

Deaths were determined by computerized linkage with National Health Service records. Death certificates were coded according to ICD9 criteria, with the coronary heart disease deaths being those with codes 410 to 414. Observations included in the first report (Thorogood et al., 1994) were those recorded through March 1993, there being more than 100,000 person-years found to be at risk by this time. Only deaths of people under 80 years of age were included.

As with the Health Food Shoppers Study, this whole cohort was healthier than average. During the follow-up, only about 38% of the expected CHD deaths occurred. The CHD death rate ratio for meat-eaters, as compared with non-meat-eaters (i.e., vegetarians, and people who ate fish but not meat), was 1.82 (95% confidence interval, 1.22–2.78); when this was adjusted for differences in cigarette smoking, body mass index, and social class, the ratio fell to 1.39 (95% confidence interval, 0.91–2.13). As it is very likely that the effect of vegetarian status depends in part on lower body mass index, including this latter variable in the model probably represents an overadjustment. The finding of a significant trend toward lower blood cholesterol values, as the frequency of meat consumption decreased (Appleby et al., 1999), offered an additional explanation for the lower CHD mortality rate for vegetarians.

Later analyses (Appleby et al., 1999; Mann et al., 1997), attempting to remove any healthy-volunteer bias, excluded those with established cardiovascular disease or diabetes at study baseline and also evaluated the effects of foods other than meat. When the first five years of the follow-up period were excluded, the death rate ratio for nonvegetarians, as compared with vegetarians, became 1.12 (95% confidence interval, 0.65–1.96), much closer to unity, but the confidence interval was very wide. If the weakening of the effect is real, this may imply that the healthy-volunteer bias was greater for the vegetarians than for the nonvegetarian controls. Perhaps less healthy vegetarians were more likely to stay out of the study.

Excluding subjects with a history of cardiovascular disease or diabetes at baseline also diminished the estimated effect of nonvegetarian status, with a death rate ratio then of 1.18 (95% confidence interval, 0.64–1.43). Excluding diabetics, however, may have removed part of the biological effect of nonvegetarianism, as Adventist data suggest that vegetarians have a lower diabetes-associated mortality rate (see Chapter 8). Thus important questions remain.

When the effects of other foods and nutrients on the risk of incident fatal CHD for nondiabetics were evaluated, some interesting results became apparent (see Fig. 10–1). More frequent consumption of eggs and cheese and greater consumption of animal fat, saturated fat, and dietary cholesterol were all associated with quite substantial and statistically significant elevations in risk. In contrast, no significant protective effects were noted for consumption of dietary fiber, fruit, salads, fish, or alcohol, although confidence intervals were wide enough to have missed moderate-size effects.

Greater nut consumption was associated with a death rate ratio of 0.87 (95% confidence interval, 0.45–1.68). As can be seen, the wide confidence interval here also allows a variety of possibilities. Peanuts are often consumed with beer in pubs. It is quite unclear how important this observation may be, but possible associations between particular foods and broader

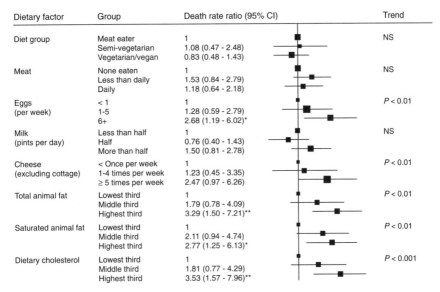

Dietary factor	Group	Death rate ratio (95% CI)		Trend
Diet group	Meat eater	1		NS
	Semi-vegetarian	1.08 (0.47 - 2.48)		
	Vegetarian/vegan	0.83 (0.48 - 1.43)		
Meat	None eaten	1		NS
	Less than daily	1.53 (0.84 - 2.79)		
	Daily	1.18 (0.64 - 2.18)		
Eggs	< 1	1		P < 0.01
(per week)	1-5	1.28 (0.59 - 2.79)		
	6+	2.68 (1.19 - 6.02)*		
Milk	Less than half	1		NS
(pints per day)	Half	0.76 (0.40 - 1.43)		
	More than half	1.50 (0.81 - 2.78)		
Cheese	< Once per week	1		P < 0.01
(excluding cottage)	1-4 times per week	1.23 (0.45 - 3.35)		
	≥ 5 times per week	2.47 (0.97 - 6.26)		
Total animal fat	Lowest third	1		P < 0.01
	Middle third	1.79 (0.78 - 4.09)		
	Highest third	3.29 (1.50 - 7.21)**		
Saturated animal fat	Lowest third	1		P < 0.01
	Middle third	2.11 (0.94 - 4.74)		
	Highest third	2.77 (1.25 - 6.13)*		
Dietary cholesterol	Lowest third	1		P < 0.001
	Middle third	1.81 (0.77 - 4.29)		
	Highest third	3.53 (1.57 - 7.96)**		

Figure 10–1 Death rate ratios (and 95% confidence intervals) for coronary heart disease for selected dietary factors. Factors are adjusted for age, sex, smoking, and social class, in subjects with no history of cardiovascular disease or diabetes at recruitment: the Oxford Vegetarian Study. The area of each square is proportional to the number of deaths from ischemic heart disease in that group. Semivegetarian was defined as eating meat less than once a week, eating fish only, or both. *$p < 0.05$; **$p < 0.01$ by Fisher's z test. *Source:* Adapted and reprinted by permission from Appleby PN et al., The Oxford Vegetarian Study: an overview, *Am J Clin Nutr* 70(Suppl):525s–531s, 1999. Copyright American Society for Clinical Nutrition.

dietary patterns always need to be considered. It is likely that a number of cultural and other dietary differences distinguish nut-eaters, or vegetarians, in different parts of the world.

The analyses described here were adjusted for age, sex, smoking status, and social class, but not for other foods. Hence, the results are probably not independent of each other. For instance, the high egg consumers may tend also to be the high cheese consumers. Data were not shown separately for men and women.

In summary, the Oxford Vegetarian Study also suggests that vegetarians are modestly protected against CHD, although confidence intervals are often wide. When considering individual foods, the main evidence was for hazards associated with consumption of animal products and animal fats, rather than for protection from fruit and salads. This contrasts with the results of the Health Food Shoppers Study, although that study collected little data on high-fat foods.

THE HEIDELBERG VEGETARIAN STUDY

In the Heidelberg Vegetarian Study, vegetarian participants from the former Federal Republic of Germany responded to an advertisement and short questionnaire that had been inserted in several vegetarian magazines in 1976 (Frentzel-Beyme et al., 1988). In 1978 a more detailed questionnaire was mailed to those who agreed to participate in the study. This later questionnaire included food-frequency questions on meats, fruits, vegetables, pasta, and dairy products, along with questions on smoking and alcohol-drinking habits, physical activity, demographic variables, and medical and family history. The questions on foods were often organized so that the names of specific vegetables, nuts, and fruits consumed could be included in responses; there were either three or five frequency categories available for the various foods.

A total of 1904 subjects (858 men and 1046 women) returned the questionnaire, these being 82.5% of those who had received them. Further questionnaires, regarding illness and changes in dietary habits, were mailed in 1982 and 1989. Vital status of subjects was determined, after 11 years of the follow-up, in May 1989, using the Registrar's Office in a subjects last place of residence. Copies of death certificates were obtained and coded according to ICD9. The expected number of deaths was calculated using age- and sex-specific mortality rates for the Federal Republic of Germany between 1980 and 1986. These were then used to determine standardized mortality ratios.

The subjects were classified according to whether they defined themselves, at the enrollment, as "strict vegetarians" who avoided fish and meat completely or as "moderate vegetarians" who would occasionally eat these foods. By these criteria, 1163 (521 men and 642 women) were called strict vegetarians, and 741 (337 men and 404 women) were called moderate vegetarians. Only 6% of the strict vegetarians were vegans, and the majority of both groups were lacto-ovo vegetarians. The study participants had a better education than the average person, and only 7% had a body mass index greater than 26, whereas this was true of 40% of the general population at the age of 55. Most subjects in the study had been vegetarians for at least five years.

The analyses here are based on the recording of 225 deaths after 11 years of the follow-up, although an earlier report had been based on 82 deaths (Frentzel-Beyme et al., 1988). A healthy-volunteer effect was noted during the first four years of the follow-up, with fewer deaths than there were in later years (Chang-Claude et al., 1992).

After 11 years, it was clear that this study group of vegetarians had a much lower mortality rate from cardiovascular diseases than other Germans. Standardized mortality rates (SMRs) for these diseases were 39% (95% confidence interval, 29%–51%) and 46% (95% confidence interval, 35%–60%) of the expectations for men and women, respectively (Chang-Claude et al., 1992). For ischemic heart disease, the SMR is stated as being about one-third of the expectation. As an attempt to exclude any possible bias from the healthy-volunteer effect, an analysis was done that excluded the first five years of the follow-up. Then the SMR for CHD among males was 0.45 (95% confidence interval, 0.24–0.77), and among females, 0.43 (95% confidence interval, 0.20–0.81), suggesting that this effect, if present, created little bias.

There were no significant differences found between strict and moderate vegetarians for all-cause, cancer, or CHD mortality, although the small number of events included makes the power of these tests very limited. The strict vegetarian men and women did experience only half the risk of CHD deaths that the moderate vegetarians did, but numbers of events are small and this result is compatible with chance alone.

The investigators also checked whether the duration of vegetarianism was important and divided the population into those who had been vegetarians for either more than 20 years, or 20 years or less (Chang-Claude and Frentzel-Beyme, 1993). Where vegetarianism was of longer duration, there was some indication of reduced CHD mortality, with a relative risk of 0.88, but the 95% confidence interval was wide (0.31–2.53), precluding any firm conclusion. It is noteworthy that only 4% of males and 3% of females in the group were smokers, as compared with 41% and 26% of the general male and female population of Germany at that time. So this explains part of the protection from CHD death found in this vegetarian study group.

In summary, this study clearly indicates that German vegetarians have a much lower risk of CHD mortality than other Germans. The exact cause of this reduction in risk is not identified here, although it is probably partly due to lower rates of smoking and partly due to dietary factors.

MYOCARDIAL INFARCTION AND VEGETARIANISM IN BANGALORE, INDIA

Two hundred patients aged 30–60, who were admitted consecutively to a coronary care unit with a diagnosis of acute myocardial infarction, were enrolled in this Indian case-control-study as the cases (Pais et al., 1996). Two hundred controls were selected from a group of outpatients attending a clinic for a general physical examination; for an eye or ear, nose, and throat evaluation; or for elective surgery for conditions unlikely to be related to CHD risk. Any individuals with evidence of previous CHD or cardiac disease were excluded from both groups. About 75% of the study participants were Hindus; about 10%, Muslims; and 16%, Christians. Many Hindus are vegetarians, and in this study 30% of cases and 42% of controls were vegetarians.

This study is included here, despite being a case-control study in design and being retrospective in the sense that diet was measured after the onset of the myocardial infarction. The major problem with retrospective studies in the present context is the possibility that the choice of vegetarian status results from having had a myocardial infarction, rather than the choice preceding the heart attack and possibly having a causal influence. However, in this study, previous diets were measured while the subjects were still in the hospital, and thus there was no opportunity for the subjects to change their diets. Moreover, their vegetarianism was usually a lifelong dedication and was usually prompted by religious factors rather than any expected effects on health.

The pertinent results indicated that nonvegetarians experienced more events as their relative risk of myocardial infarction was 1.82 (95% confidence interval, 1.54–6.67), as compared with vegetarians, and this advantage persisted after an adjustment for differences in smoking habits, blood glucose levels, and HDL and LDL cholesterol and triglyceride levels. However, after adjusting for the waist-to-hip ratio, the vegetarian advantage became nonsignificant. This again strongly suggests that the protective effect of vegetarianism acts at least partially through its effect on body weight and shape. This may be particularly important for the Indian population, as they are especially prone to abdominal obesity, reduced insulin sensitivity, hypertriglyceridemia, small dense LDL particles, and the consequences of these metabolic abnormalities (Hughes et al., 1997; Pinto, 1998; Vardan et al., 1995).

COMBINED ANALYSIS OF DATA FROM PROSPECTIVE STUDIES OF VEGETARIANS

A common problem found in the three studies just described, and to a lesser extent in the two Adventist studies from California is that of the wide confidence intervals that obscure the interpretation of some results. Thus the investigators at Loma Linda University and at Oxford University initiated a collaborative analysis of all of the available data from the prospective studies that included a high proportion of vegetarians.

The five studies included in the collaboration (Key et al., 1998, 1999a) were the Adventist Mortality Study (follow-up, 1960–1965), the Adventist Health Study (follow-up, 1976–1988), the Health Food Shoppers Study, the Oxford Vegetarian Study, and the Heidelberg Vegetarian Study. For the collaborative analysis, a total of 76,172 individuals were enrolled, 53,490 of whom were California Adventists. But more importantly, the analysis found 809,394 person-years at risk, and non-Adventists contributed 43% of these.

Deaths and person-years at risk were only included for those up to age 89, and the main analyses compared vegetarians with "nonvegetarians." For the purposes of the collaborative analysis, in four of the studies, vegetarians were defined as those who did not eat meat or fish. In the Health Food Shoppers Study, vegetarians could only be defined as those who considered themselves "vegetarian." The more detailed data collected 1.5 to 6 years after the baseline year of this last study indicated that at these times, 66% of those subjects initially claiming to be vegetarian still ate meat less than once each month. We were also able to establish whether subjects in all studies had followed the vegetarian diet for less than five years or more than five. For the Adventist studies, this required us to equate the time when vegetarians actually became vegetarian with the time of their baptism, a reasonable assumption for most.

Cigarette smoking was measured by different questions in the different studies, but in all of the studies, current smoking habits were clearly identified. Common definitions of body mass index, education, the alcohol consumption categories, and the exercise categories (more or less frequent) could be established for all of the studies except the Health Food Shoppers Study. Thus an adjustment for these covariates was possible while still including most of the data in the analysis.

Our analyses always compared CHD mortality between vegetarians and "nonvegetarians" of a particular study, and then pooled the mortality ratios using a random effects model (Der Simonian and Laird, 1986). Adjustment for the potentially confounding variables mentioned above was possible. Fatal coronary heart disease was defined by ICD9 codes 410–414 in all of the studies.

It is interesting to compare the characteristics of the subjects in the five studies (see Table 10–3). Participants in the California Adventist studies were rather older, on average, perhaps reflecting the popularity of vegetarianism among younger people in the United Kingdom and Germany. The British subjects were much more likely to be current smokers than the others, and there was a tendency in all of the studies for vegetarians to smoke less, consume alcohol less frequently, and be slightly more frequent exercisers than the "nonvegetarians." The smokers in the Adventist studies were largely the non-Adventist spouses who also enrolled in these studies. The California Adventists were more obese by 2 to 3 kg/m^2, although

Table 10-3. Characteristics of Subjects in the Five Studies of the Collaboration

Study	Diet Group	No. of Participants[a]	No. of Deaths Before Age 90	Median Age (Years)	Current Smoker (%)	Mean Body Mass Index (kg/m²)	Current Alcohol (%)	High Education (%)	High Exercise (%)
MEN									
Adventist	Nonvegetarian	5023	423	49	7.2	25.7	2.0	54.4	77.9
Mortality	Vegetarian	3971	303	51	2.9	24.6	0.7	63.3	81.2
Health Food	Nonvegetarian	2462	598	46	30.6				
Shoppers	Vegetarian	1519	385	41	20.1				
Adventist Health	Nonvegetarian	9045	1372	52	8.5	25.4	14.0	78.7	65.8
	Vegetarian	3169	362	51	0.2	23.8	0.4	86.5	71.3
Heidelberg	Nonvegetarian	304	33	45	9.9	22.1	29.4	62.8	34.8
	Vegetarian	480	58	43	4.2	21.3	14.1	56.4	40.3
Oxford Vegetarian	Nonvegetarian	2572	208	34	29.1	23.0	86.0	67.9	62.6
	Vegetarian	1603	168	33	17.5	22.0	63.2	64.8	67.4
WOMEN									
Adventist	Nonvegetarian	9257	491	50	1.2	25.1	1.6	51.6	51.9
Mortality	Vegetarian	6287	418	54	0.1	24.0	0.7	59.7	54.9
Health Food	Nonvegetarian	3626	640	45	18.0				
Shoppers	Vegetarian	2271	504	47	12.3				
Adventist Health	Nonvegetarian	11,904	1332	52	2.7	24.8	4.8	78.4	51.9
	Vegetarian	4834	498	54	0.2	23.0	0.2	85.4	54.9
Heidelberg	Nonvegetarian	370	19	49	3.2	21.3	24.9	46.6	32.8
	Vegetarian	603	75	53	2.2	20.9	7.3	43.7	37.0
Oxford Vegetarian	Nonvegetarian	3801	216	34	18.5	22.1	76.3	59.9	58.4
	Vegetarian	3071	227	32	13.4	21.3	56.5	60.1	65.4

[a]Number of subjects aged 16–89 years at recruitment for whom data on smoking and diet group were available. Data on body mass index, alcohol, education, and exercise were not available for the Health Food Shoppers study, and data on exercise were missing for women in the Adventist Mortality study. Overall, data on body mass index, alcohol, education, and exercise were available for 81.5, 83.4, 83.0, and 66.1% of subjects, respectively.

Source: Reprinted by permission from Key TJA et al., Mortality in vegetarians and non-vegetarians: a collaborative analysis of 8,300 deaths among 76,000 men and women in five prospective studies, *Public Health Nutr* 1:33–41, 1998.

this is partly explained by their older ages. Note that in all of the studies the vegetarians had a lower BMI than the "nonvegetarians" at the various locations.

The combined results (Key et al., 1999a) were a 32% (95% confidence interval, 6%–61%) increase in CHD mortality, among the "nonvegetarians" but only a nonsignificant 8% increase in risk of a fatal stroke (though with wide confidence intervals). These results were based on 2264 deaths (deaths of people over age 89 were excluded), and the analyses were adjusted for age, sex, and smoking habits.

There was evidence that the differences in effects on CHD mortality found between the studies was rather more than that expected from just random variation in the data, as indicated by a significant chi-squared test for heterogeneity. The two British studies showed less benefit for vegetarians than the other studies. One implication may be that there are fewer dietary and other differences between vegetarian and (as defined here) "nonvegetarian" study subjects in Britain than there are between similarly defined vegetarian and "nonvegetarian" California Adventists. The study that shows the least effect, the Health Foods Shoppers Study, has the least stringent definition of vegetarianism and has a long follow-up period after a single estimate of dietary habits. Thus a greater bias toward the null, or no-effect, value may be present in this study.

When this analysis was broken down by gender, the CHD death rate ratios were 1.45 (95% confidence interval, 1.19–1.79) for men and 1.25 (95% confidence interval, 1.05–1.49) for women, comparing "nonvegetarians" with vegetarians (Key et al., 1999a). Although the men appeared to obtain more protection from their diet, the difference between the sexes was not statistically significant and may be due to chance. For cerebrovascular disease mortality, the death rate ratios were 1.30 (95% confidence interval, 0.98–1.75) and 1.02 (95% confidence interval, 0.83–1.25) for men and women, respectively, again suggesting that this possible effect may be stronger in the men.

Do the effects of vegetarianism differ for people of different ages? As was true for California Adventists alone, in the combined data the benefits for both CHD and possibly cerebrovascular mortality appeared greatest for younger people (see Table 10-4). The effect of the duration of a vegetarian diet was also evaluated. Those who had been vegetarians for less than five years had a nonsignificantly increased death rate ratio of 1.20 (95% confidence interval, 0.90–1.61), whereas those who had been vegetarians for more than five years had a significantly lower death rate ratio of 0.74 (95% confidence interval, 0.60–0.90), when both were compared with "nonvegetarians." This trend was seen in all five studies. A less pro-

Table 10–4. Coronary Heart Disease Death Rate Ratios for "Nonvegetarians" versus Vegetarians by Age at Death: A Collaborative Analysis

Age at Death (Years)	Death Rate Ratio[a] (95% Confidence Interval)	No. of Deaths
<65	1.82 (1.18–2.86)	259
65–79	1.45 (1.11–1.89)	1086
80–89	1.09 (0.86–1.37)	919

[a]Death rate ratios are adjusted for age (within categories), sex, and smoking and for study using a random effects model.

Source: Adapted and reprinted by permission from Key TJA et al., Mortality in vegetarians and nonvegetarians: a collaborative analysis of 8,300 deaths among 76,000 men and women in five prospective studies, Public Health Nutr 1:33–41, 1998.

nounced trend favoring the longer-lasting vegetarian diet was also seen for cerebrovascular disease mortality.

When an adjustment was made for the potentially confounding variables— alcohol consumption, education, BMI, and exercise (in the four studies for which these data were available)—the death rate ratio of CHD for "nonvegetarian" subjects changed little, from 1.64 to 1.50 (note that these ratios are both further from the null value now that the Health Food Shoppers Study has been excluded because of missing covariate data). Moreover, removing subjects from the analysis who had a history of cardiovascular disease or diabetes (again only possible in the four studies), and thus focusing on incident CHD events, still resulted in a statistically significant increase of 32% (95% confidence interval, 3%–69%) in the CHD risk for the "nonvegetarians."

The term "nonvegetarian" used in this discussion is set off in quotation marks, because the "nonvegetarians" cited here were often not nonvegetarians or omnivores in the usual sense. In fact, most were health-conscious individuals who ate less meat than average—about one-quarter of the "nonvegetarians" ate meat less than once a week or ate only fish.

In retrospect, the attempts to include the Health Food Shoppers Study in the collaborative analysis diluted the comparison. Because of the limited characterization of meat consumption in the Health Food Shoppers Study, we were forced to adopt a very loose definition of nonvegetarians: subjects who ate any meat or fish.

Probably the most informative results of this analysis (Key et al., 1999) are revealed when the Health Food Shoppers data are omitted. Then the reference "nonvegetarian" category includes only those who eat meat at least once per week (on average, probably three to four times), a reference category similar to that commonly used in the California Adventist studies. This is compared with vegetarians, who eat no fish or meat.

The results then show a relative risk of 1.52 (95% confidence interval, 1.20–1.92) for CHD mortality among nonvegetarians, a result very similar to the California findings. The relative risk for a fatal stroke among nonvegetarians is 1.15 (95% confidence interval, 0.88–1.52).

SUMMARY

1. The results from the Health Food Shoppers and Oxford studies of non-Adventists clearly find that health-conscious subjects enjoy a substantial decrease in CHD deaths but that probably only part of this can be ascribed to lower meat consumption. Other aspects of the "health-conscious" lifestyle—such as the greater consumption of fruit, vegetables, and nuts; the lower intake of animal fats; more physical activity; better weight control; and less cigarette smoking—also play an important part, which agrees with the studies of Adventists.

2. There is good evidence, from the collaborative analysis, of lower CHD mortality among vegetarians as compared with "nonvegetarians." This is true for all and incident CHD events. The effect of vegetarianism was seen only in those who had been vegetarians for at least five years and was more evident at younger ages (below 80 years). Both men and women appeared to be protected, but men more so.

3. In fact, the main analysis of the collaborative study understates the true protection of vegetarianism as the label "nonvegetarian" for the comparison group meant only that subjects ate some meat or fish, even if only occasionally. Where the comparison "nonvegetarian" group is strengthened to mean those eating meat at least once each week, they experience at least a 50% increase in fatal CHD.

4. While the Adventist data formed a substantial proportion of the data in the collaborative analysis, the addition of the other studies produced results that generally supported the previous conclusions about vegetarian diets and CHD events. This increases our confidence in the idea that the benefits of a vegetarian diet for CHD would also apply to the general population.

11

Cancer and All-Cause Mortality among British and German Vegetarians

What is the evidence from studies of other populations that vegetarians experience different rates of cancer mortality or of mortality from all causes? The Health Food Shoppers, Oxford Vegetarian, and Heidelberg studies (see Chapter 10) addressed the risks of dying from cancer, or from any cause, among non-Adventist vegetarians. In addition, a collaborative analysis that combined the results of these studies with those of California Adventists compared cancer and all-cause mortality among vegetarian and nonvegetarian subjects.

DEATHS FROM CANCER AMONG BRITISH AND GERMAN VEGETARIANS

It is important to understand that the information presented here pertains only to those cancers that were sufficiently invasive or advanced, at the diagnosis stage, to have caused death. For most common sites, this would exclude 50% to 70% of new cancers, although for cancers that are highly fatal (e.g., cancers of the lung, stomach, and pancreas), most events are included. The only study of many vegetarians that has so far published results for all new cancers, both fatal and nonfatal, is the Adventist Health Study, and these results were discussed in Chapter 6.

A problem that pervades prospective studies of cancer is that of small numbers. As the studies of non-Adventist vegetarians are either small (the Heidelberg study) or moderately sized (the two British studies), the numbers of cancers for specific sites are also quite small, and this leads to wide confidence intervals. In the data presented below, results based on less than 10 recorded cancer deaths for a particular site are excluded.

Table 11–1. Standardized Mortality Ratios (95% Confidence Intervals) for Site-Specific Cancers: Health Food Shoppers Compared to Other British Subjects

Cancer Site	Men	Women
All cancers	0.50 (0.43–0.58)	0.76 (0.68–0.86)
Stomach	0.37 (0.18–0.66)	0.66 (0.34–1.15)
Colon and rectum	0.64 (0.42–0.95)	0.87 (0.61–1.20)
Pancreas	0.79 (0.39–1.41)	1.00 (0.56–1.64)
Lung	0.27 (0.19–0.38)	0.37 (0.23–0.56)
Breast		0.88 (0.68–1.12)
Ovary		0.90 (0.56–1.37)
Prostate	1.06 (0.71–1.52)	

Source: Adapted and reprinted by permission from Key TJA, Thorogood M, Appleby PN, Burr NL, Dietary habits and mortality in 11,000 vegetarians and health-conscious people: result of 17-year follow up, *Br Med J* 313:775–779, 1996. Published by BMJ Publishing Group.

The Health Food Shoppers Study (Key et al., 1996) recorded 451 cancer deaths during an average follow-up of 16.8 years—181 for men and 270 for women. As noted previously, this was a study of 10,977 health-conscious British men and women, many of whom were vegetarians. When comparing the recorded cancer deaths in this population with the total number expected, using national cancer mortality rates, the standardized mortality ratios for all cancers for male and female study participants, respectively, were 0.50 (95% confidence interval, 0.43–0.58) and 0.76 (95% confidence interval, 0.68–0.86). Clearly there are characteristics of this health-conscious population that have resulted in much lower mortality rates from cancer.

Results for specific cancer sites are found in Table 11–1. Although the health food shoppers had significantly lower rates than other British subjects for only cancers of the stomach, colon/rectum, and lung, it is noteworthy that mortality ratios for every cancer site for both sexes were less than 1.0, with the exception of cancer of the prostate among men and cancer of the pancreas among women. There is the possibility, as usual, of a healthy-volunteer bias, but any such effect is probably small as an earlier analysis of CHD and total mortality (Burr and Sweetnam, 1982) found only minor differences in mortality ratios when events occurring in the first year of the follow-up were excluded in order to minimize this effect.

The Oxford Vegetarian Study (Thorogood et al., 1994) recorded 164 fatal cancers during an average follow-up of about 12 years. This was a study of 6115 subjects who ate meat less than once per week. These vegetarian subjects then invited 5015 nonvegetarian friends or relatives, who ate meat once each week or more, to join the study as controls. Using mortality rates from the general British population, the researchers predicted 262.5 cancer deaths for this whole study population of 11,130 subjects, which resulted in a standardized cancer mortality ratio of 0.62 (95% confidence interval, 0.53–0.73) for all cancers. Thus, the combined group of vegetarians and nonvegetarian controls in the study experience many fewer deaths from cancer than expected.

The reduction in cancer mortality was especially evident among the vegetarians. The standardized cancer mortality ratio was 0.80 (95% confidence interval, 0.64–0.98) for the nonvegetarian controls, but 0.50 (95% confidence interval, 0.39–0.62) for the vegetarians, when both were compared with expected values in the general population. Thus, directly comparing the controls with the vegetarians, the corresponding death rate ratio was 1.61 (95% confidence interval, 1.19–2.17). An adjustment for differences in smoking habits, body mass index, and social class left this result essentially unchanged. Restricting the analysis to those who had never smoked, and adjusting for the other two factors, produced a cancer death rate ratio of 1.79 (95% confidence interval, 1.12–2.86), comparing controls with vegetarians. Restricting the analysis to deaths beyond the first five years, to allow for a possible healthy-volunteer effect, did reduce the death rate ratio comparing controls with vegetarians to 1.25, and showed a wide confidence interval of 0.76–1.67 due to the smaller number of cases.

The Heidelberg Vegetarian Study observed 58 cancer deaths during 11 years of follow-up—26 for men and 32 for women (Frentzel-Beyme and Chang-Claude, 1994). This study included only "strict" and "moderate" vegetarians, the latter being persons who ate meat or fish occasionally. When German national cancer mortality rates were applied to this population, the resulting standardized mortality ratios for cancer were 0.48 (95% confidence interval, 0.31–0.70) for men and 0.74 (95% confidence interval, 0.50–1.04) for women. Thus, as in the previous studies, there is evidence of a much lower cancer mortality rate among these health-conscious individuals when they are compared with the general population. Moreover, when the analyses were restricted to follow-up years 6 and beyond, to minimize a healthy-volunteer effect, the standardized mortality ratio for men was still 0.41 (95% confidence interval, 0.21–0.71). The corresponding ratio for women was higher at 0.90, although the confidence interval was wide (0.56–1.36).

Results were presented by cancer site, but the numbers were so small that I will mention only those for cancers of digestive organs, where there were 11 deaths among men and 9 among women. The corresponding "standardized" mortality ratios were 0.56 (95% confidence interval, 0.28–1.01) and 0.49 (95% confidence interval, 0.23–0.93). The data also showed that those who had been vegetarians for at least 20 years experienced only half the risk of cancer deaths (relative risk, 0.51, $p < .05$), as compared with those who had been vegetarians for shorter periods (Frentzel-Beyme and Chang-Claude, 1994).

In summary, these individual studies compared the cancer mortality experience of vegetarian and health-conscious individuals with that expected for the general population. In addition, the Oxford Vegetarian Study could compare the cancer experience of the vegetarians with the nonvegetarian controls in the study groups. All of the studies found that health-conscious subjects have much lower cancer mortality, also vegetarians in the Oxford study did better than the nonvegetarians. The Heidelberg study reported that the duration of vegetarianism may be important, perhaps fitting with the long period of time that it takes cancers to develop. The information on specific cancer sites was hampered by small numbers in all studies, but cancers of the digestive system, as a group, were reduced in the two studies that presented such data.

ALL-CAUSE MORTALITY IN BRITISH AND GERMAN VEGETARIANS

The number of deaths from all causes in the studies of non-Adventist vegetarians was, of course, much greater than that for CHD or specific cancers. There were 1343 deaths (666 male and 677 female recorded) in the Health Food Shoppers Study (Burr and Butland, 1988; Key et al., 1996), 404 deaths (no breakdown by sex was published) in the Oxford Vegetarian Study (Thorogood et al., 1994), and 225 deaths (111 male and 114 female) in the Heidelberg Vegetarian Study (Chang-Claude et al., 1992).

As compared with expectations based on national mortality rates, the recorded numbers of deaths allow the calculation of standardized mortality ratios for all subjects in these studies. These are shown in Table 11–2, and often take values close to 0.5. This leaves little doubt that the health-conscious subjects of these studies have a large overall mortality advantage over others in the United Kingdom or Germany. The question is why.

Table 11–2. Standardized Mortality Ratios (Comparing Study Mortality to National Mortality Data) and Death Rate Ratios (Nonvegetarians versus Vegetarians) in the Three Studies of Non-Adventist Vegetarians

Study	Men	Women
STANDARDIZED MORTALITY RATIOS		
Health Food Shoppers	0.52 (0.48–0.56)	0.60 (0.56–0.65)
Oxford Vegetarian	0.46 (0.42–0.51)	
Heidelberg Vegetarian	0.44 (0.36–0.53)	0.53 (0.44–0.64)
DEATH RATE RATIOS		
Health Food Shoppers	0.96 (0.86–1.08)[a]	
Oxford Vegetarian (meat ≥ 1/wk versus <1/wk)	1.25 (1.01–1.45)[b]	

[a]Adjusted for age, sex and smoking.

[b]Adjusted for smoking, body mass index, and social class.

One possibility is that a healthy-volunteer effect may explain this apparent risk reduction if only healthy "health-conscious" subjects volunteered for these studies, so biasing observations during the initial follow up period. However, an earlier analysis of the Health Food Shoppers Study (Burr and Sweetnam, 1982) found little change when dropping the first year of the follow-up. This suggests that if a healthy-volunteer effect exists, it is small. Similarly, in the Heidelberg Vegetarian Study, the standardized mortality ratios, when considering only follow-up years 6 and beyond, were still much reduced at 0.44 (95% confidence interval, 0.34–0.57) for men and 0.62 (95% confidence interval, 0.49–0.78) for women.

Death rate ratios comparing nonvegetarians with vegetarians, within each British study, are also shown in Table 11–2. The Heidelberg study did not enroll nonvegetarians. In the Oxford study (Thorogood et al., 1994), there was a moderate disadvantage for the nonvegetarians, with a relative risk of 1.25 (95% confidence interval, 1.01–1.45). However, if the first five years of the follow-up were excluded, the relative risk was then estimated at 1.01, but with a wide confidence interval (0.77–1.32). This may suggest that unhealthy vegetarians were originally less likely to join the study than were unhealthy nonvegetarians.

There was no evidence of higher total mortality among the "nonvegetarians" in the Health Food Shoppers Study as the death rate ratio was 0.96. This study, as noted in Chapter 10, compared those who called themselves vegetarians with health-conscious subjects who did not consider themselves vegetarians. Excluding the first year of the follow-up changed the result very little (Burr and Sweetnam, 1982). Hence the evidence that vegetarianism, defined as any meat consumption, is the cause of the lower mortality among these populations is far from convincing, but, noting the confidence intervals, a modest effect could have been missed by chance.

COLLABORATIVE ANALYSIS OF CALIFORNIA ADVENTIST, BRITISH, AND GERMAN STUDIES

As also explained in Chapter 10, the definition of a nonvegetarian is a problem in the collaborative analysis. In order to give a more biologically meaningful contrast, the results shown in Table 11–3 compare vegetarians with regular meat-eaters (thereby excluding occasional meat-eaters). The main reported results of the collaborative study diluted the "nonvegetarian" category with subjects who ate meat, though less than once per week. In addition, the meat intake of "nonvegetarians" in the Health Food Shoppers Study could not be quantified, but was probably often quite low. Thus, we also exclude data from that study in the results presented here. This is

Table 11–3. Collaborative Analysis of Deaths from Selected Cancers and All-Causes by Vegetarian Status: Death Rate Ratios (95% Confidence Intervals)[a]

Cause of Death	Vegetarians (n = 23,265)	Regular Meat-Eaters[b] (n = 31,766)
Stomach cancer	1.00	1.41 (0.83–2.38)
No. of deaths	28	38
Colorectal cancer	1.00	0.91 (0.65–1.27)
No. of deaths	71	78
Lung cancer	1.00	1.61 (1.00–2.63)
No. of deaths	26	89
Female breast cancer	1.00	1.33 (0.88–2.04)
No. of deaths	41	61
Prostate cancer	1.00	1.33 (0.83–2.13)
No. of deaths	33	51
All-cause death	1.00	1.19 (1.04–1.35)
No. of deaths	2041	3017

[a]Adjusted for age, sex, and smoking status. Data from the Health Food Shoppers Study is excluded because information on the frequency of meat consumption was not collected.

[b]Meat ≥1/wk.

Source: Key TJ, Fraser GE, Thorogood M, Appleby PN, Beral V, Reeves G, Burr ML, Chang-Claude J, Frentzel-Beyme R, Kuzma JW, Mann J, Mc Pherson K, Mortality in vegetarians and nonvegetarians: detailed findings from a collaborative analysis of 5 prospective studies, *Am J Clin Nutr* 70(Suppl):516s–524s, 1999. Copyright by American Society of Clinical Nutrition.

an attempt to use definitions from the other studies that are most comparable with those used in the California Adventist studies. Although this problem with the definition of a nonvegetarian was important for cardiovascular results, it is even more so for the endpoints of this chapter. As the real effects of meat intake on cancer and all-cause mortality may be less strong, they are more easily obscured by such a technical problem.

Cancer Mortality

As relatively few deaths were recorded for a specific cancer site in the British and German studies, and sometimes even in the larger cohorts of California Adventists, we pooled data from meat-eaters and lacto-ovo-vegetarians in four studies as a collaborative analysis of fatal cancers (Key et al., 1999a). Although this was then an analysis of 55,000 men and women, with an average follow-up period of 10.6 years, the number of site-specific cancer deaths was still less than ideal. Thus the analysis was restricted to cancers of the stomach (66 cases), colon/rectum (149 cases), lung (115 cases), breast (102 cases), and prostate (84 cases). These numbers may seem surprisingly small, but, again, these are only fatal cases. Comparisons and adjustments were always made within a particular study, and then the cancer mortality ratios were combined to form a pooled estimate using a random effects model (Der Simonian and Laird, 1986). Persons with a previous diagnosis of cancer (except nonmelanoma skin cancer), and persons 90 years of age and over, were excluded from these analyses.

Despite the wide confidence intervals, as compared with the vegetarians, the regular meat-eaters tend to have a greater risk of dying from these cancers (Table 11–3). This agrees with the finding for California Adventists, and with the results from many other studies, showing that those who eat more fruits and vegetables and less animal products generally have a lower risk. The results of this collaborative analysis are not detailed enough to point the finger specifically at meat, but at least they suggest the benefits of a dietary pattern that tends toward being vegetarian.

The one rather surprising result is that regular meat-eaters experience a little less colorectal cancer, although the result is not statistically significant. This is not consistent with the California Adventist data or with data from several other large-cohort studies (see Chapter 6). The apparent discrepancy (*1*) may be due to chance, (*2*) may occur because in these analyses we could consider only the 35% to 40% of colon cancer patients who die from their cancer, or (*3*) may occur because rectal cancers are lumped with the colon cancers in these analyses. We did not find that vegetarian status protected against rectal cancer in the Adventist data, so placing colon and rectal cancers together may dilute an effect on colon cancer alone.

There were no clear differences in these endpoints between those who had been vegetarians for less than, or greater than, five years, although confidence intervals were very wide for the shorter-term vegetarians as there were always fewer than 10 deaths for a specific cancer site.

All-Cause Mortality

Adding the data for all-cause mortality from the two California cohorts to data from the two non-Adventist studies allows a summary death rate ratio (see Table 11–3) to be formed that compares the risk for regular meat-eater to that for vegetarians, using the definitions described above. The comparison is done after an adjustment for any differences in age, sex, and smoking habits.

The summary result is a significant 19% increase in the risk of all-cause mortality among the regular meat-eaters. This is quite consistent with the results for California Adventists. Interestingly, in the collaborative analysis (Key et al., 1999a), vegetarians, fish-eaters who never ate meat, and those who ate meat but less than once each week all had about the same risk of dying from any cause. This was lower than that of regular meat-eaters.

DISCREPANCY BETWEEN RESULTS FOR CANCER AND ALL-CAUSE MORTALITY

The most striking result from the British and German studies is the great reduction in cancer and all-cause mortality for the study groups, when they are compared with the general population in those locations. It seems that these "health-conscious" populations are either self-selected for better genetic fitness, which seems unlikely, or else some of their unusual health habits do effectively reduce mortality. The challenge is to identify the active principles behind this quite dramatic effect.

The tendency toward a vegetarian diet is certainly one contender. When comparing results for nonvegetarians with those for vegetarians across studies, great care should be taken regarding the definition of a nonvegetarian. In the Health Food Shoppers Study, we can make little progress as a nonvegetarian was simply defined as a health-conscious subject who did not choose the label "vegetarian." It is not clear how much the vegetarians and nonvegetarians in this study differed in their meat consumption (Appleby et al., 2002).

The main published results from both the collaborative analysis and the Oxford Vegetarian Study were based on a classification for vegetarians and nonvegetarians that provides a quite modest difference in meat consumption between the two groups. In this situation, only small relative risks would be expected if meat were indeed hazardous, and it is difficult to achieve statistical significance with small effects. In both of these studies, however (Appleby et al., 2002; Key et al., 1999a), it was possible to define nonvegetarians (labeled "meat-eaters" in those studies) as those who ate meat at least once per week. Results then became more compatible with those for California Adventists. In summary, the British studies identified study groups with health habits, and perhaps other characteristics, that greatly reduce mortality. However, the main results reported provide only a weak test of whether meat consumption had anything to do with this.

Even when nonvegetarians were defined as those who ate meat at least once per week, the apparent advantages of vegetarianism seemed a little weaker in the Oxford study as compared with the California studies. There are several possible explanations that deserve further study, as follows:

1. Because of climatic and geographic differences, the British vegetarian diet may include fewer fruits and vegetables, or less variety, than that in California.
2. The Oxford Study (Appleby et al., 2002) has a quite long follow-up (16 years) after a single dietary assessment. Undocumented changes in diet after the study baseline will weaken associations, and we apparently observed this in the Adventist data comparing a 6- to a 12-year follow-up

(as an example see the discussion about nut consumption and heart disease in Chapter 9).

3. There is a focus on fatal cancers, rather than both fatal and nonfatal cancers, in the Oxford Study. Yet it is possible that the lifestyle associations with cancers are less evident for the more aggressive tumors that result in death. That cancers at the same anatomic site may not all have the same biology is indicated—for instance, by the quite different risk factor associations with colon cancer, according to whether or not there is a family history of this cancer (La Vecchia et al., 1999; Sellers et al., 1998).

4. Vegetarianism is a sociologically complex choice, and it is clear that vegetarians and nonvegetarians also differ according to nonmeat dietary and other, nondietary, factors. These other factors will undoubtedly differ by culture and location, yet may influence disease risk.

SUMMARY

1. Health-conscious individuals and vegetarians have distinctly lower mortality rates for cancer and all-cause mortality than the general population. This is true even after an adjustment for cigarette smoking and is probably at least partially due to their generally superior health habits, even aside from less meat consumption.

2. It seems unlikely that vegetarians experience markedly less overall cancer mortality than other health-conscious individuals who eat a little meat. However, there is suggestive evidence for some increased risk when meat is eaten once per week or more.

3. Larger studies that include fatal and nonfatal cancers, and also sizable groups who are either vegetarians or relatively heavy meat-eaters, would give further valuable information. Such studies are under way in Great Britain and California.

4. A decrease in all-cause mortality is probably conferred by vegetarianism, but of quite a modest magnitude (as was also found for Adventists alone—see Chapter 7), considering that only some causes of mortality are affected.

5. One should be very cautious when equating the statistical effect of the "vegetarianism" label with a causal role for meat consumption, unless there is control for other foods and behaviors in the analysis. Vegetarians differ from nonvegetarians in many ways apart from their meat intake, and these differences will also vary according to culture and location.

12

Risk Factors for Cardiovascular Disease and Cancer among Vegetarians

A risk factor is a trait that places a person at higher risk of developing a disease and is generally considered to have a causal link to that disease. Risk factors may be behavioral, psychosocial, physiologic, or biochemical. Well-known examples for cardiovascular disease are high-serum LDL cholesterol, hypertension, diabetes mellitus, cigarette smoking, physical inactivity, and lack of social support.

This book is of course largely concerned with the effects of diet on chronic disease. Since any effects of diet are probably mediated by physiologic and biochemical mechanisms, it would strengthen the evidence that a vegetarian diet protects against CHD and cancer if this diet were found to change physiologic and biochemical risk factors in ways that are generally thought to reduce risk. Then there would not only be a statistical association between a vegetarian's dietary habits and risk of disease but also some evidence of the mechanism that underlies the reduced risk. An understanding of mechanisms is one way to strengthen causal inference.

Hypertension, diabetes mellitus, and obesity are not only risk factors for CHD but disorders in their own right. The evidence that a vegetarian diet may affect the risk of these disorders among Adventists was considered separately in Chapter 8. In this chapter, studies of non-Adventist vegetarian groups only are described in relation to the risk of these factors. For other risk factors, studies of both Adventist and non-Adventist vegetarians are included here. Results from similar studies of vegan vegetarians are discussed separately in Chapter 13.

RISK FACTORS FOR CARDIOVASCULAR DISEASE

Effect of Vegetarian Diets on Blood Lipids

There is a reasonable expectation that vegetarians would have lower levels of total and LDL cholesterol, because their intakes of saturated fat and cholesterol are lower, and intakes of dietary fiber, phytosterols, and, in some settings, polyunsaturated fat are higher—all trends that favorably affect serum LDL cholesterol levels (Howard and Kritchevsky, 1997; Jacobs et al., 1979; Van Horn, 1997).

The effect of vegetarianism on HDL cholesterol ("good" cholesterol) is more difficult to predict. It is generally lowered by diets that have little fat and are high in carbohydrates (Albrink and Ullrich, 1986; Howell et al., 1997), but these characteristics are more typical of vegan diets than of lacto-ovo vegetarian diets. Diets containing more polyunsaturated fat than either saturated or monounsaturated fat may also slightly lower HDL cholesterol levels (Mattson and Grundy, 1985; Shepherd et al., 1978; Sirtori et al., 1986). Vegetarians, even non-Adventist vegetarians (Appleby et al., 1998; Li et al., 1999; Roshanai and Sanders, 1984; Sanders and Key, 1987; Thefeld et al., 1986; Williams, 1997), typically drink less alcohol than others, and this would be expected to result in modestly lower HDL cholesterol levels (Haskell et al., 1984). Vegetarians are often health-conscious and may exercise more than others. This has been shown to raise HDL cholesterol in vegetarians in the same way as it does in others (Williams, 1997). Vegetarians tend to be thinner than others, and this is also associated with higher HDL levels (Heath et al., 1994; Katzel et al., 1995).

Vegetarians have lower levels of both serum total and LDL cholesterol. This has been consistently found in many studies. Some of these studies have been observational in design, comparing a group of vegetarians with a group of nonvegetarians (they are usually matched by age, sex, and other factors) (Appleby et al., 1995; Armstrong et al., 1979; Berkel, 1979; Burr et al., 1981; Fisher et al., 1986; Fraser and Swannel, 1981; Gear et al., 1980; Groen et al., 1962; Haines et al., 1980; Hardinge and Stare, 1954b; Hardinge et al., 1962; Hayes, 1968; Li et al., 1999; Pan et al., 1993; Rouse et al., 1983a; Sacks et al., 1975; Simons et al., 1978; Thorogood et al., 1987; West and Hayes, 1968). One study of this type was conducted among adolescents (Ruys and Hickie, 1976), and others were done among black Adventists (Famodu et al., 1998; Melby et al., 1994). Others have evaluated vegan vegetarians who eat no animal products (these studies are treated separately in Chapter 13). There is always a concern that factors aside from diet will differ among vegetarians and omnivores, and that these may have caused any lipid differences. If the groups are well matched, however, evidence of a dietary effect on blood lipids can be strong.

Table 12–1. Differences in Serum Cholesterol between the Vegetarian and Nonvegetarian Seventh-day Adventist Members of 233 Pairs

| Type of Nonvegetarian | No. of Pairs | Mean Serum Cholesterol Levels (mg/dL) | | p |
		Nonvegetarian	Vegetarian	
MFF < 1×/mo	61	183	188	>.20
MFF < 1×/wk (>1×/mo)	47	192	182	>.05
MFF 1–2×/wk	48	200	181	<.01
MFF ≥ 3×/wk	77	207	188	<.01
Total	233	196	185	<.01

MFF, meat, fish, or fowl.

Source: Reprinted with permission from West RO, Hayes OB, Diet and serum cholesterol levels: a comparison between vegetarians and non-vegetarians in a Seventh-day Adventist group, *Am J Clin Nutr* 21:853–862, 1968. Copyright by American Society for Clinical Nutrition.

As one example of such a study, West and Hayes (1968) compared 233 Adventist nonvegetarians with 233 Adventist vegetarians in Washington, D.C. The matching was done with respect to the specific church subjects attended, sex, age (within five years), marital status, height, weight, and an occupational classification. The nonvegetarians were grouped into four categories ranging from those who ate meat less than once each month through those eating meat more than three times weekly.

Those who ate meat once a week or more had serum cholesterol levels that were, on average, 19 mg/dL ($p < .01$) higher than those for the vegetarians (Table 12–1). The potential confounding effects of the matched variables were removed by the study design as they were always equal in the different nonvegetarian-vegetarian comparisons. This, of course, does not isolate meat alone as the causal agent, as other dietary and unmatched nondietary factors may also differ between vegetarians and nonvegetarians.

Lipid levels were also compared among 1344 meat-eaters (more than once per week), 136 fish-eaters (fish, but not meat, more than once per week), 374 semivegetarians (meat or fish less than once per week), 1785 strict vegetarians (but excluding vegans), and 134 vegans (who ate no animal products) in the Oxford Vegetarian Study (Appleby et al., 1995). This study is notable for its large number of subjects and a detailed division into different categories of vegetarian/fish/meat consumption. As compared with meat-eaters, the proportionate levels of total and HDL cholesterols for other dietary categories are shown in Table 12–2. Total cholesterol levels were significantly lower in all non-meat-eating categories, but particularly so for vegans, where the difference was 16% to 18%. By contrast, there were no significant differences for HDL cholesterol. In an attempt to isolate the effect of meat, the investigators adjusted for the other significant dietary factors that were also related to blood lipid levels. After an adjustment for dietary fiber and cheese (for men), and for type of fat spread, di-

Table 12-2. Mean Age-Adjusted Ratios (Standard Errors in Parentheses) of Cholesterol Concentration by Sex: Blood Cholesterol Levels of Other Categories Divided by Those of Meat Eaters

Diet	Total Cholesterol		HDL Cholesterol	
	Men	Women	Men	Women
Meat-eater	1.00	1.00	1.00	1.00
Fish-eater	0.93 (0.027)	0.96 (0.019)	1.08 (0.039)	1.05 (0.026)
Semivegetarian	0.92 (0.019)	0.95 (0.012)	1.04 (0.026)	1.00 (0.015)
Vegetarian	0.92 (0.010)	0.92 (0.008)	1.01 (0.014)	0.99 (0.010)
Vegan	0.84 (0.023)	0.82 (0.017)	1.04 (0.035)	0.98 (0.025)

Source: Reprinted with permission from Appleby PN, Thorogood M, McPherson K, Mann JL, Associations between plasma lipid concentrations and dietary, lifestyle and physical factors in the Oxford Vegetarian Study. *J Human Nutr Diet* 8:305–314, 1995.

etary fiber, and tomatoes (for women), the average effect of eating meat at least five times weekly was an elevation of serum total cholesterol by 8.6% in men and 8.8% in women.

Similar results hold true for subjects of African descent. Melby et al. (1994) compared 66 vegetarians with 56 semivegetarians (one to three servings of meat per week) and 45 nonvegetarians. All subjects were African-American Seventh-day Adventists. The vegetarians consumed 13% fewer calories than the nonvegetarians, and had lower intakes of saturated fat, potassium, and sodium. As expected, they also had significantly lower values for the waist/hip ratio. Perhaps as a consequence of some of these factors, there were significant differences between dietary groups for total cholesterol (181.5, 189.2, and 208.5 mg/dL for vegetarians, semivegetarians, and nonvegetarians, respectively), and LDL cholesterol (119.7, 127.4, and 139.0 mg/dL), but not for HDL cholesterol. Other work has compared vegetarian and nonvegetarian African Adventists in Nigeria (Famodu et al., 1998), with very similar results.

If it is conducted well, an experiment has a stronger study design than an observational study, as subjects have their diets controlled by the investigators, other factors being kept constant. Two such studies are those conducted by Sacks et al. (1981) and Cooper et al. (1982). Both confirm results from observational work. In the Sacks study, 21 strict vegetarians (but not necessarily vegans), after a two-week control diet (usually vegetarian), incorporated 250 g of beef daily into their diet, under supervision. This was added without changing total calories, by reducing the intake of other foods. Finally, two weeks were again spent eating the control diet. During the meat-eating phase, blood total cholesterol rose, on average, 19% (140 mg/dL, rising to 166 mg/dL), and then fell to 137 mg/dL while on the control diet ($p = .01$). There were no significant changes in HDL cholesterol (31 mg/dL, 32 mg/dL, and 31 mg/dL) during the three study phases and no change in mean body weight. Thus, this study isolates the effects that swapping meat for vegetarian foods has on blood lipid levels.

In the Cooper study, 15 subjects were randomly assigned to either an experimental vegetarian diet that contained no animal products except skim milk or a control diet that closely approximated the usual intake in the United States. After three weeks, the subjects switched to the contrasting diet for the final three weeks. The subjects prepared their own food but were given assistance with meal planning and recipes by study nutritionists. During the vegetarian period, 30% fewer calories were consumed, although weight decreased by only 1.6 lbs, on average, during this time. Serum total, LDL, and HDL cholesterol levels were 140.0, 93.2, and 33.4 mg/dL, respectively, on the vegetarian diet, whereas on the control diet they were 160.0 ($p < .01$), 109.2 ($p < .025$), and 37.1 (NS) mg/dL, where the p values refer to the contrast between the two diets. Although the vegetarian diet decreased total and LDL cholesterol levels, it is not clear what role the lower total energy intake might also have played. As many vegetarians do eat fewer calories, this may still be considered a proper test of the vegetarian hypothesis.

In summary, the evidence that vegetarians have lower total and LDL cholesterol levels is convincing, and it is very likely that part of this effect is due to the absence of meat. The effects of a vegetarian diet on HDL cholesterol (or the closely associated apolipoprotein A) are less certain but are minimal or absent in most studies (Appleby et al., 1995; Melby et al., 1994; Pan et al., 1993; Thorogood et al., 1987), but not all (Berkel, 1979; Fisher et al., 1986). Adventists as a group, including both vegetarians and nonvegetarians, tend to have lower HDL cholesterol levels than non-Adventists (Berkel, 1979; Fønnebø, 1985, 1988; Fraser et al., 1987). At least part—perhaps all—of this effect may be due to their avoidance of alcohol (Belfrage et al., 1973; Haskell et al., 1984). Although there is evidence that lean red and white meats in the diet need not raise blood cholesterol levels (Davidson et al., 1999; Scott et al., 1994), many nonvegetarians prefer the flavor of fattier meats. As the blood cholesterol-raising effect of meats is largely related to the meat fat, if meats are to be eaten, the use of leaner meats would seem prudent, but it is unclear whether this choice would also reduce risks that meat-eating may also pose for cancer, hypertension, diabetes, and possibly arthritis.

Effect of the Vegetarian Diet on Blood Pressure

High blood pressure is an established and potent risk factor for atherosclerotic disease. During the course of normal day-to-day activities, blood pressure varies constantly and at times substantially. Physical activity, anxiety, and room temperature are some factors that may provoke these short-term changes. Any research protocol must then establish consistent environmental conditions, as well as a rigorous measurement technique to properly compare blood pressures in different experimental situations.

Even under appropriate experimental conditions, blood pressure may vary a good deal for no apparent reason. One consequence is that it is not easy to prove that an experimental factor, such as diet, has truly changed the blood pressure. Considerable, apparently random, variability results in less statistical power. Despite these problems, there is a sizable literature that compares blood pressure levels between vegetarians and nonvegetarians. As for blood lipids, observational studies here are also usually comparisons between free-living vegetarians and nonvegetarians. Other studies experimentally impose well-controlled dietary conditions on the study subjects. Comparisons of blood pressure levels between vegetarian and nonvegetarian Adventists are discussed in Chapter 8. Results of these studies are generally consistent with the findings cited in this chapter. Unless stated otherwise, the fourth Korotkoff sound (K4) is used for diastolic blood pressure in the following descriptions.

The evidence clearly indicates that vegetarians have lower blood pressure than nonvegetarians. Three observational and several experimental studies are briefly described here as a sample of this evidence. In one of these studies, blood pressures were measured for 116 men and women living in communal households in the greater Boston area, and these people mainly ate food from vegetable sources and had done so for at least three years. These were compared with blood pressures from a randomly selected group of nonvegetarian controls from the Framingham study, who were matched by age and sex with the vegetarians. The systolic and diastolic blood pressures of the controls were 119 and 77 mm Hg, respectively, whereas for the vegetarians; equivalent values were 108 ($p < .001$) and 63 ($p < .001$) mm Hg (p values refer to the comparison between the groups). The vegetarians, as is often the case (see Chapter 8), were, on average, 15 kg lighter, and this may be one mechanism that explains their lower blood pressures (Stamler, 1991).

However, there is evidence that the lower body mass index in vegetarians is not the only determinant of the blood pressure differences. For instance, Rouse et al. (1983a) compared blood pressures between 98 Adventist lacto-ovo vegetarians and 113 Mormon omnivores in Perth, Australia. They found that the vegetarians had systolic blood pressures that were lower by 8.2 mm Hg ($p < .01$) in men and 8.6 mm Hg in women, and diastolic pressures were lower by 6.2 mm Hg ($p < .05$) in men and 7.9 mm Hg ($p < .01$) in women. When an adjustment was made for differences in body mass index, significant differences remained but of a smaller magnitude. Systolic blood pressures were then lower by 5.6 mm Hg ($p < .05$) in men and by 5.8 mm Hg ($p < .05$) in women. The diastolic pressures were 3.5 mm Hg ($p = NS$) lower in vegetarian men and 5.9 mm Hg ($p < .05$) lower in women. The implication is that the body mass index difference accounted for some, but not all, of the blood pressure difference.

A similar study in a different setting found similar results. A total of 98 confirmed vegetarians were compared with 98 nonvegetarians, who were matched with the vegetarians by age and sex; all were living in Israel (Ophir et al., 1983). The vegetarians showed consistently and significantly lower blood pressure levels, such that only 2% of the vegetarians were hypertensive (defined as $\geq 160/95$), whereas this was true for 26% of the omnivores. Comparisons within categories of body weight (to adjust for this factor) did not substantially change this result. It was noted that sodium excretion was quite similar for the two groups, whereas potassium excretion (and therefore intake) was significantly higher in the vegetarians, a finding also reported by several others (Armstrong et al., 1979; Ophir et al., 1983; Rouse et al., 1983b, 1984).

Results of other observational studies comparing vegetarians with non-vegetarians have been cited (Armstrong et al., 1979; Burr et al., 1981; Haines et al., 1980; Li et al., 1999; Sacks et al., 1974). Although one British study (Burr et al., 1981) did not find lower blood pressure levels in the vegetarians, the other studies support the findings described above. The "vegetarian effect" on blood pressure may not be present before the adult years as blood pressure levels in Adventist children and adolescents were not lower than those of their non-Adventist peers (Harris et al., 1981; Kuczmarski et al., 1994).

As for the diet–lipid comparisons, experimental studies allow closer control over the study variables and, if randomized, reduce the risk of confounding by factors other than the exposure of interest—in this case, the vegetarian diet. However, as such studies are often smaller and may have restrictive criteria of inclusion and exclusion, they are often less representative of a broad range of subjects.

One of the first experiments to test the effect of meat-eating on blood pressure was conducted by Donaldson at Loma Linda, California, in 1926. For 13 days, five men (normal students) were fed a lacto-ovo vegetarian diet, and then for 16 days, beef, mutton, and fish were introduced, to produce a diet at the same caloric level as the first diet, although protein changed from 10% to 20% of calories. On the vegetarian diet, blood pressure levels averaged 107/62, and on the meat diet they were 120/66 (K5 was used for diastolic blood pressure). Although interesting, this study had no separate control group (subjects served as their own controls), so other uncontrolled environmental changes could, in theory, have been important. Intake of other foods must also have changed to accommodate the meat.

The study by Sacks et al. (1981) described above, with respect to blood lipid changes, also demonstrated a significant 3 mm Hg elevation in systolic blood pressure when a daily 250 g of meat was added to the diet. However, the smaller rise in diastolic blood pressure did not achieve statistical significance. Whether it was the added meat that changed the blood pressure or the loss of vegetarian foods that were eliminated to keep calories constant is unclear.

A group of investigators from Perth has also actively pursued the diet–blood pressure connection (Rouse et al., 1983b) and has demonstrated that blood pressure fell after a change to a vegetarian diet. These researchers randomly assigned 59 healthy omnivorous subjects to either a control omnivorous diet for 14 weeks or to one of two lacto-ovo vegetarian/omnivorous diet groups who crossed over from 6 weeks of a lacto-ovo vegetarian diet to 6 weeks of the omnivorous diet, but in reverse order. Blood pressure levels for the control group did not change, but in the other groups they fell, on average, 5 to 6 mm Hg systolic and 2 to 3 mm Hg diastolic (statistically significant) during the vegetarian period (Fig. 12–1). The dashed lines in the figure all trend downward, and these represent time periods where a vegetarian diet followed either an omnivorous or a control diet. By contrast, the two heavier solid lines trend upward, and these depict time periods where the omnivorous diet followed the vegetarian diet. This was after an adjustment for age, body mass index, heart rate, weight

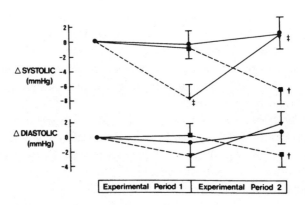

Figure 12–1 Mean changes in resting blood pressures measured in the laboratory. *Source:* Reproduced by permission from Elsevier Science, from Rouse IL et al., Blood-pressure lowering affect of a vegetarian diet: controlled trial in normotensive subjects, *Lancet* 1:5–10, 1983.

change, and baseline blood pressure. Body weight and urinary sodium and potassium did not differ significantly during the dietary periods. In a study of identical design, but one conducted among 58 mildly hypertensive subjects, Margetts et al. (1986) found a significant 5 mm Hg fall in systolic blood pressure with the vegetarian diet, but the 1.2 mm Hg fall in diastolic blood pressure was not statistically significant.

The results described here have led most investigators to conclude that vegetarians have modestly, but significantly, lower blood pressure levels than omnivores. It is unclear whether the lack of meat in the vegetarian diet is the active principle or whether other unique characteristics of this diet (e.g., more polyunsaturated fat, dietary fiber, and potassium) may play a part. Subsequent studies that were conducted to test these and other ideas are now summarized. The physiologic mechanisms underlying a vegetarian effect on blood pressure are not well understood, although in one controlled experiment, Sciarrone et al. (1993) again showed that the vegetarian diet lowered blood pressure, but also that this effect was associated with lower catecholamine and renin activity levels in those with the greatest drops in blood pressure. Rouse et al. (1984) compared blood and urine levels of a number of vasoactive compounds that may affect blood pressure in 47 vegetarian–omnivore pairs matched for age, sex, and body mass index. Vegetarians again excreted more potassium than nonvegetarians, but sodium excretion was similar in both groups. There were no significant differences in resting or post-stress (mental and physical) levels of noradrenalin, adrenalin, cortisol, or renin; or in resting levels of angiotensin II, thromboxane B_2; or in other urinary prostaglandins. The one significant difference was that the blood pressure response to the cold pressor test (one hand in ice water for 2 minutes) was much less ($p < .01$) in vegetarians than in the controls.

A series of controlled dietary experiments among small groups of subjects was subsequently conducted, largely by groups of investigators from Boston, and Perth, in an attempt to identify the foods or nutrients responsible for the blood pressure differences. Several of these studies involved changing dietary fat—in particular, the ratio of polyunsaturated to saturated fatty acids (P/S ratio)—and observing the effect on blood pressure. However, these changes were achieved in different ways.

Two experiments were reported together in the same publication by Sacks et al. (1984a). The first included 19 subjects and was designed to check the effects of reducing saturated fat (from 21 to 10 g per day), dietary cholesterol (from 398 to 69 mg per day), and protein (from 74 to 53 g per day), by using a low-fat diet in a crossover design. Intake of polyunsaturated fat, carbohydrates, and dietary fiber did not change, and the P/S ratio increased due to the reduced saturated fat. The second study measured the effect of adding an egg each day to the diet, thus raising cholesterol intake. The 17 subjects were blinded to this supplement as the egg was incorporated with other cooked foods. In neither case was there any significant change in blood pressure. However, potassium excretion (per gram of urinary creatinine) was higher in the low-fat diet of the first study. In neither study were there changes in body weight or sodium excretion.

Another crossover experiment (Margetts et al., 1984) measured the effect of markedly changing the dietary P/S ratio by both reducing saturated fats and increasing polyunsaturated fats (P/S ratio changed from 0.30 to 1.05). The linoleic content of the plasma rose, as expected, during the higher-P/S-ratio dietary periods. The only dietary macronutrients that changed during the study were the proportions of total fat derived from these two types of fatty acid. Body weight did not change significantly, and neither were blood pressure levels significantly affected by these changes.

In a somewhat similar study, Sacks et al. (1987a) replaced about one-third of the intake of calories from saturated fat with either polyunsaturated fat or carbohydrates for six weeks in a randomized double-blind, crossover protocol. A difference here is that the 21 subjects were mildly hypertensive. They ate their usual diet except that they were required to add either an 8-oz portion of yogurt or a 12-oz specially prepared milkshake that contained the different levels of the fatty acids or carbohydrates. Fasting plasma fatty acids changed significantly in the expected directions during the study. Again, there were no significant changes in blood pressure. Sacks et al. (1987b) next compared the effects of equivalent quantities of dietary linoleic acid and the monounsaturated oleic acid during four-week dietary periods in an isocaloric design, where other macronutrients, body weight, and urinary excretion of sodium and potassium did not change. They found no significant effect on blood pressure.

In contrast to these studies, two Finnish experiments also varied the dietary P/S ratio over a period of several weeks and did detect changes in blood pressure. The usual Finnish diet is quite fatty, and in the first study (Puska et al., 1983) the intervention consisted of a low-fat (23% of calories) diet with a high P/S ratio (about 1.0). After a 2-week baseline phase, 57 couples ate the experimental diet for six weeks, before reverting to their usual diet for another 6 weeks. During the study phases, food records showed that the P/S ratio changed from 0.27 to 0.98 and back to 0.29, with this being achieved by markedly lowering saturated fat intake and slightly raising polyunsaturated fat intake. Protein also went up a little with the low-fat intervention; intake of monounsaturated fats fell; and total calories decreased by 20%, although body weight changed by only about 1 kg, on average. Urinary sodium and potassium did not change significantly during the intervention and switchback phases. The systolic blood pressure was 7.2 mm Hg lower ($p < .001$) and the diastolic was 4.0 mm Hg lower ($p < .001$) on the low-fat diet.

In the second study, Puska et al. (1985) changed the P/S ratio for 12 weeks either from 0.2 to 0.9 or from 0.2 to 0.4 in two separate intervention groups, and then there was a final observation period of five weeks, when subjects reverted to their usual diets. The first group consisted of 41 subjects, and the second of 43. Saturated fat intake fell markedly during the lower-fat period in both groups, and polyunsaturated fat intake increased markedly in the first group only, to produce the P/S ratio of 0.9. Intake of monounsaturated fats, total fat, and dietary cholesterol also fell greatly with the interventions. A fall in the serum cholesterol level provided some evidence of good compliance with the lower-fat diets. In the group with the greater P/S change, blood pressure levels fell by 4 mm Hg systolic and 6 mm Hg diastolic during the intervention, and then rose by 5 mm Hg systolic and 3 mm Hg diastolic during the switchback (all statistically significant). Body weight fell by 1.7 kg over the course of the study, but this was not related to the diet type. There were relatively minor changes in urinary sodium and potassium that are probably not biologically important. The group with the more modest change in P/S ratio with the intervention experienced blood pressure changes that were also statistically significant and of only a slightly lesser magnitude.

We turn now from the null effect, or the confusing data on the effects of dietary fatty acids, to the possible effects of different proteins on blood pressure. Once again, the evidence suggests no effect. The level of vegetable protein was markedly changed in a study (Sacks et al., 1984b) of 18 vegetarians that used a crossover design. During one six-week dietary period, subjects consumed high vegetable-protein patties, and during another period, low-protein rice patties were provided. These were in addition to the subjects' usual diets. Dietary protein rose from 63 to 119 g per day with the high-protein supplement. Total calories also were higher with this diet, but body weight did not change significantly, nor did the intake of other macronutrients. There were no significant effects on blood pressure.

The quality of dietary protein was systematically changed in another West Australian study (Prescott et al., 1988) by comparing the effects of nonmeat protein with those of meat protein in a randomized parallel group design, with 50 subjects being divided into two dietary groups. There was a 4-week "run-in" period, followed by 12 weeks of the experimental diet. Subjects were pair-matched by sex, age, weight, and sitting systolic blood pressure. Aside from protein, dietary factors were balanced between the two groups. There were no significant changes in body weight during the study. Blood pressures tended to be 1 to 2 mm Hg higher in the nonmeat group, although these differences were not statistically significant.

A characteristic of most vegetarian diets is an increased intake of dietary fiber, this being contributed by extra fruits and vegetables. The relationship between the intake of dietary fiber and blood pressure has not been intensively investigated and is complicated by the many different chemical forms of fiber, and its origin from different food groups—in particular, vegetables, fruits, and whole grains. However, a number of studies have not been able to demonstrate significant effects.

A series of small experiments (Brussaard et al., 1981; Stasse-Wolthuis et al., 1980) were conducted at the Agricultural University at Wageningen, the Netherlands. These evaluated the effects of consuming fiber from different food sources (28–37 g/day of dietary fiber as compared with 18 g/day for the control diet, each being consumed for a period of five weeks). Each dietary group contained about 15 subjects. Body weight, total energy, and other nutrients stayed relatively constant, although potassium excretion increased significantly with the high-fiber diets. There were no significant changes in blood pressure. Another, larger crossover trial (Fehily et al., 1986) in England compared blood pressure levels for four-week periods during which 201 subjects were encouraged to eat either a high-cereal-fiber diet (31 g/day) or their usual diet of 19 g/day in total fiber during a control period. Total energy intake, intake of other macronutrients, and body weight did not change significantly during the study. Blood pressure also did not change significantly.

Perhaps the best study for testing the fiber–blood pressure hypothesis was undertaken by the West Australian group (Margetts et al., 1987) and involved 88 healthy omnivores in a randomized crossover design. There were two six-week experimental periods, in which subjects were given either high- or low-fiber biscuits (that looked and tasted the same). The fiber was taken from bran, whole-meal flour, bananas, and apricots, and this changed fiber intake from about 15 to 58 grams per day. Body weight did not change consistently, total fat was a little lower, and total energy intake was a little higher with the high-fiber diet. Potassium and magnesium excretion was substantially increased by the added fiber. Despite this, there were no blood pressure changes that could be ascribed to the high-fiber diet.

Although I will not review the literature connecting potassium consumption to blood pressure levels here, a relatively weak negative association has been observed in many trials involving hypertensive and normotensive individuals. A meta-analysis of these results (Whelton et al., 1997) found an overall reduction of 3.11 mm Hg (95% confidence interval, −1.91 to −4.31 mm Hg) in systolic and a reduction of 1.92 mm Hg

(95% confidence interval, -0.52 to -3.42) in diastolic blood pressure with the use of potassium supplementation.

The literature discussed above represents one of the more frustrating chapters in preventive cardiology research. While results from both observational and experimental studies agree that vegetarians have significantly lower blood pressure levels, it has so far proved impossible to determine the mechanisms involved or the dietary variables that are responsible.

Some of the reasons for these difficulties can be understood, and speculation is possible regarding others. Repeated blood pressure measurement yields exceedingly variable results, both in the short term, and also during the several weeks of a typical study, when there is usually a gradual medium-term fall in average pressure levels, even with no intervention. The latter is presumably due to the subjects' increasing familiarity with procedures and the study staff. However, it introduces yet another component of variance that is to be distinguished from any effects of diet.

Many studies have not had the statistical power to detect differences in blood pressure of the order of 3 to 7 mm Hg. The more powerful studies were those from Western Australia, where often 60 to 90 subjects were involved, and all subjects contributed to the measured effect of each diet in a crossover design. However, the results from these studies, in relation to dietary fat, protein, and fiber, were uniformly negative.

It seems quite probable that dietary fat is not the active principle. Changing fat in the diet does not happen in isolation. None of these studies were "metabolic ward" studies in which subjects were fed all of their food. Rather, they were free-living individuals who made complex changes in their diet, primarily to alter the intake of dietary fats, for instance, but which no doubt also involved compensatory changes in the intake of non-fatty foods as well. The latter, uncontrolled changes may differ in different societies and could potentially affect blood pressure in different ways. Vegetarians eat more fruits and vegetables than others. These foods contain numerous phytochemicals whose biological action is poorly defined. Some of these may be important for blood pressure control.

I speculate that the lower blood pressure levels in vegetarians probably result from several mechanisms. These include a lower body mass index and higher potassium intake, but also other unknown factors that may each contribute only 1 to 2 mm Hg to a blood pressure lowering. Hence these factors are very difficult to detect. It is also possible that variables act more strongly in combination than individually. There is little direct evidence to support such effect modification in this context, except to note that many factors differ simultaneously between vegetarian and omnivore diets. The results of the large DASH study (see Chapter 8) are relevant to this discussion; although the DASH diet was not a vegetarian one, it minimized meats and emphasized fruits, vegetables, and nuts. The effects in lowering blood pressure were strong and easily detected, but again the active components could not be individually identified.

The Vegetarian Diet and Risk of Obesity

Obesity is clearly a potent risk factor for CHD (Manson et al., 1995; Rimm et al., 1995). However, it has not been so clear whether obesity has an independent effect, or whether increased risk occurs only because obese individuals are more likely to have elevated LDL and lower HDL cholesterol levels and are more likely to be diabetic and hypertensive. If the second option is true, then obesity would still be an important cause of CHD, but acting through these other factors.

The alternative is that obesity increases the risk of CHD beyond its effects on these well-established risk factors. The answer seems to be that this is so, but that effects mediated through traditional risk factors account for much of the increased hazard. Both the Nurses' Health Study (Manson et al., 1990) and the Health Professionals Follow-up Study (Rimm et al., 1995) found that associations with CHD were attenuated, but did remain important, after an adjustment for the traditional risk factors mentioned above. Similar findings have been reported from the Adventist Health Study for nonfatal myocardial infarction (Fraser et al., 1992a).

It is widely established that, on average, vegetarians have substantially lower BMI values than nonvegetarians have. This is true for the Adventist Mortality and Adventist Health studies, as described in Chapter 8. Large studies of non-Adventist vegetarians and omnivores in the United Kingdom also found consistent and impressive differences in body mass index between vegetarians and others (Key and Davey, 1996; Key et al., 1999b; Thorogood, 1995; Appleby et al., 1998). For instance, the European Prospective Investigation into Cancer and Nutrition in the United Kingdom (Key and Davey, 1996) collected data on 6850 meat-eaters, 3776 eaters of fish (but not meat), 8827 vegetarians, and 1652 vegans. A comparison of body mass indices is shown in Figure 12-2. Mean values of BMI and the percentage of obese subjects are consistently lower among the vegetarians.

Undoubtedly, part of the protection that vegetarians obtain from CHD comes about because they are thinner. However, no single risk factor, such as obesity, entirely explains their decreased risk. This is clear because the collaborative analysis of five prospective studies of vegetarians still found that they were significantly protected from CHD (relative risk, 0.66; 95% confidence interval, 0.55–0.79), even after adjusting for body mass index (Key et al., 1999a).

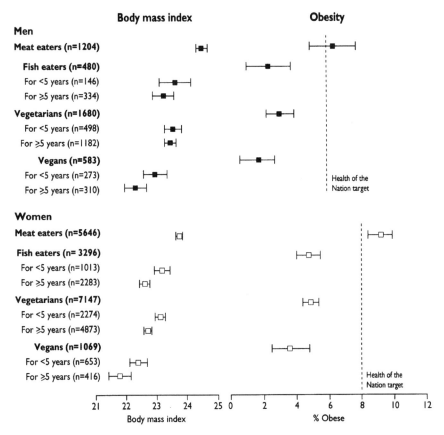

Figure 12–2 Mean (95% confidence interval) body mass index and percentage of subjects who were obese by type of diet (values are adjusted for age). *Source:* Reprinted with permission from Key T, Davey G, Prevalence of obesity is low in people who do not eat meat, *Br Med J* 313:816–817, 1996. Published by BMJ Publishing Group.

Effect of Vegetarian Diet on Blood Coagulation and Viscosity Variables

The majority of myocardial infarction cases involve a coronary thrombosis, in which one of the coronary arteries is obstructed by a blood clot. Usually this occurs at the site of an unstable, cholesterol-rich atherosclerotic plaque. Hence, it is not surprising that the blood levels of a number of factors involved in normal blood clotting have proven to be risk factors for CHD. In particular, these include fibrinogen, factor VII, and lower levels of natural "clot-busters" or fibrinolysins (Pahor et al., 1999). Thus, it is of interest to determine whether levels of these factors are affected by diet.

The investigators in the Northwick Park Heart Study, a prospective study done in England, identified 50 local vegetarian subjects and compared them with 282 of their study's participants (Haines et al., 1980). After an adjustment for differences in age and skinfold thickness, the vegetarian males and females both had significantly lower levels of factor VII, but not of fibrinogen. Somewhat paradoxically, fibrinolytic activity and antithrombin levels were also lower in the vegetarians. The investigators speculated that a low-risk population may have less need for the latter factors that are activated in the presence of clotting and existing artery disease.

A study comparing vegetarian and omnivorous Buddhists in Taiwan (Pan et al., 1993) did not demonstrate significant differences in most of the blood-clotting factors that they measured. These included fibrinogen, factors VIIc and VIIIc, and plasminogen. The level of antithrombin III, a fibrinolytic factor, was higher in vegetarian men, but not in women.

In Nigeria, Famodu et al. (1999) compared 36 vegetarian with 40 nonvegetarian Adventists and found the vegetarians to have significantly lower levels of plasma fibrinogen and increased fibrinolytic activity, as measured by euglobulin lysis time. In Chile, Mezzano et al. (1999) matched 26 vegetarians with omnivorous controls by age, sex, and socioeconomic status. Plasma levels of all factors synthesized in the liver were lower in the vegetarians, but this included both the procoagulant fibrinogen, factor VII, and the anticoagulant, antithrombin III. By contrast, extrahepatic factors, such as tissue plasminogen activator and plasminogen activator inhibitor, did not differ between the dietary groups. In Australia, Li et al. (1999) compared 18 high-level meat-eaters with 60 moderate-level meat-eaters, 43 lacto-ovo vegetarians, and 18 vegans. They found no differences in blood fibrinogen, factor VII, or antithrombin III between the lacto-ovo vegetarians and the meat-eaters.

Two studies have evaluated platelet function in vegetarians and nonvegetarians, with rather surprising results. Both Li et al. (1999) and Mezzano et al. (1999) found that the vegetarians had significantly greater platelet aggregability with a variety of stimuli (e.g., collagen, ADP, arachidonic acid, epinephrine), though not with the same stimulants in both studies. However, an earlier study could not detect a difference (Fisher et al., 1986) in platelet function between vegetarians and omnivores. The fatty acid composition of platelets varies markedly between vegetarians and nonvegetarians in ways that can be predicted from their diets. There is less saturated fatty acid, more n-6 polyunsaturated fatty acid, and less n-3 fatty acid in the platelets of vegetarians (Agren et al., 1995; Fisher et al., 1986; Li et al., 1999). Possibly the lower $n3:n6$ fatty acid ratio may explain any tendency toward increased aggregability.

So, as seems quite common in dietary research, the results with respect to coagulation factors are quite confusing. The studies are often small, and if we consider a nonsignificant result to be neutral rather than negative, it seems that blood fibrinogen and factor VII levels may be lower in vegetarians, but it is quite unclear whether thrombolytic factors, such as antithrombin III, are higher or lower. The functional test—euglobulin clot lysis time—employed by Famodu et al. (1999) did quite strongly indicate greater fibrinolytic activity in the Nigerian vegetarians.

When trying to interpret these results, we must also recognize that vegetarians in different parts of the world, and in different socioreligious groups, may be very different from each other in ways apart from their avoidance of meat. The results discussed here can only suggest certain trends and probably indicate that future research should endeavor to establish consistent results within well-defined groups of vegetarians, before seeking to generalize findings to other such groups. Whether trends that may be considered adverse, such as increased platelet aggregability (if confirmed), are truly adverse effects in this special group also needs to be established. Given the low risk of CHD in vegetarians, any adverse effects are clearly more than counterbalanced by other beneficial influences. It is possible that the lowering of blood LDL cholesterol is a primary requirement for risk reduction, and when this is accomplished, contrary forces are less influential.

Rheology is the study of blood stickiness or viscosity. The major contributor to blood viscosity is the proportion of the blood composed of red blood cells, known as the packed cell volume. The viscosity of the fluid portion of blood, known as the plasma, is also important, and the protein fibrinogen is the main contributor to this viscosity component. Both of these viscosity factors are less well known risk indicators for CHD events (Ernst, 1995; Koenig et al., 1998b). Greater blood viscosity increases the probability of thrombosis and also increases shear forces at the artery wall, which may lead to atherosclerosis.

There may be less blood viscosity in vegetarians. A total of 48 German vegetarians were compared with a group of omnivorous controls of similar ages (Ernst et al., 1986). In men and women, independently, the packed cell volume was lower in the vegetarians than in the controls. Plasma viscosity was also significantly reduced in the vegetarians, although a weakness is that this analysis did not adjust for a difference in the proportion of women between the vegetarians and the control groups. Hemoglobin levels or red blood cell counts have sometimes also been reported by others as modestly lower in vegetarians (Gear et al., 1980; Li et al., 1999), which supports the packed-cell-volume findings for the German vegetarians.

Diabetes Mellitus in Vegetarians

There is reason to suspect that diabetes may be less frequent among vegetarians, because vegetarians are less obese (see Chapter 8) and because the vegetarian diet would usually have a lower glycemic index (Jenkins et al., 1995). This means that the diet contains fewer foods that stimulate insulin production, a situation that correlated with lower rates of incident diabetes mellitus in the Nurses' Health Study (Salmeron et al., 1997). In addition, vegetarians may have enhanced insulin sensitivity, which could be due to their lower iron stores (Hua et al., 2001).

The evidence for Adventists (see Chapter 8) is that the vegetarians do have a lower risk of diabetes, and this is largely because they are less obese. Information about the frequency of diabetes among non-Adventist vegetarians is difficult to find. A follow-up of the Health Food Shoppers Study in the United Kingdom (Key et al., 1996) calculated standardized mortality ratios for diabetes mellitus of 0.35 for men (95% confidence interval, 0.10–0.90), and 0.20 for women (0.04–0.59), when comparing the health-conscious study group with others in the United Kingdom. A more recent update (P.N. Appleby, personal communication, 2002) combines data from both the Oxford Vegetarian and Health Food Shoppers studies and divides the results into vegetarian and nonvegetarian study subjects. The standardized mortality ratio for vegetarians (as compared with the reference population of England and Wales) is 0.29 (95% confidence interval, 0.12–0.56) and for the nonvegetarians it is 0.24 (95% confidence interval, 0.11–0.45). There is thus no clear evidence of a difference between vegetarian and nonvegetarian health-conscious groups, but both differ greatly from the general population and confidence intervals are wide. Diabetes on the death certificate is probably a poor surrogate for incidence of diabetes, however.

An interesting, but somewhat anecdotal, report describes how established diabetics may attain better control of blood sugar and be able to reduce (or even discard) medications if they follow a relatively strict vegetarian diet (Nicholson et al., 1999). The question of treatment for an established disease is not the same as preventing the disease in the first place, but it is probably related. Evidence of better control in established adult-onset diabetics with a vegetarian diet certainly provides some hope of preventive potential as well.

Other Cardiovascular Risk Factors among Vegetarians

Whether a vegetarian diet changes the levels of newer lipid risk factors, such as lipoprotein (a) (Fortmann and Marcovina, 1997), LDL particle size (Grundy, 1997), and triglyceride-rich lipoprotein remnants (Hodis, 1999), does not seem to have been studied. However, dietary fat intake does affect LDL particle size in those who are genetically predisposed to forming smaller particles (Krauss and Dreon, 1995), and may also affect the concentration of triglyceride-rich remnants as these two problems are related (Otvos, 1999). Hence it may well be that a lower-fat vegetarian diet would produce beneficial changes here, too.

Atherosclerosis is known to have a prominent inflammatory component, and recently certain serum markers of inflammation, particularly C-reactive protein (Pahor et al., 1999), have been shown to predict a higher risk for CHD events. Mezzano et al. (1999) compared levels of C-reactive protein for 26 healthy vegetarians and for 26 omnivores, who were matched according to age, sex, obesity, and socioeconomic status; they found no significant differences, but confidence intervals were extremely wide.

However, the vegetarians did have higher levels of blood homocysteine than the omnivores (13.5 as compared with 9.55 μmol/L, $p < .005$). This rather surprising result occurred despite higher levels of blood folate and pyridoxine in the vegetarians, as might be expected. However, the vegetarians had lower levels of blood vitamin B_{12}, and the higher levels of blood homocysteine correlated with this variable. A contrasting result has been found in vegans who frequently supplement with vitamin B_{12} (Haddad et al., 1999a) and is described further in Chapter 13.

Blood homocysteine levels have sometimes (Bostom and Selhub, 1999; Robinson et al., 1998), but not always (Kuller and Evans, 1998), predicted higher risk of CHD. Elevated homocysteine levels are reduced by higher intakes of the B vitamins—folate, pyridoxine, and B_{12} (McCully, 1998). Vegetarians typically have higher blood levels of folate and pyridoxine (Haddad et al., 1999a; Mezzano et al., 1999; Sanders and Key, 1987), but sometimes lower levels of B_{12} (Hokin and Butler, 1999; Mezzano et al., 1999). The balance of these effects on levels of homocysteine in vegetarians clearly needs more study, particularly in view of the findings (described above) of Mezzano et al. (1999).

RISK FACTORS FOR CANCER

While there are a number of widely known behavioral and environmental risk factors for cancer (e.g., cigarette smoking, alcohol consumption, certain occupations), physiologic and biochemical indicators of increased risk are less widely established. The emphasis here is on risk factor changes that may result from particular dietary habits, and that in turn will change the risk of developing cancer. Identification of such risk factors would help us understand how diet may influence risk. The blood levels for certain vitamins, minerals, phytochemicals, and hormones are thought to influence the risk of cancer in animals, and possibly in humans. Several of these could theoretically be changed by dietary habits. In the section below, the evidence indicating that these factors predict the risk of cancer is briefly described, followed by any comparisons of their levels among vegetarians and omnivores.

Relationship between Obesity, Cancer, and the Vegetarian Diet

A recently completed meta-analysis of the larger prospective and case-control studies of cancers of the breast, colon, endometrium, prostate, kidney, and gallbladder evaluated the nature of any relationship between cancer and obesity (Bergstrom et al., 2001). Significantly increased risks from higher values of body mass index were found for cancers of the breast (postmenopausal only), colon, prostate, endometrium, and kidney. While the increased risk in overweight subjects (BMI between 25 and 30) was 15% or less for some of these sites (breast, colon, and prostate), risk increases of 59%, 36%, and 34% were observed for cancers of the endometrium, kidney, and gallbladder, respectively, when the overweight were compared with the thinner subjects. Broadly similar findings were reported from a cohort of 28,129 obese Swedes (Wolk et al., 2001) when their rates were compared with those expected from the whole country.

Among the common cancers, breast and colon cancer are consistently related to obesity. For instance, in the Iowa Women's Health Study, Folsom et al. (2000) found not only a 30% higher risk of all cancers combined ($p < .001$) when they compared extreme quartiles of BMI, but also substantially increased risks for breast, colon, and uterine cancer for those who were more obese. A large study of deaths from colon cancer found a strong relationship between body mass index and risk, especially among men (Murphy et al., 2000). Further support is given by the Adventist cohorts where relatively overweight Adventists were at a significantly greater risk of cancers of the breast and colon (Fraser and Shavlik, 1997b; Mills et al., 1989b; Phillips and Snowdon, 1985; Singh and Fraser, 1998).

The reasons for these associations are not entirely understood, and probably differ for cancers at different sites. However, postmenopausal women who are more obese have higher levels of estrogen, produced by conversion from adrenal steroids in the additional adipose tissue (Siiteri, 1987). Obesity is also associated with higher levels of insulin (Bogardus et al., 1985; Folsom et al., 1989; Jernstrom and Barrett-Connor, 1999), which is a probable promoter of tumor growth (see the following discussion).

As described in this chapter under cardiovascular disease risk factors, and for Adventists in Chapter 8, there is no doubt that vegetarians are significantly thinner, on average, than others. This probably accounts in part for the lower risk that has been found among vegetarians for several of these malignant tumors.

Phytoestrogens, Cancer, and the Vegetarian Diet

Phytoestrogens are compounds from plants that have chemical similarities to estrogens and may compete at binding sites with natural estrogens, thus having an antiestrogenic effect; in larger quantities, phytoestrogens may manifest their own mildly proestrogenic action. Two classes of such substances are isoflavones and lignans.

Isoflavones are polyphenolic compounds that, for practical purposes, are found only in soy foods. The main isoflavones in these foods are genistein and daidzein. Animal-feeding studies using isoflavones have shown a decreased incidence of some hormone-related tumors (Barnes, 1995), and there is some evidence (see Chapter 6) that people who consume more soy foods have lower rates of breast cancer and possibly prostate and colon cancers. Indeed, it is claimed that the markedly lower rates of breast and prostate cancer in the Far East are due to the much greater consumption of soy products in these areas (Messina et al., 1994).

Lignans are another class of weakly estrogenic polyphenols, principally enterodiol and enterolactone, that are formed from precursors in a variety of plant foods by the action of colonic bacteria. Sources of these precursors include, in particular, linseed (flaxseed), but also other seeds, cereals, grains, fruits, and vegetables (Thompson et al., 1991). Both lignans and isoflavones also have antioxidant properties (Wei et al., 1995).

Limited evidence suggests that vegetarians have high levels of both isoflavones and lignans in body fluids, and this would not be surprising, as they typically eat more of the foods that provide these substances. Adlercreutz et al. (1986) compared the excretion of enterolactone, enterodiol, daidzein, and its metabolite, equol (see Table 12–3), between omnivorous

Table 12-3. Urinary Excretion of Lignans and Isoflavonic Phytoestrogens in Young Women with Different Habitual Diets (Geometric Means, nmol/24h)

	Omnivores	Lactovegetarians
BOSTON WOMEN		
Enterolactone	2050	4170
Enterodiol	280	740
Daidzein	320	1260
Equol	69	100
HELSINKI WOMEN		
Enterolactone	2460	3650
Enterodiol	203	368
Daidzein	219	275
Equol	102	64

Source: Reprinted with permission from Adlercreutz H, Fotsis T, Bannwart C, Wahala K, Makela T, Brunow G, Hase T, Determination of urinary lignans and phytoestrogen metabolites, potential antiestrogens and anticarcinogens in urine of women on various habitual diets, *J Steroid Biochem* 25:791–797, 1986.

and lactovegetarian premenopausal women in Finland and Boston. As can be seen, the excretion of these substances was a good deal higher among the vegetarians, particularly those in Boston. These results were later extended by a similar comparison between 10 vegetarian and 10 omnivorous postmenopausal Finnish women, with very similar results (Herman et al., 1995).

Thus, although replication of this evidence would be valuable, it seems probable that the cells of vegetarians are bathed in higher concentrations of antioxidant phytoestrogenic substances. If both animal and basic science work are reflected in the human experience, some protection against certain cancers would be expected.

Folic Acid, Dietary Antioxidants, Cancer, and the Vegetarian Diet

Methylation of DNA plays an important role in gene regulation. Folate is an essential cofactor in the production of *S*-adenosylmethionine, the primary methyl donor in the body. In rodents a chronic deficiency of this cofactor reduces methylation of the DNA cytosine and may thereby contribute to the loss of normal controls on proto-oncogene expression (Dizik et al., 1991). Moreover, a few human studies associate lower levels of blood folate with an increased risk of colon cancer or adenoma (Editorial, 1994; Giovannucci et al., 1993a; Slattery et al., 1999). Vegetarians generally have higher folate intakes and higher blood levels of folate (Haddad et al., 1999a; Mezzano et al., 1999; Sanders and Key, 1987), due to their greater consumption of fruits, cereals, legumes, and leafy green vegetables. This may contribute to a lower incidence of certain cancers among Adventists and other vegetarians.

As oxidants can damage cellular DNA, it has long been speculated that antioxidant substances play an anticarcinogenic role (Byers and Perry, 1992). Antioxidants in the diet, aside from the phytoestrogens, include other flavonoids, vitamin C, the carotenoids, and vitamin E. Although research in animals suggests that higher blood levels of many of these substances may reduce the risk of cancer, evidence for humans is not convincing, or even particularly suggestive. However, more human research is needed. It is reasonable to suspect that blood levels of many of these substances would be higher in vegetarians, but as the risk factor status of common dietary antioxidants is not established, these data are not discussed here in detail.

Vitamin D, Calcium, Cancer, and the Vegetarian Diet

Vitamin D and its metabolites have an antiproliferative and differentiating effect in laboratory work using breast cancer cells (Lipkin and Newmark,

1999). Thus, vitamin D tends to drive cells to a more stable state of development and may reduce the risk of the cellular disorganization and unrestrained multiplication that are characteristic of malignancy. It has been demonstrated among human subjects that vitamin D suppresses proliferation and invasion by malignant prostate cells (Blutt and Weigel, 1999; Ingles et al., 1998; Schwartz et al., 1997). These actions of vitamin D are probably mediated by levels of vitamin D cellular receptors and possibly by the stimulation of insulin-like growth-factor binding proteins (Rozen et al., 1997).

Some experimental studies have reported that calcium supplementation reduces colonic proliferation in predisposed human subjects (Bostick et al., 1995), but other studies have not (Gregoire et al., 1989). Nevertheless, in epidemiologic work, rates of colon cancer have often been found to be lower when calcium intake is higher (Garland et al., 1985; Kato et al., 1997; Sellers et al., 1998). In contrast, for prostate cancer, Giovannucci (1998) has suggested that calcium intake may increase risk. He hypothesizes that 1,25-OH vitamin D is a protective principle, and it is widely known that levels of this vitamin are reduced by intake of calcium and phosphorus (found largely in dairy products), which would, under his hypothesis, then increase the risk of prostate cancer (Chan et al., 1998a; Giovannucci et al., 1998). There is some evidence to support such an effect (see Chapter 6).

Whether the intake of calcium or blood levels of vitamin D can yet be considered risk indicators for certain human cancers is not clearly established. However, there is no good reason to suspect a greater intake of calcium in vegetarians (Weaver and Plawecki, 1994) or that vitamin D levels would be higher. In fact, dietary vitamin D intake is lower in some vegetarian diets that minimize dairy products, but this may be less relevant as the major factor affecting vitamin D status is often exposure to sunlight. Dietary intake is important for bone health, at least, only when exposure to sunlight is inadequate (Henderson et al., 1987).

Blood Levels of Sex Steroids in Women, Cancer, and the Vegetarian Diet

Risks of cancers of the female breast and of the ovaries depend somewhat on lifetime exposure to sex steroids as estimated by the use of hormonal supplements (Beral et al., 1999; Collaborative Group on Hormonal Factors in Breast Cancer, 1996, 1997; Hankinson et al., 1995), and, in the case of breast cancer, on blood levels of endogenous estrogens (Cauley et al., 1999; Hankinson et al., 1998b; Key, 1999; Pike et al., 1993; Thomas et al., 1997) and also on years of menstruation (Henderson et al., 1996).

Vegetarians probably have a later age at menarche, and, in adult life, possibly lower levels of estrogens. A study of 230 white non-Hispanic girls in Southern California, who experienced menarche during the study, recorded their dietary habits at study baseline (Kissinger and Sanchez, 1987). The study population was drawn from Seventh-day Adventist and public schools in Southern California. Those in the highest quartile of the use of meat had an average age at menarche of 12.45 years, whereas menarche for those in the lowest quartile (vegetarians) occurred at 12.96 years ($p < .025$), about 6 months later. As compared to those who ate no meat analogues (many are soy based), those in the highest quartile had an average age at menarche that was delayed by 9.4 months ($p < .001$; mean age was 13.22 years). High levels of nut, grain, and bean consumption were also associated with significantly older ages at menarche by at least five months.

Levels of endogenous estrogens during menstrual years have sometimes, but not always, been reported as lower in adult vegetarians than in omnivores. When Armstrong et al. (1981) compared 46 premenopausal vegetarians with 47 nonvegetarians, they found that, in the vegetarians, total urinary levels of estrogens and levels of estriol, and plasma prolactin were significantly lower, and the level of plasma sex hormone-binding globulin was significantly higher. Another, smaller study (14 vegetarians and 9 nonvegetarians) of premenopausal women found similar differences (Shultz and Leklem, 1983). Plasma levels of estrone and estradiol-17β (drawn at the midluteal phase of the cycle) were significantly lower in the vegetarians. Goldin and Gorbach (1988) also found significantly lower blood estrogen levels in premenopausal vegetarians than in omnivorous women.

However, a large study comparing pre- and postmenopausal vegetarians with omnivores in the United Kingdom did not find significant differences in levels of either estrogen or sex-hormone binding globulin (Thomas et al., 1999). Nevertheless, trends were in the direction of lower levels of estrogens and higher levels of sex-hormone-binding globulin in the vegetarians. The analysis indicated that any true differences could probably be accounted for by differences in body mass indices between the dietary groups.

Two studies of menstruating teenage vegetarian and omnivorous girls did not find differences in estrogen levels. Gray et al. (1982) compared 23 vegetarians with 26 subjects who ate meat at least weekly. No differences were found in levels of estrogens or of prolactin measured on the same days (days 11 and 22) of the menstrual cycle for each girl. Another study of 75 Adventist adolescent girls (35 vegetarians, 40 nonvegetarians) also found no significant differences in estrogen levels in a multivariate analysis (Persky et al., 1992).

The possibly lower levels of blood estrogens in premenopausal adult vegetarians may be related to their lower levels of fat consumption. In support of this, a meta-analysis of 13 studies provides quite strong evidence that higher-fat diets are associated with higher levels of blood estradiol in both pre- and postmenopausal women (Wu et al., 1999). Moreover, vegetarian women excrete greater quantities of estrogen in their feces, and this has also been correlated with lower blood levels of estrogen (Goldin and Gorbach, 1988).

There is some evidence that consumption of soy isoflavones can decrease blood concentrations of ovarian hormones (Lu et al., 2000) and raise those of sex-hormone-binding globulin (Pino et al., 2000). However, others found effects only on luteal-phase estradiol levels in Asian women, but not in non-Asian women, and found no effects on hormone-binding globulin (Wu et al., 2000).

Thus, the lower incidence of breast and ovarian cancer seen in Adventist women may be due, in part, to a modestly later menarche and to lower levels of blood estrogens that are not evident until the postteen years. Soy products, other phytoestrogen-containing foods, a lower fat intake, and less obesity may all play roles in producing these differences in hormone levels. More research is necessary.

Existing data from men do not clearly support associations between levels of male sex hormones (androgens) and the risk of prostate cancer (Nomura et al., 1988; Signorello et al., 1997). Further, there are no clear-cut differences in blood levels of these hormones when vegetarians and omnivores are compared (Allen et al., 2000; Hill and Wynder, 1979; Key et al., 1990). Thus, there is currently little support for the idea that lower rates of prostate cancer among Adventist vegetarians are mediated through changes in blood levels of androgens.

Insulin, Insulin-Like Growth Hormones, Cancer, and the Vegetarian Diet

Insulin and insulin-like growth hormones stimulate the growth of cancerous tissues in the laboratory (Resnicoff et al., 1995; Toretsky and Helman, 1996), and this raises the possibility that they may also do so in the intact organism. The blood levels of insulin-like growth factor 1 seen in the Physicians' Health Study were positively related to the risk of colon cancer, prostate cancer, and premenopausal breast cancer found in a prospective analysis (Chan et al., 1998b; Hankinson et al., 1998a; Ma et al., 2000). Insulin itself is probably a promoter of colon cancer, in particular (Giovannucci, 1995), and some have claimed that a higher level of blood insulin or of insulin-related factors increases the risk of this cancer (McKeown-Eyssen, 1994; McKeown-Eyssen and the Toronto Polyp Prevention Group, 1996; Singh and Fraser, 1998).

There is little information about blood levels of insulin or insulin-like growth factors in vegetarians as compared with others. As vegetarians may have greater insulin sensitivity (Hua et al., 2001), their carbohydrate metabolism can probably be handled with lower blood insulin levels. A recent analysis of data from the United Kingdom (Allen et al., 2000) found that blood insulin-like growth factor 1 in vegan men was 9% lower than in either other vegetarians or omnivores ($p = .002$). Clearly, more evidence is needed to support this finding and to decide whether it is biologically significant.

Proliferative Activity of the Colonic Mucosa, Colon Cancer, and the Vegetarian Diet

It has long been thought that an expansion of the proliferative compartment of epithelial cells within colonic crypts is a risk factor for future colonic neoplasms and malignancy. Such increased activity has been documented for individuals at higher risk of colon cancer. The work of Lipkin et al. (1985) clearly indicates that there is much less colonic mucosal proliferative activity in vegetarian Adventists than in nonvegetarian but health-conscious subjects, or in those with a family history of colon cancer, or in those with sporadic colonic adenomas.

However, recent results (Sandler et al., 2000) raise doubts as to whether rectal mucosal proliferation is a useful prospective indicator of colorectal neoplasia. Hence the status of colonic or rectal cell proliferation as a risk indicator will be decided by future research. The significance of there being less mucosal proliferative activity among vegetarians is uncertain, but this finding does raise the possibility that it is an early indicator of their lower risk.

SUMMARY

Cardiovascular Disease

1. Vegetarians are less obese than omnivores. This is associated with a lower risk of cardiovascular disease, resulting from effects on blood lipids, and lower risks of diabetes and high blood pressure. However, there may be other unknown mechanisms whereby obesity decreases risk independently from these intermediaries.
2. Vegetarians have lower values of serum total and LDL cholesterol than omnivores. This has been established in both observational and experimental studies and is in accord with expectations based on the nutrient content of these diets.

3. Serum HDL levels are not consistently lower in lacto-ovo vegetarians than in omnivores. Adventists may have slightly lower levels, perhaps due to their avoidance of alcohol, but the biological significance of this is not known.

4. Vegetarians have lower blood pressure levels, and this is beyond the decrease accounted for by their lower levels of obesity. Both observational and experimental studies have confirmed this result.

5. The components of the vegetarian diet responsible for lower blood pressure are not completely understood. Despite many experimental studies, clear effects of different fatty acids, dietary fiber, and proteins from different sources have not been demonstrated. A number of studies now indicate that greater potassium intake is associated with modestly lower blood pressure levels, and vegetarians often consume more potassium. It has also long been known that obesity is a powerful determinant of blood pressure levels, and vegetarians are less obese. One study suggests that lower values of catecholamines and less renin activity may play a part.

6. The results of studies comparing coagulation and fibrinolytic variables for vegetarians with those for others are often conflicting. There is preliminary evidence of lower values of fibrinogen, and of factor VII, but greater platelet aggregability, among vegetarians, but all of this needs further study. Vegetarians are a heterogeneous group, and the influences of other, perhaps nondietary, factors may contribute to disagreements among study results. Vegetarians probably have lower blood viscosity, mainly due to slightly lower levels of hemoglobin and packed cell volumes. Lower levels of fibrinogen, when present, will also reduce plasma viscosity.

7. Diabetes mellitus is probably less common in vegetarians. Most of the evidence for this comes from studies of Adventists (see Chapter 8).

8. One study finds higher blood homocysteine levels for vegetarians (correlating with their lower blood vitamin B_{12} levels), despite their higher intake of folate. Supplementation with vitamin B_{12} should overcome this problem (see Chapter 13). This interesting finding needs confirmation and would not be expected in most lacto-ovo vegetarians, who usually obtain sufficient amounts of vitamin B_{12}.

Cancer

1. That vegetarians are thinner than omnivores also has implications for cancer. In particular, thinner persons have lower risks of breast, colon, endometrial, and, probably, other cancers.

2. Vegetarians probably have higher blood levels of isoflavones and lignans, which are both phytoestrogens. A modest body of evidence suggests that this may protect them against prostate, breast, and colon cancers.

3. Vegetarians often have higher blood levels of folic acid and of antioxidant vitamins, obtained from plants. There is evidence that folate may protect against colon cancer, but there is still little credible evidence of protection against cancer from the antioxidant vitamins.

4. Blood levels of vitamin D and calcium intake may be risk indicators for several cancers. However, vegetarians probably do not have different values from others for these factors.

5. Vegetarian women may have lower levels of estrogens in their blood and higher concentrations of sex-hormone-binding globulin. In addition, menarche is modestly, but significantly, delayed among California vegetarian teenagers. Thus, lifetime exposure to estrogens may be reduced, and if so, this would result in lower risks of breast, and perhaps ovarian, cancers.

6. Insulin and insulin-like growth hormones are promoters of tumor growth. Due to the reduced adipose tissue in vegetarians, one might expect they would have lower values of blood insulin, but there is as yet little direct evidence of this.

7. A possible preclinical indicator of risk for colon cancer is increased colonic or rectal mucosal proliferative activity, as seen in a biopsy. Colonic proliferative activity appears to be much less prevalent among Adventist vegetarians.

13

Risk Factors and Disease among Vegans

Vegans avoid all animal products in their diet, even eggs and dairy products. The reason for these choices is often animal rights rather than the expectation of better health. One might, however, predict that certain risk factors would have even more favorable values for vegans than for lacto-ovo vegetarians since the intake of saturated fats, cholesterol, and sodium is lower still in vegans, and their consumption of dietary fiber and potassium is greater. If a lacto-ovo vegetarian diet is beneficial, do vegans gain even further benefits? Evidence that addresses this question is presented in this chapter.

My intention is not to establish the nutritional adequacy of the vegan diet in terms of recommended daily allowances for nutrients and vitamins, but, in keeping with the rest of this book, to focus on the risk for common chronic diseases. However, a vegan diet is nutritionally adequate if certain precautions are taken (see Chapter 15), and these have been succinctly reviewed by the American Dietetic Association (ADA Reports, 1997).

In comparison with lacto-ovo vegetarians, vegans, in some settings at least, consume less total energy and generally obtain a greater percentage of calories from carbohydrates, and less from fats (particularly saturated fats), and show a higher ratio of dietary polyunsaturated fats to saturated fatty acids (Famodu et al., 1999; Li et al., 1999; Toohey et al., 1998). In addition, vegan diets contain very little vitamin B_{12} without supplements (Rauma et al., 1995a), but the level of fiber and folate consumption is often high, especially if expressed as a percentage of calories (Famodu et al., 1999; Roshanai and Sanders, 1984; Toohey et al., 1998). Intake of antioxidant vitamins, and their serum levels, may be much higher in vegans than in omnivores (Rauma et al., 1995b), but it is not certain whether there are consistent differences between vegans and lacto-ovo vegetarians (Toohey et al., 1998).

RISK FACTORS FOR CHRONIC DISEASE IN VEGANS

A vegan diet can produce important short-term changes in risk factors (Mc-Dougall et al., 1995), and this raises the possibility also of longer-term beneficial effects.

Obesity in Vegans

Vegans usually have lower body weights for a particular height than other vegetarians. This was clearly true in a report from the United Kingdom, where 1652 vegans were compared with 8827 other vegetarians, all of whom were recruited for the European Prospective Investigation into Cancer and Nutrition (EPIC) (Key and Davey, 1996). Vegan men and women had BMI values at least one unit (kg/m^2) lower than those of other vegetarians (see Fig. 12–2). However, Australian vegans examined by Li et al. (1999) were only marginally thinner than Adventist lacto-ovo vegetarians. Also, Adventist vegans in Nigeria were a good deal thinner than lacto-ovo vegetarians, although this difference was not statistically significant (Famodu et al., 1998), and vegans studied by Haines et al. (1980) were reportedly thinner than the other vegetarians. Further, a group of 18 vegan Adventists in California were significantly thinner (BMI of 22.9 kg/m^2) than lacto-ovo vegetarians (BMI of 24.7 kg/m^2) (Calkins et al., 1984). Other studies comparing Adventist vegans with lacto-ovo vegetarians also reported similar results (Haddad et al., 1999a; Toohey et al., 1998).

Blood Lipids in Vegans

Vegans do have clearly lower levels of total and LDL cholesterol as compared with omnivores, as expected (Burslem et al., 1978; Fisher et al., 1986; Roshanai and Sanders, 1984; Sanders et al., 1978; Sanders and Key, 1987). Comparisons of HDL cholesterol between vegans and omnivores have sometimes (Burslem et al., 1978; Fisher et al., 1986), but not always (Roshanai and Sanders, 1984; Thorogood et al., 1987), found lower values in the vegans.

Cholesterol levels have also been lower in vegans than in lacto-ovo vegetarians in most studies that have examined this question. Thorogood et al. (1987) compared the blood cholesterol levels of 114 British vegans with those of 1550 other vegetarians. They found lower total cholesterol (165.6 as compared with 188.4 mg/dL), and lower LDL cholesterol (88.0 as compared with 105.8 mg/dL), when they adjusted for age and sex. Values of HDL cholesterol did not differ between the two vegetarian groups.

A few other smaller studies have also made such comparisons. For example, 10 vegans, 15 lacto-ovo vegetarians, and 25 omnivores matched by age and sex were compared by Fisher et al. (1986), who reported mean blood cholesterol values of 134.7, 150.3, and 172.9 mg/dL, respectively, for the three diet groups, and differences between both vegetarian groups and the omnivores were statistically significant. The two vegetarian groups could not be formally compared as they were not matched by age and sex. A similar comparison for HDL cholesterol found values of 36.1, 45.0, and 49.5 mg/dL for the three groups. There were no significant differences in blood triglyceride levels. Thus the ratios of total to HDL cholesterol were 3.73, 3.34, and 3.49, respectively, suggesting a slightly higher risk for the vegans when we use these criteria, due to their lower HDL cholesterol levels.

Many years ago, Hardinge et al. (1962) compared serum total cholesterol levels between vegans and lacto-ovo vegetarians in California and found the levels to be substantially lower in the vegans. Li et al. (1999) in Australia compared 18 vegans with 43 lacto-ovo vegetarians. There were no significant differences in either LDL or HDL cholesterol levels, although the HDL levels were 2.7 mg/dL lower in the vegans. In Nigeria, 8 vegans were compared with 28 lacto-ovo vegetarians, and total cholesterol levels were 173.7 mg/dL in the vegans and 185.3 mg/dL in the lacto-ovo vegetarians—not a significant difference. Haines et al. (1980) also state that the vegans in their small study had lower values of serum cholesterol than other vegetarians, but they give no data.

From these small data sets, it also appears that the expectation of blood cholesterol levels even lower in vegans than those for nonvegan vegetarians, due to their totally plant-based diet, is met. As HDL cholesterol levels may also be lower, more evidence is needed about risk, and results may differ for different study groups. Unfortunately, the small number of vegans in most of these studies makes statistical significance difficult to achieve. Whether a tendency toward lower HDL values is fully balanced by lower total cholesterol levels, when we calculate the ratio of total to HDL cholesterol ratio, is unclear. The biological consequences of the lower HDL cholesterol that may accompany a higher intake of polyunsaturated fats, for instance, is also unclear. Recent animal work suggests that lower HDL levels in this situation do not necessarily indicate a reduction in reverse cholesterol transport, for instance (Spady et al., 1999).

Blood Pressure in Vegans

As blood pressure levels are lower in vegetarians than in omnivores, it is possible that this tendency is manifest to an even greater extent in those adhering to the more extreme vegan diet. By far the best and most extensive descriptive data on this question come from the Oxford University portion of the European Prospective Investigation into Cancer and Nutri-

Table 13–1. Age and BMI-Adjusted Mean Blood Pressure Values in Different Dietary Groups: The European Prospective Investigation into Cancer and Nutrition (EPIC)

		Age-Adjusted			Age and BMI-Adjusted		
	Diet Group	N	Systolic	Diastolic	N	Systolic	Diastolic
Men[a]	Meat-eaters	3015	133.5	81.3	2893	132.9	80.9
	Fish-only	331	128.3	78.6	316	129.0	78.9
	Non-vegan vegetarians	881	128.6	78.3	836	129.9	79.1
	Vegans	302	126.1	76.7	291	127.2	77.5
Women[a]	Meat-eaters	9196	125.6	77.1	8812	125.0	76.6
	Fish-only	1669	122.7	75.0	1587	123.5	75.5
	Non-vegan vegetarians	3295	123.6	75.7	3181	124.3	76.2
	Vegans	496	121.8	74.1	484	123.1	74.9

BP, blood pressure.

[a]Differences between dietary groups all have $p < .001$, except for systolic pressure adjusted for BMI in women, where $p = .0029$.

Source: Key T (personal communication) used with permission.

tion. Key and his collaborators (personal communication) studied 12,211 meat-eaters 2000 who ate only fish, 4176 nonvegan vegetarians, and 798 vegan vegetarians. As shown in Table 13–1, there are highly statistically significant differences between these dietary groups for both men and women, and for both systolic and diastolic blood pressures. The blood pressure levels in the meat-eaters were always the highest, and those in vegans were always the lowest. The fish-eaters had blood pressure levels at least as low as the nonvegan vegetarians, and generally a little lower. Vegan vegetarians had lower blood pressure levels than nonvegan vegetarians, and these differences were all statistically significant ($p < .05$) for both systolic and diastolic pressures, except BMI-adjusted systolic pressure for women ($p = .13$).

An adjustment for differences in BMI consistently shrank the blood pressure differences between dietary groups a little, but the original trends, and similar statistical significance, remained. Thus, besides BMI, other factors must contribute to the blood pressure differences. It is also interesting that the fish-eaters do not suffer the same blood pressure consequences as the meat-eaters, presumably indicating that blood-pressure-raising factors present in an omnivorous diet are not present in the fish-eating diet.

Other published comparisons of the blood pressure levels of vegans and other vegetarians are generally much less satisfactory because of the small number of subjects involved. Australian vegans studied by Li et al. (1999) had systolic and diastolic blood pressures that were not significantly different from those of lacto-ovo vegetarians in the same study. The blood pressure levels of Nigerian vegans (Famodu et al., 1998) were modestly lower than those of lacto-ovo vegetarians in the same study, but there were only eight vegans in it, and statistical significance was not achieved. The study group reported in Haines et al. (1980) contained 27 vegans and 23 lacto-ovo vegetarians. No details are given, but it is stated that the vegans were thinner and had lower blood pressure values than lacto-ovo vegetarians; however, these differences were not statistically significant.

Aside from the EPIC results, descriptive comparisons between vegans and omnivores, rather than vegans and nonvegan vegetarians, are rather unimpressive, and two of three observational studies found no significant differences (Famodu et al., 1998; Li et al., 1999; Sanders and Key, 1987). However, the studies' numbers were small, and blood pressure levels were indeed often a little lower in the vegans. An uncontrolled intervention trial, where 29 hypertensives in Sweden agreed to adhere to a vegan diet for one year, is of interest, as there were substantial drops in blood pressure levels with this intervention (Lindahl et al., 1984). Blood pressure levels dropped from an average of 151/88 to 142/83 mm Hg (systolic change, $p < .01$; diastolic change, $p < .05$).

In summary, there is good evidence that blood pressure levels in vegans are lower than those of lacto-ovo vegetarians in the EPIC study, and this is only partly explained by the tendency toward lower body weight in the vegans. The results of other comparisons between vegans and either lacto-ovo vegetarians or omnivores are hampered by small numbers, but they do not clearly differ from the EPIC results. This raises the possibility that some factor or factors, which take more extreme values in vegans than in other vegetarians, lower blood pressure levels.

Coagulation Factors for Vegans

The Australian study referred to several times above (Li et al., 1999) also compared a number of coagulation factors, including fibrinogen, factor VII, antithrombin III, and platelet function, between vegans and lacto-ovo vegetarians. None of these factors were significantly different between the two groups, but when compared with omnivores, factor VII levels were significantly lower in the vegans. Fibrinogen levels in the Nigerian vegans were significantly lower than those in omnivores and nonsignificantly lower than levels in lacto-ovo vegetarians (Famodu et al., 1999). However, it is interesting that platelet aggregability in this study was greater for vegans (and for lacto-ovo vegetarians) than for omnivores, which is potentially an adverse situation.

Thus, on the basis of the very sparse amount of available evidence, there are no clear differences in the values of these factors between vegans and lacto-ovo vegetarians, but there are possibly some differences between vegans and omnivores. More evidence is clearly needed.

Other Risk Factors for Vegans

Although one study noted that vegetarians have higher levels of homocysteine than others (Mezzano et al., 1999), this undoubtedly resulted from the lower serum levels of vitamin B_{12} in the vegetarians in this study. In contrast, a comparison of 25 California vegans and 20 nonvegetarians (Haddad et al., 1999a) found no differences in serum homocysteine levels (8.0 in nonvegetarians and 7.9 in vegans). However, there were also no significant differences in serum vitamin B_{12} levels between these dietary groups, as many subjects used supplements. Blood levels of folate, which lowers homocysteine levels, were significantly higher in the vegans. In the same study, hematocrit levels, an important determinant of plasma viscosity, did not differ between vegans and nonvegetarians.

CHRONIC DISEASE INCIDENCE AND MORTALITY IN VEGANS

The published studies on the disease experience of vegans are based on very small numbers of events and confidence intervals are wide, so results are not definitive. Hence only the presence or absence of major additional effects beyond those of the lacto-ovo-vegetarian diet can be evaluated.

The collaborative study (cited earlier) of five cohorts of vegetarians collected data on 573 vegans below the age of 90 (Key et al., 1999). The relative risks for ischemic heart disease deaths and deaths from all causes for vegans and for other vegetarians, when compared to omnivores, are shown in Table 13–2. These analyses are adjusted for age, sex, and smoking status (never or formerly smoked; current light or current heavy smoker), using a random effects model.

Data from the Health Food Shoppers Study are not included in the upper part of the table, as all the data necessary to clearly establish that a subject was a vegan were not collected in this study. Then the results shown for vegans, in the upper part of the table, are based on only 17 ischemic heart disease deaths and 68 deaths from any cause. If it is assumed that all nonvegetarians in the Health Food Shoppers Study were regular meat-eaters and that vegetarians who did not consume dairy products were in fact vegans, then this study could be included in the analysis. This increased the number of "vegans" to 1146, with 165 deaths being recorded. Results, when these subjects are included, are shown in the lower part of the table.

Table 13-2. Mortality Ratios (95% Confidence Intervals in Parentheses) of Vegans Compared with Other Vegetarians and Nonvegetarians in the Collaborative Analysis of Prospective Studies of Vegetarians[a]

Cause of Death	Nonvegetarians	Non-vegan Vegetarians	Vegans
EXCLUDING HEALTH FOOD SHOPPERS STUDY			
Ischemic heart disease	1.00	0.66 (0.52–0.83)	0.74 (0.46–1.21)
All causes	1.00	0.84 (0.74–0.96)	1.00 (0.70–1.44)
INCLUDING HEALTH FOOD SHOPPERS STUDY (HFSS)[b]			
Ischemic heart disease	1.00	NA	0.89 (0.65–1.24)
All causes	1.00	NA	1.06 (0.81–1.38)

NA, not available.

[a]All analyses adjusted for age, sex, and smoking status.

[b]Assumes that nonvegetarians in HFSS were regular meat-eaters and that vegetarians who ate no dairy foods were vegans.

Source: Key TJ, Fraser GE, Thorogood M, Appleby PN, Beral V, Reeves G, Burr ML, Chang-Claude J, Frentzel-Beyme R, Kuzman JW, Mann J, McPherson K, Mortality in vegetarians and nonvegetarians: detailed findings from a collaborative analysis of 5 prospective studies, *Am J Clin Nutr* 70(Suppl):516–524, 1999. Copyright by American Society for Clinical Nutrition.

Although confidence intervals are quite wide, there is nothing in Table 13–2 to suggest any advantage for the vegans when they are compared with other vegetarians for either numbers of deaths from all-causes or deaths from ischemic heart disease. The numbers of cancer and stroke events, although found in the original report, are too small for a meaningful analysis.

The disease experience of vegans has also been separately evaluated in the California Adventist studies. Although numbers are again much smaller than might be ideal, there is the advantage of being able to evaluate all-cause mortality, ischemic heart disease deaths, cancer deaths, and deaths from other causes, with no upper age limitation. This combines the data from the Adventist Health and Adventist Mortality studies in stratified proportional hazards analyses, where the strata refer to the two studies. One consequence of combining the two studies is that vegetarians must be defined as those eating meat less than once per week (rather than per month), as this is a limitation of the questions asked in the earlier study. The absence of eggs and dairy foods in the diet is of course added as a criterion when defining vegans.

Subjects at the baseline of either study who had reported a previous case of cancer, CHD, arthritis, or stroke are excluded from these analyses, as it seemed possible that some Adventists who had already developed these problems may then choose to follow church recommendations very rigorously, and, as part of this, become vegans. Hence for these subjects, the

Table 13–3. Relative Risks (95% Confidence Interval in Parentheses) of Death among Vegans and Others in a Combined Age- and Sex-Adjusted Analysis of the Adventist Mortality and Health Studies: Both Sexes Combined

Cause of Death	Omnivores	Lacto-ovo Vegetarians	Vegans
Coronary heart disease	1.00	0.82 (0.74–0.92)	0.81 (0.56–1.79)
Cancer	1.00	0.78 (0.68–0.90)	1.14 (0.73–1.78)
Other	1.00	0.93 (0.86–1.01)	0.76 (0.56–1.05)
All causes	1.00	0.87 (0.82–0.92)	0.84 (0.68–1.04)

baseline disease would have caused the veganism, rather than the reverse being true. Leaving such people in the analysis may have incorrectly elevated mortality rates in vegans due to higher death rates in those with chronic disease.

There were 668 vegans identified in the studies following the exclusions cited above, and during the follow-up, 91 deaths—29 from CHD, 21 from cancer, and 41 from other causes—were recorded. Results of the proportional hazards analyses are shown in Table 13–3.

As expected, lacto-ovo vegetarian Adventists had significantly lower mortality than omnivore Adventists, whether the cause of death was CHD, cancer, or death from all causes. However, although vegans had lower risks of death from CHD, other causes, and all causes than did the lacto-ovo vegetarians, differences were small. In addition, confidence intervals were wide, no doubt due to the small number of vegans included. If results for vegans are compared with those for the lacto-ovo vegetarians, there were no differences even close to significance, except for the possible excess of cancer mortality among vegans ($p = .10$). This may be a chance difference or, if real, may imply either a higher risk of new cancers among vegans or a poorer survival rate after a diagnosis of cancer. There is no good reason to suspect either, although lifestyle factors that affect survival after a cancer is diagnosed are poorly understood. An adjustment of these analyses for baseline BMI, BMI-squared, and hypertension changed the results in only minor ways.

Clearly, the existing evidence cannot provide definitive answers to these questions, except to indicate that veganism does not appear to result in either dramatic protection or increased risk when compared with other vegetarian diets. Whether important, but more modest, differences are indeed present must await further research. Presently funded studies of vegetarians in the United Kingdom and California should provide better information in the future.

SUMMARY

1. Vegans are thinner than other vegetarians.
2. Levels of total blood cholesterol and of blood LDL cholesterol are lower in vegans than in other vegetarians. HDL levels may also be lower, but the evidence is not consistent.
3. Blood pressure levels in vegans appear to be modestly, but significantly, lower than those in other vegetarians. This statement is based mainly on a large British data set.
4. Data on other risk factors are too sparse to allow meaningful comparisons between vegans and others.
5. Conclusions about disease events among vegans are also hampered by the low numbers of subjects in studies. But it seems unlikely that there are large differences in disease experience between vegans and other vegetarians. Studies that include more vegans would be necessary to detect any small or moderate differences. The California Adventist results did raise the possibility of higher cancer mortality in vegans (with a borderline statistical significance), but this needs confirmation from other studies to carry much conviction.

14

Changing a Population's Diet: A Behavioral View of the Adventist Experience

HELEN HOPP-MARSHAK, KITI FREIER, AND GARY FRASER

Although Americans, on average, have made definite changes toward a more healthful diet over the last 20 to 30 years, these have been relatively modest, despite the strong media and governmental focus on diet and its health effects. Recently, for instance, the U.S. Surgeon General declared obesity to be a national epidemic. As described in Chapter 1, Adventists tend to make food choices that are quite different from those of their non-Adventist neighbors. Moreover, they began doing this many decades before there was any credible scientific evidence to demonstrate the benefits.

What made this behavioral change possible in a diverse and geographically dispersed group? Are there lessons here that may be helpful for others who wish to make similar changes? It is possible to find explanations for Adventists' success with dietary changes and maintenance that are based on theories from the behavioral sciences. While there are no data that directly address this question in regard to Adventists, research on similar issues in other study groups provide some likely explanations.

Different models are used to explain behavior or behavioral change. While these may emphasize different areas, they build on each other. Considering different models is important to see the different ways in which a type of behavior can be maintained or changed. According to a value system model, the religious beliefs of Adventists influence their lifestyle. A social influence model would explain that the subculture to which Adventists belong helps support and maintain the healthy lifestyle chosen by individuals. Figure 14–1 suggests determinants and pathways in both the initiation of new health-related behaviors and their maintenance. Both values and social influences are undoubtedly important in the initiation and maintenance of the Adventist lifestyle, which includes not only an emphasis on diet and physical activity but also the avoidance of any mind-altering or addictive substances such as alcohol and tobacco.

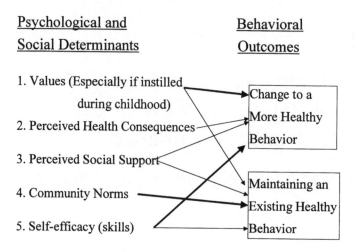

Figure 14–1 Determinants of initiation and maintenance of healthy behaviors.

THE VALUE SYSTEM EXPLANATION

If one wishes to change a behavior and this becomes part of the individual's values, morals, or belief system, the motivation and the likelihood of success are strengthened. The energy behind the motivation is increased by the value or meaning that the change has acquired. Research demonstrates that with religious values, an especially powerful influence comes from the accompanying moral obligation (Ortberg et al., 2001).

After a successful change, it is necessary to maintain the new behavior over the long term. Is belief in a value system that encourages adoption of healthful behaviors also important in this respect? Research from the behavioral sciences indicates that this is often the case, although other factors also play roles (Ajzen and Fishbein, 1980). When a behavior is embedded in a value system, it is more resistant to change since it has become an important part of the identity of the individual. Internalization of these values, particularly if this happens early in life, will also enhance maintenance. In this chapter we will discuss the influence of one's home culture, which further illuminates the importance of values for both initiation and maintenance.

An emphasis on a healthy lifestyle is one of the defining features of the Seventh-day Adventist religion and is very much a part of members' value systems. Adventists are encouraged to adopt a lifestyle that promotes health and well-being. The underlying belief is that one's body is the "temple of God" (I Cor. 6:19, 20) and should be kept in a condition that respects this view.

THE SOCIAL INFLUENCES EXPLANATION

Several models from the behavioral sciences identify social factors that are important determinants of behavior. Two, in particular, have gained recognition because of their ability to predict behavior and to identify factors that, when used in interventions, do produce behavioral change. These two models are called the theory of planned behavior (Ajzen, 1991; Ajzen and Fishbein, 1980) and the social learning (or, sometimes, cognitive) theory (Bandura, 1997). There is also a relatively new approach to behavior change that focuses on a sense of community and on the importance of altering the social and physical environment to achieve both behavior change and its maintenance. Can these somewhat overlapping constructs explain the health-related behavior of Adventists?

Theory of Planned Behavior

This theory (Ajzen, 1991) was developed as an extension of the theory of reasoned action and focuses on three key determinants of the intention to perform a behavior:

1. Attitudes or feelings about the consequences of performing a behavior— e.g., decreased risk of heart disease (positive), or the need to avoid certain foods (negative)
2. Subjective or group norms that influence a person's perception of what other important people think of this behavior, and how important it is to comply with these expectations—e.g., a family expects one to comply with a particular diet, and how much does one care what the family thinks one should do?
3. The perceived ease or difficulty of adhering to this behavior—e.g., How easy does one think it is to find vegetarian recipes, resist social pressure, etc?

These three factors are important when we try to understand and predict intentions, and, in turn, intentions are the best (though imperfect) predictors of subsequent behaviors such as particular exercise and dietary habits (Godin and Kok, 1996).

How might this theory of planned behavior help explain the lifestyle of Adventists? Attitudes toward particular health behaviors are influenced by beliefs about their consequences. If being an Adventist fosters a positive attitude toward healthful living through a greater emphasis on the benefits of such a lifestyle—which is highly probable—then this would encourage the adoption of these healthy behaviors. The subjective or social norms of the Adventist community would also promote these habits as long as a member wishes to behave as his Adventist peers and family suggest. Finally, being part of the Adventist community would usually enhance perceptions of control over, and ability to perform, the health behaviors by providing resources such as recipes, cooking skills, and easily prepared and affordable foods.

Social Learning Theory

There is considerable evidence that a primary determinant of behavior is perceived self-efficacy: the belief that one is capable of performing a particular behavior in specific situations and locations once the intention is formed (Bandura, 1997). This is the primary construct of the social learning (or cognitive) theory. The confident feeling that one's efforts to engage in a behavior will be successful is a better predictor of future behavior than is past behavior. Thus this feeling of confidence is an important factor explaining why people do or do not initiate or sustain behavior change. For instance, Schwarzer and Renner (2000) found that people who had a higher degree of self-efficacy, or confidence, in their ability to eat a low-fat/high-fiber diet were more likely to consume such a diet in the future than were those who lacked this confidence.

There are many factors that can enhance this belief in self-efficacy, including practice in performing the behavior, as well as seeing others perform the behavior and receive benefits from it (Bandura, 1997). There is also undoubtedly a collective or group self-efficacy—the confidence that the group collectively has in its shared goals (Triandis, 1989).

How might greater self-efficacy, or confidence, help explain the unusual success that Adventists have with dietary change and maintenance? Growing up in an Adventist family, living in an Adventist community, or even simply attending church with fellow members on a regular basis, will—by example and experience—engender confidence in and comfort with this lifestyle. Many Adventists (and other religious groups) also benefit from the belief that prayer results in divine assistance in the effort to change entrenched behaviors.

Social and Community Support

Research in the behavioral sciences indicates that strong feelings of social support and community are important for initiating and maintaining behaviors. As discussed in Chapter 9, there is considerable research documenting the importance of types of social support that depend on interpersonal relationships. It is especially apparent that the perception of support, even if this support is needed only occasionally, can improve physical and mental health (Berkman and Breslow, 1983; Penninx et al., 1996).

Effective interpersonal social support systems enable the successful initiation of new behaviors, as well as the long-term maintenance of established behaviors.

Behavior is also influenced by the broader social and physical environment in which people live (Bracht, 1990). Thus, complementing a focus on interpersonal social support, supportive characteristics of the community are also critical to the long-term maintenance of health behaviors. The community approach argues that permanent behavioral change is best achieved by changing the community standards (norms) of approved behavior.

Most commonly, the immediate families and closest friends of Adventists are Adventists, too. Thus the support obtained from these individuals (see Chapter 1) will tend to reinforce and support the desired behaviors. Many Adventists live in "Adventist communities" that may surround medical, educational, administrative, or commercial health food institutions. There is undoubtedly social pressure against deviating too far from community values. Even meat-eating Adventists would rarely if ever bring a meat dish to a church potluck. Most Adventists attend church each week, and this period of meeting with the church community can also be used very effectively for education and persuasion.

HOME CULTURE AND VALUES

It is clear that parents' values influence the nature and maintenance of values and belief systems of their children (Grusec, 1997). Research on parenting and its relationship to childhood development shows that moral, prosocial behavior and values are instilled at a very early age and that these early social forces have a lifelong influence on the child (Schuck and Bucy, 1998). Parents' values and beliefs thus importantly shape their children's development, despite other influences from our heterogeneous society.

A particular subculture that defines the parents' core values, such as a religious group (or any other group) may promote meaning for children and will help to form a particular worldview. This will shape a child, even within a larger social system that may not support the same values. Parental transmission of values tied to spirituality will have an even stronger effect in that they support a core belief system. Thus, if health is tied to this belief system, as it is within the Adventist culture, children are likely to continue to embrace their parents' dietary and health behaviors as adults.

This idea is supported by the results of the Valuegenesis Study, which documented the values of Adventist youth (Dudley and Gillespie, 1992). Some 11,000 Adventist young people were asked how much they agreed with specific Adventist church recommendations and standards. Health-related issues comprised six of the seven standards that were most clearly supported by these young people. Of this group, 92% agreed with not using illegal drugs, 91% agreed with not using tobacco, 88% agreed with not drinking beer or liquor, 85% agreed with daily exercise, 74% agreed with not drinking wine, and 73% agreed with not eating "biblically unclean meats." These data support the fact that health is a core value in the Adventist belief system and as such its value is transmitted to children from birth. This results in very stable support for these behaviors despite potentially contradictory influences exerted by peers or the broader society.

Other studies have found that messages from parents about what is appropriate behavior may be so strong that even when children are exposed to different attitudes and experiences, they will usually revert to ingrained or habitual choices (Witt, 1997). Values that are also based on a religious belief system are probably even stronger and more enduring as they are supported not only by parents but also by the larger church community. Thus the community's home, cultural, and social systems may work together. If a "village" raises the child, behaviors will be more stable and enduring.

Implications for Behavioral Change among Non-Adventists

Could other religious groups, societies, clubs, even communities, be equally effective in promoting behavioral change? This indeed seems possible. The maintenance of health and the avoidance of disease by use of preventive activities can form a natural part of Christianity, Judaism, Islam, and possibly other religions. Other societies and community groups may also see the promotion of a healthful lifestyle among their members as a valuable focus. Then value systems and behaviors could be changed if a focus on health was one defining feature of the group.

Many begin to value a change in health habits if they are persuaded by reports of scientific data such as those cited in this book. However, it is a common experience that, following a change in values, good intentions alone will not succeed in changing behavior. As illustrated by the models described in this chapter, when the group culture supports a belief in clear benefits, defines standards of behavior, and then provides skills and opportunities to improve self-efficacy, success becomes much more likely. The perception that one's performance is being observed and compared with community values may also be motivating. The teaching of the necessary skills becomes easier when one belongs to a supportive and focused club, group, or society. If these values can be instilled early in life, long-term maintenance of the behavior standards is more likely. Thus communities or groups that desire to promote change should also develop this as a value system for their children.

Other groups, both religious and nonreligious, have been successful in maintaining or promoting difficult and complex changes in health-related behaviors. For example, many Hindus are vegetarians or at least do not eat beef. Most Muslims do not use alcohol or tobacco, or eat pork. Certain Jewish groups do not eat pork and carefully prepare other flesh foods. Mormons do not use tobacco or alcohol. Vegetarian societies in the United Kingdom, the United States, and many other countries, are very active. Many of their members may already have been vegetarians when they joined, but even these benefit from the group support and the sharing of skills and knowledge that these societies afford. Motives in some of these latter cases often have had little to do with improving health, but the ability of a closely knit, value-driven group to successfully motivate and sustain difficult changes is still apparent.

SUMMARY

1. For generations, Adventist have adhered to dietary and other health behaviors that are very different from society norms.
2. Probable explanations include (*1*) the high value that is placed on health; (*2*) positive attitudes about the benefits of such behaviors; (*3*) the knowledge that important individuals (e.g., friends, family) expect this behavior; (*4*) the fact that the necessary skills, education, and foods are readily available; (*5*) the existence of a supportive community; and (*6*) the fact that for many, these values were instilled early in life and are thus enduring.
3. Tying such values to a religious belief system gives them special meaning and force.
4. Members of other organizations and religious groups could use similar methods to produce positive behavioral changes if good health became highly valued by the group.

15

Shifting to a Vegetarian Diet: Practical Suggestions from a Nutritionist

ELLA HADDAD

With a new understanding and appreciation of the health benefits of vegetarian diets, some are motivated to make changes in this direction. How is this accomplished? Is it difficult?

The term vegetarian encompasses a range of dietary practices. Although "vegetarian" is not consistently defined in the scientific literature, the following definitions are commonly used:

> *Lacto-ovo vegetarians* do not eat meat, poultry, fish, or seafood, but do consume milk, dairy products, and eggs.
>
> *Lactovegetarians* have a similar diet but exclude eggs.
>
> *Vegans* (sometimes also called strict, pure, or total vegetarians) avoid all animal products including dairy, eggs, and possibly honey. They may also refuse to wear furs, leather, silk, or wool.
>
> *Semivegetarians* (or partial vegetarians) include some animal foods, such as fish and poultry, in the diet. They often avoid red meat.

It is not difficult or complicated to plan appealing and nutritionally adequate vegetarian meals. The same steps of food selection, preparation, and presentation that are used in conventional diets are necessary for vegetarians. Meals should be both tasty and nutritionally adequate. Here are some useful guidelines that are generally consistent with the most recent position paper issued by the American Dietetic Association (Messina and Burke, 1997).

GUIDELINES

Choose a Variety of Plant Foods

While vegetarian diets are typically defined by the exclusion of meat or other animal products, a healthy vegetarian diet is one that incorporates a wide variety of plant foods. Eating more plant foods infuses the diet with an abundance of vitamins and photochemicals. There are dozens of different grains, legumes, vegetables, fruits, nuts and seeds from which to choose. Variety involves the selection of different items from within each food group on a day-to-day, week-to-week, and season-by-season basis. In addition to the need for variety, food selection must also be balanced. This requires that foods be selected from all the food groups, thereby avoiding overemphasis on a single food or food group. An eating pattern that incorporates a variety of plant foods is more likely to meet nutritional needs.

Ensure Adequate Calories to Meet Energy Needs

A diet restricted in food amounts can limit the intake of essential nutrients. Although many adopt the vegetarian lifestyle to facilitate weight control, obtaining adequate amounts of energy to support growth or maintain weight is critical for some individuals, such as young athletes, growing children, pregnant and lactating women, and the elderly. This is because plant foods are generally low in fat and high in noncaloric fiber. Fruits and vegetables also have a higher water content than animal foods, which are generally high in fat and calorically dense. It is often necessary for vegetarians to eat larger quantities of food in order to obtain enough calories to meet energy needs. Plant foods that have higher caloric and nutrient density include nuts, nut butters, seeds, dried fruits, avocados, and olives. Vegetable oils, such as olive or canola oil, may also be used in moderation to provide energy and essential fatty acids.

Reduce Intake of Foods That Provide Few Nutrients

When adopting a vegetarian diet, it is also important to limit the intake of foods that have added sugar and discretionary fat. Sugars include not only table sugar but also brown sugar, honey, syrup, and high-fructose corn syrup. Sugars and sugar-containing foods supply calories but are limited in nutrients. Discretionary fat is that obtained from full-fat dairy products and fat added to foods during their preparation or consumption.

Although vegetarian diets tend to be lower in total fat, saturated fat, and cholesterol than traditional diets, it is possible for a vegetarian to actually consume more saturated fat and cholesterol than the average meat-eater. This occurs when generous amounts of whole milk, regular ice cream, high-fat cheese, fried foods, and chips are consumed on a regular basis.

VEGETARIAN FOOD GUIDE

A convenient and practical method for planning meals is to follow a daily food guide. Food guides provide the framework for selecting both the kinds and amounts of foods that together provide a nutritionally satisfactory diet. They assign foods to groups on the basis of similarity in composition and nutritive contribution. The Vegetarian Food Guide Pyramid (Figure 15–1), which was developed by a team of nutrition scientists, is a useful guide for the various vegetarian eating styles, whether they might be the lacto-ovo

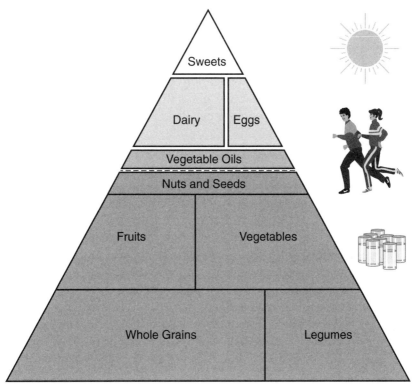

Note: A reliable source of vitamin B_{12} should be included if no dairy or eggs are consumed.

Figure 15–1 Vegetarian food guide pyramid. *Source:* Haddad EH, Sabaté J, Whitten CG, Vegetarian food guide pyramid: a conceptual framework, *Am J Clin Nutr* 70(Suppl): 615s–619s, 1999. Copyright by American Society of Clinical Nutrition.

vegetarian or vegan style, low in fat or higher in fat (Haddad, 1994; Haddad et al., 1999b). Foods in the broader base of the pyramid should be eaten in larger quantities, whereas those toward the smaller apex of the pyramid are to be eaten occasionally or not at all. The food groups, typical serving sizes, and the recommended number of daily servings that make up a balanced vegetarian diet, are shown in Table 15–1. Because energy and nutrient requirements of individuals differ, a range in the recommended number of daily servings is given for each group. Those with low energy needs may select the minimum number of servings in the range for their daily intake, whereas those with higher energy needs should select more servings from each group. If the principles of variety and caloric adequacy are adhered to, eating at least the minimum recommended number of daily servings from each food group ensures adequate nutrition for most individuals.

Whole Grains

Whole grains include the major staples—wheat, rice, and corn—as well as oats, barley, rye, millet, and the vast array of products made from flour and grains, such as breads, breakfast cereals, pasta, noodles, tortillas, and crackers. Whole grains are the foundation of the vegetarian eating style and provide energy, protein, B vitamins, minerals, phytochemical content, and fiber. Choose six or more servings per day of mostly whole-grain breads and cereals.

In the milling process, the bran and germ are separated from the starchy endosperm, and the latter is ground into flour. Nutrients and phytochemical content are not evenly distributed throughout the grain; because the higher concentrations are in the outer part of the grain, refining results in reduced nutrient and phytochemical content. Although some refined and processed grains may be enriched or fortified with selected nutrients, whole grains are a better choice since they provide a wider range of minerals, antioxidant nutrients, fiber, lignans, and phenolic compounds than are found in refined grains.

This does not mean that refined grains, or their products, must be avoided altogether. The inclusion of some refined-grain foods provides interest for the diet and may be helpful in meeting caloric needs of those not able to consume sufficient amounts of the bulkier whole grains.

Legumes

Legumes are a large family of plants distinguished by their seed-bearing pods. From an agricultural perspective, the 13,000 species of legumes come

Table 15–1. The Vegetarian Food Groups: Suggested Plan for Vegetarian Meals

Food Group	Foods	Servings per Day	Typical Serving Size
Whole grains	Grains (wheat, rice, corn, oats, barley, rye, millet, triticale, and sorghum); cooked and ready-to-eat breakfast cereals; bread, tortilla, macaroni, pasta	6 or more	1 slice bread or 1 small roll; $1/2$ bun or bagel; $3/4$ cup (1 oz) ready-to-eat cereal; $1/2$ cup cooked cereal, rice, or pasta; 1 medium tortilla
Legumes, beans, and peas	Beans, peas, lentils, garbanzos	3 or more	$1/2$ cup cooked dry beans, lentils, or slit peas
Soy foods	Soybeans, tofu, tempeh, soy yogurt, meat substitutes		$1/2$ cup tofu, soy foods, textured soy protein, or meat substitutes
Soy beverage	Fortified (calcium, vitamin D, etc.) soy beverage		1 cup fortified soy beverage
Vegetables	Potatoes, yams, corn, broccoli, green beans, carrots, spinach, squash, zucchini, tomatoes, lettuce, mushrooms, asparatus, cauliflower, cabbage, brussels sprouts, squash, kale, bok choi, waterchestnuts, artichoke, jicama, eggplant, seaweed, lettuce, peppers, celery, onions, etc.	4 or more	$1/2$ cup cooked vegetable; 1 cup raw vegetable or salad; $3/4$ cup vegetable juice
Fruits	Apple, apricot, banana, blackberry, blueberry, boysenberry, cantaloupe, fig, grapefruit, grape, honeydew melon, kiwi, mandarin, mango, melons, orange, papaya, peach, pear, persimmon, pineapple, plum, raspberry, strawberry, tangerine, watermelon, etc.	3 or more	1 medium apple, orange, banana; $1/2$ cup cooked or canned fruit; $3/4$ cup fruit juice

(continued)

Table 15–1. The Vegetarian Food Groups: Suggested Plan for Vegetarian Meals *Continued*

Food Group	Foods	Servings per Day	Typical Serving Size
Nuts and seeds	Almond, Brazil, cashew, coconut, hazel, macadamia, pecan, pine, pistachio, walnut, flax, pumpkin, sesame, sunflower, etc.	1 or more	$1/4$ cup (1 oz) almonds, walnuts, or seeds; 2 tablespoons peanut butter, almond butter or tahini
Vegetable oils	Avocado, olives, olive oil, nut oils, seed oils, plant oils, margarine, butter, sour cream, cream cheese, mayonnaise, salad dressing, etc.	Optional	1 teaspoon vegetable oil or margarine; 2 teaspoons salad dressing
Dairy	Milk, buttermilk, yogurt, cottage cheese, cheese, ice cream, kefir, etc.	Optional	1 cup nonfat or 1% milk or yogurt
Eggs		Optional	1 egg (limit yolks to 3 per week)
Sweets	Table sugar, honey, molasses, jam and jelly; soda, sweetened beverages, and sweetened fruit drinks; sorbet; sherbet; cake, cookies, pie, muffins, brownies, sugary rolls, candy	Optional	

in two classes: grain legumes, such as beans and peas grown primarily as protein staples; and oilseeds, such as soybeans and peanuts, which are grown for both their oil and protein content. Since the nutrient profile of peanuts is similar to that of tree nuts, peanuts are usually placed in the nut group. For the purpose of vegetarian dietary guidance, the legume food group includes three distinct, nutritionally important groups of food: cooked dry beans and peas, meat substitutes, and fortified soy-based milk alternatives.

Cooked beans and peas

Dry beans and peas have been a dietary staple since biblical times. Although the different varieties of beans (pinto, kidney, navy, lima, black, mung) and peas (garbanzos, split peas, black-eyed peas, lentils) vary widely in color, size, taste, and shape, their nutritional compositions are similar. Cooked dry beans and peas are a dense source of protein, remarkably low in fat, high in soluble fiber and B vitamins, and a substantial source of minerals. The protein content of beans is generally between 20% and 30% of energy. Choose one or more servings per day. A serving of cooked beans (approximately 90 g or half a cup of cooked beans) provides approximately 7 to 8 g of protein. The soluble fiber in beans and peas is effective in lowering cholesterol and modulating blood sugar levels (Messina, 1999).

Some individuals are reluctant to eat beans because of possible intestinal gas formation. Beans contain several oligosaccharides that are indigestible because humans lack the enzyme α-galactosidase. Proper soaking, rinsing, and cooking can rid beans of 90% of their gas-producing sugars. For those unaccustomed to eating legumes, beans can be introduced gradually in small amounts. Canned cooked beans (preferably without the pork!) are generally better tolerated.

Soybeans and soy-based foods

Soybeans are higher in protein and fat than other beans and this protein has the highest quality of any vegetable protein. Choose one or more servings per day. Soy-based foods include soy beverages, soy yogurt, soy cheese, tofu, tempeh, soynuts, and soy-based meat substitutes. Tofu is a cheese-like curd made from soybeans and is an ingredient in many oriental dishes. Other products made from soybeans are textured vegetable protein and some meat substitutes.

Recent studies have shown that an intake of approximately 25 g of soy protein, as obtained in 4 oz of tofu, lowers blood cholesterol. Soybeans are unique among the legumes because they are a concentrated source of the isoflavones genistein and daidzein, which have weak estrogen-like activity and may provide other health benefits, such as a reduced risk of certain cancers (Messina, 1999).

Soy-based and other meat substitutes. Meat substitutes are generally commercially prepared foods made from either soybeans, wheat protein, peanuts, or other plant protein sources. They are sometimes called meat analogues. Some are made to look and taste like different types of meat. There are analogues that mimic sausages, hot dogs, hamburgers, fish, and chicken. Textured vegetable protein (TVP) has the texture of ground meat and can indeed be substituted for ground meat in recipes. Some products are made exclusively from plant foods, while others may contain egg albumin or dried milk solids or whey. Some are supplemented with vitamin B$_{12}$ and other nutrients. These products are not essential to the vegetarian diet but are enjoyed by many vegetarians for the sake of variety, convenience, and ease of preparation.

Fortified soy-based milk alternatives. If milk and other dairy foods are avoided, it is desirable to use an appropriate milk alternative. A milk can be made from soybeans by cooking, grinding, and squeezing the beans, then processing to remove some troublesome enzymes. This milk is commonly chosen as a dairy milk alternative. The choice is especially important for children, adolescents, pregnant and lactating women, and the elderly, whose intake of protein, calcium, and vitamin D may otherwise be marginal. In Western diets, dairy products supply approximately three-quarters of the calcium and are an important source of protein and vitamin D. Because of this, it is recommended that milk alternatives such as soymilk provide 5–7 g of protein per serving, and that they be fortified with calcium (250–300 mg per cup) and vitamin D (400 IU per quart).

Other Vegetables

The word *vegetable* has, through common usage, come to apply to those plants or parts of plants that are served either raw or cooked as part of the main course of a meal. Vegetables (four or more servings per day), along with legumes and grains, are at the center of the vegetarian plate. With the exception of starchy vegetables such as potatoes, sweet potatoes, yams, corn, carrots, and green peas, most vegetables contain relatively little carbohydrate. Vegetables as a group contain generous amounts of vitamins, minerals, antioxidants, and phytochemicals. Phytochemicals are natural substances, found only in plant foods, that probably protect the body's cells from damage and disease. Vegetables provide protein, fiber, calcium, iron, and trace minerals and are eaten raw, cooked, or juiced.

Fruits

The fruit group (three or more servings per day) includes not only fresh fruit but frozen, dried, and canned fruit, as well as fruit juices. Fruits tend to be higher than vegetables in carbohydrates. Although their nutrient content varies, most fruits provide important amounts of fiber, vitamins A and C, minerals, antioxidants, and phytochemicals.

Nuts and Seeds

Nuts, the dried fruits of trees, include almonds, walnuts, hazelnuts, macadamia nuts, pecans, pine nuts, and pistachio nuts. Although, botanically, peanuts are a legume, they are commonly included in this group because they resemble nuts in their nutritional makeup. Dried seeds, such as sesame, pumpkin, squash, sunflower seeds, and flaxseed, also belong to this group. Nuts and seeds (one or more servings per day) may be eaten either raw or dry roasted or may be added to foods. They may also be ground and used as butters or spreads. It is preferable to avoid nut products that are fried in fat or highly salted.

The nutritional contribution of nuts and seeds to plant-based and vegetarian diets is substantial. They are an important source of protein; B vitamins, such as niacin; vitamin E; magnesium and iron; and trace minerals such as zinc, copper, manganese, and selenium, which would otherwise tend to be present at low levels in a vegetarian diet. Nuts and seeds are also a source of unrefined "healthy" unsaturated fat providing essential fatty acids and energy necessary for plant-based eating patterns. A unique characteristic of walnuts and flaxseed is their relatively high content of the essential omega-3 fatty acid called alpha linolenic acid.

Vegetable Oils (Optional)

Vegetable oils provide essential fatty acids and are good sources of energy. Because they are refined products, very energy dense, and with only some of the beneficial characteristics of the parent foods, they should be used in moderation. Choose monounsaturated oils such as canola and olive oil, or polyunsaturated oils such as corn, safflower, or sunflower oil. Select soft or tub margarines with oil listed as the first ingredient on the label. Avoid tropical oils (coconut oil, palm kernel oil, palm oil), as these are much more highly saturated, and also avoid hydrogenated fats, which all tend to raise blood cholesterol levels.

Nuts, avocados, olives, olive oil, and canola oil are high in monounsaturated fat. Sources of omega-3 polyunsaturated fatty acids are walnuts, flaxseed, canola oil, soy oil, soy foods, and wheat germ.

Dairy (Optional)

If milk or dairy products are consumed, it is best to use low-fat or nonfat varieties such as skim milk and low-fat cheeses. If milk or dairy products are not consumed, select a fortified milk substitute (as noted). Milk and dairy foods are important sources of calcium, protein, and vitamin B_{12} for lactovegetarians. Milk is often fortified with vitamin D.

Eggs (Optional)

Eggs provide an inexpensive source of high-biological-value protein. However, because of the high cholesterol content of egg yolks (213 mg per yolk), health-related dietary recommendations suggest limiting egg yolks to 2 to 3 per week. Egg whites contain no fat or cholesterol.

Sweets (Optional)

Foods with substantial amounts of refined sugar belong in this group. In addition to added sugar, many sweets and desserts also contain flour, butter, margarine, hydrogenated fat or oil, eggs, cream, or other processed and refined ingredients, or ingredients with a high proportion of saturated fat. Except for calories, their nutrient contribution to the diet is low. Sweets and desserts should be consumed in moderation and should be limited when weight maintenance or weight loss is desired.

HOW TO MAKE THE TRANSITION TOWARD A VEGETARIAN DIET

Breaking away from an eating style that is rooted in habit, culture, and tradition takes effort and time. Some people like to make rapid changes, while others take a more gradual approach. The gradual approach allows time to find new ways to meet dietary and nutrient needs. The goal is to make changes that one can live with and that are nutritionally sound.

Meal planning as a vegetarian involves rethinking the concept of meat as the entree or main dish. In Western societies, meal planning centers around meat or a meat entree. For vegetarians there are other entrees. Most commonly, these are prepared from commercial meat substitutes, grains, starchy vegetables, beans, and other legumes or from soy and soy products. These foods are hearty, satisfying, and versatile. Vegetarian meals are often planned around combinations of vegetables and grains. Examples include pasta and vegetables, or, in particular, legume and grain combinations, such as beans and rice. The suggestions that follow can help you make a smoother transition.

Make a List of Vegetarian Meals That You Currently Enjoy

This first step calls for examining your current diet. You can do this by thinking about your eating habits and by keeping a food diary for a few days. What do you usually have at each meal? Where do you usually eat your meals? Make a list of your favorite dishes and meals that are vegetarian ones and build from these as a foundation. Plan to eat a vegetarian meal several times a week using foods that you know and enjoy.

Add More Vegetarian Meals by Revising Favorite Recipes

Identify your favorite recipes that are meat-based and change them to vegetarian dishes. For example, meat sauce for spaghetti can be changed to a marinara sauce or a vegetable sauce. Textured vegetable protein, tofu, or commercial meat substitutes may be used in recipes instead of ground beef.

Expand Your Options by Finding New Foods and New Recipes

In the long run, many varied foods keep vegetarian diets healthy and interesting, even though some of the foods may initially be new. Become actively involved in finding new foods and learning how to prepare them. A plethora of vegetarian cookbooks, magazines, pamphlets, and recipes can be obtained at bookstores, at the library, and on the Web (Melina et al., 1995; Messina et al., 2001; Sabaté, 2001). Experiment with vegetarian recipes that fit your tastes. To improve your cooking skills, you may want to participate in cooking classes. Such classes are offered by local vegetarian groups, health promotion programs, or food and nutrition departments at colleges and universities. Experiment with cuisines of other cultures.

Have Convenience Foods and Quick Meals Easily Available

Many vegetarian meals can be made without investing much time in the kitchen. Vegetarian convenience foods and meals are readily available at your local market and specialty stores. Take time to stock your cupboard and freezer with supplies necessary to prepare meals in a hurry. Among the staples that you will find useful are these: ready-to-eat whole-grain cereals fortified with vitamin B_{12}; quick-cooking whole-grain cereals; whole-grain breads and crackers; canned beans, such as kidney, pinto, black, and white beans; canned vegetarian soups or soup mixes; frozen vegetables; tomato sauce; canned or frozen meat substitutes; and nuts and seeds.

Make a List of Vegetarian Meals You Can Eat away From Home

An inventory of vegetarian options at nearby carry-out places, cafeterias, and restaurants can be very helpful. The cuisines of the world are an inspiring example of how plant foods are transformed into delicious meals. Since many ethnic groups eat little meat, you can benefit from the cultural and culinary diversity of ethnic restaurants and markets. Check the meatless offerings at Ethiopian, Middle Eastern, Chinese, Vietnamese, Thai, and Indian restaurants.

NUTRITIONAL CONSIDERATIONS

Protein

It is commonly assumed that the major concern about vegetarian diets is insufficient protein. Vegetarians who consume milk, dairy products, or eggs generally obtain more than enough protein to meet their needs. Obtaining adequate protein may occasionally be a problem for those who avoid all animal foods if the recommended quantities of cereal grains, legumes, soy foods, and nuts are not regularly eaten.

The important difference between protein of vegetable origin and of animal origin is the concentration of indispensable amino acids that they contain. These amino acids occur in milk, milk products, eggs, and meat in proportions similar to the needs of the body. The amounts of protein and concentrations of specific amino acids in some foods of vegetable origin are inadequate if consumed as the only source of protein, particularly among infants and children. The exception to this is soy protein. Soy protein products (soy flour, soy isolate) do contain the essential amino acids in a pattern similar to that of other high-quality proteins. Soy protein, as the sole or major source of protein, is adequate to promote growth and development in infants and children, along with sufficient energy and other essential nutrients.

Studies have shown that mixtures of plant protein foods can be of high protein quality. This is because the amino acid deficit of one plant protein can be corrected by combining it with another complementary plant food that contains adequate amounts of the amino acid in question. For example, although legumes are low in sulfur-containing amino acids and cereal grains are low in lysine, legumes in combination with cereal grains provide protein of a quality similar to that obtained from animal foods.

Planning vegetarian diets has in the past appeared difficult to some because of this complementation principle. Nutrition scientists now believe that it is not necessary to consume complementary proteins at the same time or during the same meal (Young and Pellett, 1994). It is the total quantity of protein and amino acids in a variety of foods, consumed over the course of the day, that ultimately determines protein adequacy. Individuals who avoid milk, dairy, and eggs should eat grains, nuts, legumes, or soy foods daily, in the amounts recommended. If total protein needs are met by a variety of plant foods containing protein, complementation will occur naturally. Specific combinations of foods at one meal are not necessary.

Vitamin B$_{12}$

Vitamin B$_{12}$ is found naturally only in foods derived from animals and actually comes from certain bacteria that the animals have eaten. Vegetarians who consume milk and eggs usually ingest adequate amounts of the vitamin unless their intake of these foods is limited. Fermented soy foods such as tempeh and miso, along with sea vegetables, are sometimes cited as containing B$_{12}$. In fact, these foods are not reliable sources and may actually interfere with B$_{12}$ absorption. Vegans who avoid all animal foods need a regular and reliable source of the vitamin, which can either be cobalamin-supplemented food(s) or vitamin preparations. Some common foods that are supplemented with vitamin B$_{12}$ are certain brands of nutritional yeasts, most ready-to-eat breakfast cereals, most meat analogues, and some milk alternatives.

Vitamin D

In the United States, milk is fortified with vitamin D. Individuals who avoid milk need a supplementary source of vitamin D, especially in northern latitudes where there is less exposure to sunlight. Vitamin D–fortified foods from plant sources include commercial dairy-free margarines, some ready-to-eat breakfast cereals, and vitamin D–fortified milk alternatives.

Calcium

Calcium is widely distributed in the plant kingdom. However, except for dark green leafy vegetables, no single food is a particularly rich source of this mineral. While individuals who consume milk and dairy products can easily meet their needs for calcium, intake may be low in diets that are solely plant-based. It is helpful that the fractional absorption of calcium from low-oxalate greens (e.g., kale) is higher than that of milk (Weaver et al., 1999). Nevertheless, in addition to eating calcium-rich greens (broc-

Table 15–2. A Sample Vegetarian Menu

Foods	Adult Female	Adult Male
BREAKFAST		
Oatmeal	$1/2$ cup	$1^1/2$ cup
Fat-free milk or fortified soy beverage	1 cup	$1^1/2$ cup
Raisins	1 tablespoon	2 tablespoons
Whole wheat toast	1 slice	2 slices
Almond butter	1 tablespoon	2 tablespoons
Banana	1 medium	1 medium
Tea, coffee, herbal tea (unsweetened)	As desired	As desired
LUNCH		
Vegetarian burger sandwich		
Whole-wheat bun	1 medium	1 medium
Vegetarian burger patty	3 ounce	3 ounce
Lettuce	2 leaves	2 leaves
Tomato	2 slices	2 slices
Mustard	2 teaspoons	2 teaspoons
Apple	1 medium	1 medium
Calcium fortified fruit juice	1 cup	1 cup
DINNER		
Lentil stew with tomatoes, onions, celery	1 cup	$1^1/2$ cup
Brown rice	$1/2$ cup	1 cup
Broccoli	$1/2$ cup	$1/2$ cup
Salad greens	1 cup	1 cup
Chopped walnuts	2 tablespoons	2 tablespoons
Oil and lemon dressing	1 tablespoon	1 tablespoon
Dinner roll		1 medium
Soft margarine		1 teaspoon
Fresh strawberries	1 cup	1 cup
Low-fat frozen yogurt, tofu ice cream or sherbet	$1/2$ cup	$1/2$ cup
NUTRIENT ANALYSIS		
Calories	1600	2200
Protein (g)	58	85
Total fat (% calories)	25	27
Saturated fat (% calories)	3	4
Vitamin D (μg)	2.7	5.4
Calcium (mg)	1200	1600

Note: The sample menu meets or exceeds the Daily Reference Intake (DRI) for nutrients except for vitamin B_{12}. Nutritional analysis software used is Food Processor (version 7.5), ESHA Research, Salem, Oregon.

coli, Chinese cabbage, kale, mustard greens, turnip greens, parsley), individuals who avoid milk should regularly consume other calcium-rich foods such as calcium-precipitated tofu, calcium-fortified milk alternatives, or calcium-fortified fruit juice. Thus, vegan children, adolescents, and women may need additional calcium, either as a fortified food or as a supplement, if their dietary intake of calcium is low. It may be prudent for some to take 400 to 600 mg of supplemental calcium per day.

Iron

Concerns about iron nutrition in vegetarians center on the fact that heme (meat) iron is more readily absorbed than are plant (nonheme) sources of iron. Some plant foods contain inhibitors of iron absorption, such as phytates in whole-grain cereals; however, the absorption of nonheme iron is substantially enhanced by ascorbic acid. In developed countries, iron deficiency is not more prevalent among vegetarians than among omnivores. Iron is widely distributed in plant foods, and fruits and vegetables are good sources of ascorbic acid. Plant foods rich in iron include legumes, seeds and nuts, green leafy vegetables, dried fruits, and enriched- and whole-grain products.

A SAMPLE VEGETARIAN MENU

An example of a vegetarian menu for one day is given in Table 15–2. We have structured this to approximately fit the guidelines described above. Notice the nutrient analysis in the lower part of the table. It is evident that this would provide a day of interesting and satisfying meals. Yet it is only one of many possible combinations. Such a diet can easily be much more interesting than that consumed by most nonvegetarian Americans.

CONCLUSION

Vegetarian diets can be planned for both nutrient adequacy and superb taste. A bonus is that they also reduce the risk of chronic disease. To assist with meal planning, it is desirable to follow a food guide. The transition to a vegetarian diet can be accomplished by becoming knowledgeable about the many food choices that are available and the resources for additional education and support. Cultivate a sense of adventure when trying new foods and new recipes.

SUMMARY

1. A wide variety of food choices is easily achieved in a vegetarian diet, and this is important for nutritional balance.
2. Vegetarians (and others) should avoid higher-calorie foods that contain few other beneficial nutrients. Higher-calorie vegetarian foods with excellent content of vitamins and other phytochemicals include nuts, seeds, dried fruits, avocados, and olives.

3. The vegetarian food guide pyramid is based on grains and legumes. Other important food groups include vegetables, fruits, nuts, and seeds.
4. Combinations of whole grains and legumes, eaten during the same day, provide high-quality protein, as do soybeans eaten alone.
5. Vegan diets need vitamin B_{12} supplementation. Unless sun exposure is optimal, vitamin D supplementation may also be necessary for those who avoid milk. Where all animal foods are avoided, children, adolescents, pregnant and lactating women, and the elderly should take special care with the adequacy of protein, vitamin D, and calcium intake.

16

The Challenge of
Nutritional Epidemiology

Fifty years of dietary research have shown that the disease experience and risk factor status of vegetarians often differ markedly from those of others. This almost invariably seems to be in the direction of lower risk. The question of which specific nutrients or foods, either used or avoided by vegetarians, affect the risk of chronic disease has been much more difficult to answer. It will be clear to the reader that despite decades of research, what is not known still far outweighs what is known with confidence. There are many "maybes" and "probables," and rather fewer "almost certains."

This situation must raise questions about the adequacy of the research methods being used to define the effects of particular foods or nutrients, and indeed the methodologic challenge is quite severe. Diet is a complex matter that involves choices among hundreds or even thousands of foods. These each contribute dozens of well-known nutrients/vitamins/minerals in different combinations, and this is aside from the large number of phytochemicals that, though often poorly defined chemically, may possess important biological activity.

The complexity of diets presents analytic challenges on several fronts. First, we expect study subjects to provide accurate or at least useful information about what they eat. Yet it is clear that the ability of most people to accurately summarize what they routinely eat is limited. In addition, accurate information about the nutrient content of particular foods is not always available. The Department of Agriculture database (U.S. Department of Agriculture, 2003), for instance, is very extensive, but different varieties of certain vegetables may differ in nutrient/vitamin content. Maturity of the product and storage time can also be important. Then there are the many phytochemicals whose content in particular foods is poorly characterized. This has been brought forcefully to our attention when we try to understand the effect of nut consumption in lowering blood cholesterol and reducing the risk of CHD. For most nuts, little is known of their constituents beyond major macronutrients, vitamins, and minerals.

Thus, it is a fact of life in observational nutritional epidemiology that the data we deal with will often have extensive errors. The effects of these errors will cascade through the analysis, degrading the accuracy of the assessment of individual dietary intakes, as well as the estimated effects of dietary habits on disease risk. Newer methods of statistical analysis should help with this problem in the future. In the meantime, there is the need for guidelines to minimize the risk of forming incorrect conclusions that depend on the errors rather than on the true evidence. Some fairly standard guidelines of this sort were described in Chapter 6.

Kushi et al. (1988) have demonstrated that for most nutrients, vegetarians had smaller within-person or greater between-person variances—characteristics that improve the accuracy of measurement and increase the range of contrasting diets within the group, thereby increasing statistical power (White et al., 1994). The between-person variance among California Seventh-day Adventists is also particularly wide (G.E. Fraser, unpublished calculations), reflecting the great diversity of dietary habits within this group. Studies among these populations probably allow the evaluation of individual foods, nutrients, and their effects with greater clarity and cost-effectiveness than is usually the case. Although one may then expect studies of vegetarians to be more efficient per person studied, the problems just described will still be present, though to a somewhat lesser degree.

Many vegetarian diets happen to be relatively low in cholesterol, saturated fats, and sodium but relatively high in dietary fiber, unsaturated fats, and potassium—all attributes that many authoritative health-professional organizations consider to be healthy. Thus, there is a valuable opportunity to directly test the health effects of a dietary pattern that is similar to, or somewhat better than, those that are often recommended.

Given the variable quality of the evidence in nutritional epidemiology, what practical application can be taken from the results presented in this book? By necessity, most of the data come from observational studies rather than clinical trials. How far can these studies be trusted?

Results from careful observational studies about the effects of other traditional risk factors (such as blood lipids and blood pressure) have generally been confirmed in subsequent clinical trials. If there are consistent results from several well-conducted observational studies, strong conclusions are possible that may form the basis for behavioral recommendations. This is particularly so when there is also some understanding of the biological mechanisms involved and if the effect appears to be quite strong. Even where the evidence is thought to be only suggestive, this may still form a basis for action in motivated individuals, particularly as the dietary changes suggested by this research usually have no known or suspected adverse effects and there is a some real prospect of benefit.

With these caveats in mind, brief summaries of the stronger findings from the preceding chapters are presented below, along with some comments on their practical implications for the population at large. Some indication is given regarding the degree of confidence with which particular findings can be viewed. These are personal opinions, but they are based on the available evidence.

FINDINGS FOR DIET AND CARDIOVASCULAR DISEASE

Vegetarian diets typically include foods contributing more dietary fiber, polyunsaturated fats, folate, antioxidant vitamins, and other antioxidant substances, but less saturated fats and cholesterol.

Vegetarians clearly have lower levels of serum total and LDL cholesterol than omnivores, and values in vegans are lower still. HDL cholesterol levels are not consistently different in vegetarians but may be lower in vegans than in omnivores, and also in Adventists (who avoid alcohol).

The evidence that vegetarians and particularly vegans have modestly lower levels of blood pressure is convincing, though the reasons for this are only partly understood.

Vegetarians are consistently less obese than omnivores, a trend even more pronounced in vegans, but this is only a partial explanation for their lower blood pressures. That vegetarians are thinner is an important observation in a society experiencing an epidemic of obesity and the associated cases of poor health.

There can be little doubt that vegetarians experience much lower rates of CHD events, a major benefit in a society where this is the single most common cause of death, and an important source of morbidity. In a relative sense, this advantage is seen especially at younger ages, although among Adventists, at least, it is evident to an important extent in men throughout their life and in women up to their eighth or ninth decades. Thus it is premature morbidity and mortality, in particular, that is reduced. Presumably, this is a consequence of the improved risk profile described in this book.

The cardiovascular disease experience of Adventists and other vegetarian populations can be interpreted as a large-scale demonstration of the benefits that accrue from the type of dietary changes recommended by the American Heart Association (Nutrition Committee, AHA, 2000) and by other similar bodies. This experience also raises the possibility that diets going beyond the published guidelines will provide even greater protection. Most nonvegetarians who read this book will not easily become vegetarians, as long-held dietary habits are difficult to change. However, many will be able to further decrease their consumption of meats, and, in their place, eat more fruit, vegetables, nuts, cereals, and legumes, with little difficulty.

Others may be more interested in knowing if there are particular foods they could emphasize, without making more major dietary changes, and still hope to gain some protection from these changes. This is where the evidence is less clear, but some suggestions can be made. The daily consumption of small quantities of nuts is very likely to provide some protection against CHD, as is the consumption of whole-grain cereals and breads. Added to this, reduced intake of saturated fats, particularly those in meats, is likely to be protective.

Other foods for which there is some evidence of benefits include fish, fruit, fiber, and plant sources of unsaturated fats. Further studies will provide additional evidence, but it is unlikely that moderate changes in the consumption of these foods will prove harmful and it is very likely that one or more will finally prove to have been beneficial.

FINDINGS FOR DIET AND CANCER

The risk factor concept is not nearly as well developed in cancer as in cardiovascular epidemiology, but some tentative conclusions can be drawn. Vegetarians typically have higher blood levels of phytoestrogens, folate, and other antioxidant substances—factors that protect against cancer in animals. Possibly relevant to female genital cancers is the observation that menarche is delayed in teenagers who either are vegetarians or eat meat analogues (often based on soybeans) more frequently. In addition, blood levels of natural estrogenic compounds are probably a little lower in adult vegetarian women. Greater lifelong exposure to natural estrogens modestly elevates the risk of breast and possibly ovarian cancer and may explain some of the excess risk for omnivores. That vegetarians are, on average, thinner than omnivores also decreases the risk of certain cancers, probably because of the resulting lower levels of both blood insulin and endogenous estrogens in the vegetarian, postmenopausal women.

The evidence that the frequency of cancers at some sites is lower for vegetarians comes almost entirely from studies of Adventists. These are probably the best studies available at present, however. The collaborative analysis of several prospective vegetarian studies was restricted to fatal cancers. This is a problem not only because fatal cases do not represent all cancers at a particular site, but also because the lower numbers of such cancers decrease statistical power. It was also difficult to find a biologically appropriate definition of a nonvegetarian in the collaborative study.

The incidence of cancers at many body sites is decreased for Adventists, but for some sites it is not clear whether this is due to vegetarianism, or even whether it relates to dietary habits. A vegetarian diet involves much more than the absence of meat, so whether differences in cancer incidence are due to meat intake or to other factors is a complex question, although some tentative conclusions are possible. In fact, there are indications that reduced meat consumption is connected to lower risk of some cancers. Within the Adventist population, there are five sites—the colon, bladder, ovaries, pancreas, and prostate—at which vegetarian Adventists experienced fewer new cancers than nonvegetarian Adventists to a statistically significant extent.

The evidence that vegetarian as compared with nonvegetarian, Adventists have a lower risk of colon cancer is strong. Moreover, it appeared that the meat (both red and white meat) was one important active principle that increased risk for the nonvegetarians. An adjustment for a variety of other foods did not change this result. Several other large studies have also found evidence that meat consumption is hazardous for risk of colon cancer. Similarly, the California Adventist data implicated meat as an important risk factor for ovarian and bladder cancer, and this did not seem to be confounded by other dietary factors. However, studies with larger numbers of cases would increase confidence in these results. Although the evidence suggested that meat and fish may play a role in prostate cancer, the effect was not quite statistically significant in a multivariate analysis, although its estimated magnitude was quite large. Again, bigger and better studies are needed. The decreased risk of pancreatic cancer among vegetarians appeared to be largely due to their greater intake of legumes and fruit, rather than the absence of meat.

The identification of other individual foods that may change the risk of cancers can only be tentative, partly because of the relatively small numbers of cancer cases of a particular type that are usually available in a particular study and also because of the measurement errors that frustrate nutritional epidemiologists. Aside from meat, there is, however, suggestive evidence for a number of other foods.

Many research studies make it clear that fruit and vegetables, as a group, are associated with decreased frequency of many cancers, including those of the lung, stomach, colon, and, probably, the pancreas, breast, and bladder (Potter, 1997a). This protection may result from chemicals distributed widely throughout the plant kingdom. Phytoestrogens such as isoflavones and lignans, folic acid (a cofactor in the methyl-donor system), or antioxidants such as the flavonoids, carotenoids, vitamin C, and vitamin E, may have protective roles. However, strong evidence for implicating most of these factors in human carcinogenesis is lacking, although that for isoflavones and folate is most interesting. Whatever the active chemical factors might be, the lower rates of certain cancers among vegetarians are no doubt in part related to their greater consumption of fruits and vegetables, and for some cancers this may be more important than the avoidance of meat.

The consumption of legumes may decrease the risk of colon cancer, although the rather scanty evidence from prospective studies, aside from the Adventist Health Study, is conflicting. Potential mechanisms have been described. Legumes may also protect against prostate and pancreatic cancer, according to multivariate evidence from the Adventist Health Study. There is little prospective evidence available from other studies that would either support or detract from these findings. The consumption of legumes, in our experience, is particularly difficult to measure accurately as beans may be included in many diverse dishes, and subjects have difficulty in summarizing this information. Thus research results relating to legumes (including those for California Adventists) need to be treated with some caution.

Much more work is necessary, but consumption of soy products may decrease the frequency of new prostate and breast cancers. If so, this is probably related to the high content of phytoestrogenic isoflavones in soy. The frequency of both prostate and breast cancers is much lower in Asia, where soy is consumed in larger quantities.

Some studies, including the Adventist Health Study, have found evidence that tomatoes may protect against prostate cancer, perhaps due to their content of the antioxidant known as lycopene. Analyses from the Adventist Health Study also find a strong protective association between greater consumption of tomatoes and the risk of epithelial ovarian centers.

Those who wish to reduce cancer risk by identifying specific foods to include or avoid, without taking a broader approach to dietary change, will have a difficult time finding conclusive evidence to guide them. However, suggestions would be to increase the intake of legumes, fruits, tomatoes, and soy products and to decrease the consumption of meats. There are no known hazards associated with such choices, and probably several of these changes will finally turn out to have been beneficial.

FINDINGS FOR DIET AND LIFE EXPECTANCY

Adventist vegetarians in California live substantially longer than other Californians. Estimates show an extra 9.5 and 6.2 years, respectively, for males and females. California Adventists, particularly vegetarian Adventists, are probably the longest-lived population that has yet been formally described. Within the Adventist population, vegetarian men live longer than their non-vegetarian counterparts by 2.1 years, and for women the difference is 1.8 years. This is despite the fact that the nonvegetarian Adventists eat meat only three times weekly on average.

These extra years for vegetarians are undoubtedly due to a number of factors that differ between vegetarians and nonvegetarians, aside from meat consumption. However, even after adjusting for differences in exercise habits, nut consumption, and obesity, we found that the vegetarian men still lived 1.53 years longer, and the women lived 1.51 years longer, than the nonvegetarians. Presumably, much of this increased life expectancy is then due to the avoidance of meat. While the extra fruit and vegetables consumed probably also play a part, we could find no direct evidence to support this in the Adventist data. The British experience, when we study the health of vegetarians and other health-conscious individuals, was that their mortality rates were greatly lower than those for the general population, which is thus consistent with the results for California Adventists.

The dietary factors implicated in longevity differences among the Adventists were meat-eating, nut consumption, and dietary and other habits that prevent overweight. The combined effects of diet apparently account for a difference of 4.5 to 5.7 years in life expectancy.

Opinions will differ as to the value of extra years of life, but many would agree that the addition of 4 to 6 years, resulting from prudent dietary choices, is an extraordinary benefit, as long as a high quality of life is maintained. There are no data that directly compare the quality of life among vegetarians at a given age with that of omnivores, but there are some indications that this is probably higher in the vegetarians. The alternative conclusion would be that the vegetarians experience the same deterioration in the quality of life as others do, but that they somehow manage to survive for a number of extra years in a state of poor health. This seems unlikely as analyses from the California Adventist data have shown that at the same ages, the vegetarian Adventists use health services less frequently and take fewer medications than nonvegetarians Adventists. Further, cardiovascular disease, cancer, diabetes, arthritis, and hypertension embrace most of the disorders that impair quality of life among the elderly. Yet these are the medical conditions that, at a given age, are experienced less frequently by vegetarians. It is also relevant that in a nonvegetarian population, Vita et al. (1998) showed directly that better health habits were in fact associated with a better quality of life among elderly subjects.

Whether vegans experience better health and greater life expectancy than lacto-ovo vegetarians cannot be definitely established by the existing data. Although they probably have modestly lower levels of blood LDL cholesterol and blood pressure, and definitely lower body mass index, than other vegetarians, it is unclear whether this translates to a reduced risk of chronic disease and mortality. The evidence that exists does not suggest major differences.

Readers who are vegetarians should be comforted by the knowledge that their nontraditional dietary habits have some important advantages for health and longevity. Although many questions remain, the evidence in favor of many of these benefits is overwhelming. Interested nonvegetarian readers will almost certainly also gain some health benefits by making the transition to a vegetarian diet or at least moving in this direction.

SUGGESTIONS FOR FUTURE RESEARCH

Since so little is known with certainty about the effects of specific foods and nutrients on health, the list of important research questions could be very long. The next few paragraphs concentrate on questions about common foods, important nutrients, and those that studies of vegetarians may address more clearly.

General Questions

Although this book presents information about the probable effects of diet on heart disease, cancer, diabetes, hypertension, arthritis, obesity, and life expectancy, it is quite likely that habitual diet choices may also affect the risk of osteoporosis, dementia, other neurologic disorders, inflammatory bowel disease, peptic ulcers, thyroid disease, renal failure, and perhaps autoimmune disorders. Little prospective evidence exists, yet these are common disorders that result in much morbidity and urgently need further study to identify possible dietary links with risk.

When comparing vegetarian and nonvegetarian diets, it is important to clarify the role of meat as compared with differences in consumption of fruit, vegetables, grains and nuts. The existing evidence does allow some conclusions, but confidence intervals are often wide in multivariate analyses, and the effects of measurement errors are unclear. In a similar vein, it has been difficult to distinguish the effects of red and white meats on health, or even whether there is a distinction.

Claims that soy products influence the risk of cardiovascular disease, certain cancers, osteoporosis, and even Alzheimer's disease have drawn much publicity. Although some preliminary epidemiologic evidence supports this assertion for breast and prostate cancers, most research to date has only documented effects of soy foods on risk factors. Given the complexity of an intact organism, with many competing effects and homeostatic mechanisms, there is a leap in promoting the idea of improving a known risk factor to that of preventing a disease. More research is necessary. In the United States, vegetarians are a convenient research population. They consume more soy products than others because soy is a good source of protein.

Cardiovascular Disease

Whether the lower HDL cholesterol levels observed for Adventists actually increase their risk of CHD is an intriguing question. This may also be related to the counterintuitive observation that in international comparisons, many populations at lower risk for CHD have lower levels of HDL cholesterol (as well as lower LDL cholesterol). The effect of a particular HDL cholesterol value may depend strongly on levels of other risk factors, or dietary habits, but this is poorly understood.

The effect of nut consumption in reducing the risk of CHD is much greater than that expected from the amount of LDL cholesterol lowering produced by the nuts. Is this due to associated factors (e.g., other dietary habits) or to nonfat elements within the nuts that reduce the risk in other ways?

Whether fruit consumption reduces the risk of CHD is controversial. There may be a threshold effect, such that increasing consumption above a low level increases protection, but additional protection is not seen beyond a moderate level of intake. Studies of vegetarians (and others), outside a high fruit-eating area such as California, may address this matter more effectively.

It is likely that whole grains and cereals reduce the risk of CHD. However, it is not at all clear whether this is due to their content of dietary fiber, folate, antioxidant vitamins, tocotrienols, phytoestrogens, or other factors.

Results from studies of Adventists suggest that meat consumption increases the risk of CHD, especially in younger and middle-aged women and in men of all ages. Further support from other studies would be useful. Does white meat increase risk also? Is it the saturated fat, the lack of dietary fiber, and/or other factors that cause this effect?

The possible role of folate, flavonoids, and other antioxidants in decreasing the risk of CHD needs further support. A problem has been the fact that often indices of these factors are also good measures of other factors that are well represented in fruits and vegetables. Thus, it is difficult to isolate the effect of one factor and to be sure it is not mixed with that of another.

Alcohol in modest doses appears to be protective for CHD, but it is not established that alcohol would further decrease the risk for vegetarian populations or for others at low risk.

Cancers

That meat consumption can increase cancer risk is still not widely accepted and this assertion does need further support. Aside from the probable effect of meat consumption in increasing the risk of colon cancer, and a possible effect on the risk of prostate cancer, it may also increase the risk at certain less common cancer sites (the bladder and ovaries), according to the Adventist data. Larger studies should help clarify this situation. The British studies of vegetarians do not clearly support these conclusions. Is this just an artifact due to the relatively low meat intake found for the non-vegetarian comparison group in some studies, the exclusion of nonfatal cancers, or the smaller numbers, or are there really geographic and cultural differences?

Our studies (and those of others) suggest a special role in cancer prevention for certain other foods. These include fruits, tomatoes, cruciferous vegetables, possibly soy foods, and other legumes. Future larger studies with high-quality dietary data should help clarify these tentative conclusions. Other vegetables may also have beneficial effects, but the evidence is less clear or even conflicting. These include the onion family, whole grains, and other good sources of flavonoids (e.g., berries), phytoestrogens, and folate.

The role of dietary calcium is presently a controversial one as some evidence suggests that it increases the risk of prostate cancer among men, but decreases the risk of colon cancer. Studies of populations that contain many vegetarians should be helpful as vegetarians often have an especially wide range of calcium intake. Some stricter vegetarians have low levels of intake as they consume few dairy products, while others use calcium supplements, and so have average or even high calcium intake levels.

Life Expectancy

We have identified five factors (three of which are dietary, or related to diet) that appear to influence life expectancy. Undoubtedly, there are others awaiting a confirmation. An important unanswered question involves the extent to which these factors do or do not improve the quality of life at a given age. This has real implications for both the desirability of the extra years, and the costs for those years to the health system.

Effects of most risk factors appear to diminish in old age, but we found this not to be so for nut consumption in California Adventists. This needs confirmation and clarification from larger studies of very elderly subjects. It is also unclear whether changes in health behavior that occur in middle-aged or older subjects are still effective. It could be that the apparent effects we observe at these older ages are just the result of a diminishing influence of dietary patterns present when subjects were younger, and that this reduced pathophysiology at that time. Studies that run long enough to record ages when changes in dietary habits took place would allow more informative analyses.

Genes

Finally, with the recent advances in our understanding of the human genome, there is at least the potential for greatly refining the predictive ability of epidemiologic studies. Most investigators consider it very likely that the effects of even established risk factors are not at all uniform across individuals. We all have at least slight differences in our body chemistry, much of which depends on individual genetic makeup. These differences may result in foods being metabolized at different rates or even into different chemical products. Hence it is entirely possible that when there is an overall 25% reduction in risk of some disease in those eating a particular food, two or more very different effects may be blended. For instance, there may be 30% of the population with some particular genetic characteristic who experience an 80% reduction in risk when eating the food, while the remaining 70% get no benefit from it at all. It would then be much more efficient to concentrate preventive efforts using this food on the 30% who will benefit, if they can be identified. Whether such different effects in different genetic subgroups will prove to be common is not yet certain.

Appendix

The Epidemiologic Studies of Adventist Health:
Their Design, Size, and Number of
Disease Events

A BRIEF HISTORY OF THE MAJOR HEALTH STUDIES OF ADVENTISTS

Although Adventists have long been convinced of the benefits of their special lifestyle, it was not until the early 1950s that the first scientific studies (Hardinge and Stare, 1954a, 1954b) were conducted to document the validity of this belief. Around this same time, with the Framingham Heart Study in its infancy and the seminal work of Ancel Keys and his colleagues attracting more attention, medical scientists developed an interest in dietary fats and blood cholesterol, and their effects on cardiovascular disease. Consequently, Adventists became an attractive group in which to test these theories, particularly those associating diet and the absence of cigarette smoking with risk of both cardiovascular disease and cancer.

In 1958, Drs. Frank Lemon and R. T. Walden received funding from federal sources to conduct a large epidemiologic study of nearly 23,000 Adventists in California. The researchers, based at Loma Linda University—a Seventh-day Adventist institution in southern California, continued collecting data intensively through 1965, and others continued follow-up less formally until 1985. This study was labeled the Adventist Mortality Study. The Adventist Mortality Study found that, overall, of 100 non-Adventist California men who died of cancer at a particular age, only 60 Adventist men of the same age died of cancer; Adventist women had a risk of 76% as compared with their similar-aged counterparts. Death from coronary disease among Adventist men as compared to non-Adventist men was 34% less; and for Adventist women, 2% less at the same ages. Of course, even Adventists eventually die, and the causes of death (irrespective of age) in Adventists and others is a different question that is addressed in Chapter 4.

In 1974, Drs. Roland Phillips and Jan Kuzma, also researchers from Loma Linda University, received funding from the National Cancer Institute to conduct a second large study of diet, cigarette smoking, and risk of cancer, again among California Adventists. The study began in 1974, and the scientists continued collecting data on both fatal and nonfatal events from this population through 1982, with a subsequent follow-up study of deaths only, through 1988.

In 1980, I received funding for a cardiovascular "add-on" to this cancer study from the National Heart, Lung and Blood Institute, and later, funding from the National Institute of Aging, for a variety of demographic studies using the large data bank already in place at Loma Linda University. This second group of studies that began in the 1970s is collectively labeled the Adventist Health Study.

At present, Loma Linda University has received funding to develop a yet larger cohort study of both black and white California Adventists. This will take advantage of what has already been learned, using new methods and technologies to help answer an increasing list of questions associating diet—or other aspects of lifestyle—with risk of chronic disease.

Starting in the 1970s, a number of other studies, often based outside the United States, have also examined both the causes of death and the risk-factor profile of Seventh-day Adventists. The interest that funding agencies have shown in these studies is a reflection of the conviction among health professionals that diet is one of several powerful influences that alter the risk of chronic disease. Other factors include cigarette smoking, alcohol consumption, exercise, and psychosocial variables. Adventists differed from the general population in all of these areas—generally in a direction thought to be protective against many diseases—but more evidence was needed.

This group, which is well integrated into American society, presents an opportunity to test many theories by making comparisons between their health and that of the general population. However, this objective is not as straightforward as it sounds. Clearly, one must compare like with like in terms of other unalterable risk factors for disease, such as age and gender. In addition, education is now known to be strongly associated with many chronic diseases, and differences between the educational status of Adventists and others may distort comparisons if analyses are not thoughtfully planned.

It is also not fair to compare the disease experience of a voluntary study group with that of the whole general population. Persons volunteering for epidemiologic studies are widely known to be more healthy than others. This dilemma needs careful handling in comparisons between voluntary Adventist study groups and others. Such comparisons could be global, comparing all Adventists with non-Adventists, or may compare non-Adventists with subgroups of Adventists (such as vegetarian Adventists or those with high levels of social support). Either volunteer groups should be compared with other such groups, or else special steps should be taken in the analyses to ensure a fair comparison.

The remainder of this Appendix gives details of the design of several studies that have been conducted to evaluate the health of Adventists, both in California and other countries. Results from these studies are found in various chapters of this book.

DESIGN OF THE ADVENTIST MORTALITY STUDY

In 1958, the goal was to enroll all California Seventh-day Adventists in a study cohort (Dysinger et al., 1963; Lemon et al., 1964; Lemon and Walden, 1966; Lemon and Kuzma, 1969; Phillips, 1975; Phillips et al., 1978, 1980a). Although church membership rolls existed, they did not include demographic information, even such as age. A free weekly official church newspaper is mailed to all Adventists, and the printers therefore had a comprehensive list of names and addresses. Using this list, five copies of a questionnaire were mailed to each household with a request that the head of household enroll all Adventist household members. Three repeat mailings were sent to those who did not respond. An additional method of enrollment used a responsible member from each of the 341 churches (often the church pastor) to make public announcements over a period of several weeks and to distribute questionnaires.

Using these methods, 47,866 individuals were enrolled. However, it became clear that the existing registration and mailing lists included inactive or unavailable members. Church clerks and pastors were asked to provide an independent count of active members and did so for churches that included 91% of the total membership. Using this amended count as a denominator, study investigators estimated that 88% of active and "available" members had been enrolled.

The questionnaire was extremely brief by present standards and asked about gender, date of birth, length of church membership, race, marital status, place of birth, occupational and residence history, and a general statement concerning health. The intention was to calculate mortality rates according to levels of some of these demographic variables and then to compare them to similar rates for other Californians.

In 1960, a total of 21,380 of the above individuals, and an additional 6,150 Adventists who did not previously enroll, all over the age of 29 years, volunteered to complete a second four-page questionnaire. Thus, a total of 27,530 subjects formed this study population. The study was conducted with the assistance of Dr. E. C. Hammond, and the questionnaire was identical to that used in his American Cancer Society (ACS) Prospective Study of one million persons from the general population that also began in 1960 (Hammond, 1966). The Adventists were members in 198 of the 351 Adventist congregations in California. Volunteers from each congregation were responsible for enrolling 10 to 20 adult local members, all of whom were members of five households. The volunteers also agreed to report each year from 1960 to 1965 on any deaths in their congregations, as one objective was to calculate death rates in Adventists, and another was to find whether Adventists with different health habits experienced different mortality.

To further help in the search for all fatalities between 1960 and 1965, church clerks were asked to complete a brief form that gave essential information necessary to identify deceased study subjects on the state death records. As a routine part of their work, these clerks also provided brief details of deceased members to the central church offices. Thus comparisons between study data and these reports were made. Finally, notifications of deaths were also identified by annual or semiannual mailings to study subjects. These methods enabled researchers to obtain death certificates from the California Department of Public Health. The cause of death was given by the "underlying" cause of death on the death certificate. A death certificate includes both immediate and underlying causes of death, as assigned by the certifying physician. The underlying cause is the basic medical problem, possibly initiating a chain of events leading to death. For instance, advanced cancer may cause pneumonia; the latter then being the immediate cause, but the cancer is the underlying cause of death. After six years of follow-up, the vital status (i.e., living or deceased) of more than 98% of study participants was established.

In a less formal extended follow-up from 1966 to 1976, an individual's vital status was ascertained only by computer linkage with the California State Death Tapes. Evidence from a substudy suggested that 93% of deaths were detected from these tapes. Adjustments were made to mortality rates to account for the undetected deaths and also to allow for the 3% to 6% of the total deaths estimated to occur out of state—the proportion of these increasing with duration of follow-up (Kuzma and Beeson, 1981).

The American Cancer Society questionnaire included questions on personal health, a limited exercise and dietary section, and data regarding other risk factors. Thus this information allowed some analyses within the Adventist group, comparing Adventists with differing demographic attributes and behaviors. However, the endpoint could include only fatal (rather than all incident) events, as nonfatal cancers and heart attacks were not sought.

The earliest reports from the Adventist Mortality Study were from all or portions of the original 47,866 subjects who completed only the first brief questionnaire (Lemon and Walden, 1964, 1966). Subsequently, a subset of the 27,530 subjects who completed the more extensive American Cancer Society questionnaire were included in the most complete and

Table A–1. Adventist Mortality Study (AMS): Age-Gender Structure of the Population More Than 35 Years of Age in 1960 Who Completed the American Cancer Society (ACS) Questionnaire

Age	California Adventist AMS Study Participants		California Non-Adventist ACS Study Participants	
	Male	Female	Male	Female
35–44	2,254	3,569	4,764	11,876
45–54	2,015	3,443	23,015	25,499
55–64	1,497	3,131	13,599	15,177
65–74	1,369	2,848	6,248	8,156
75–84	812	1,500	1,582	2,347
85+	169	333	137	326
All ages	8,116	14,824	49,345	63,381

informative published analyses of this population (Kuzma and Beeson, 1981; Lemon and Kuzma, 1969; Phillips et al, 1978, 1980a, 1980b). These were the 22,940 respondents over age 34 years in 1960. Table A–1 shows the age and sex breakdown for this latter group and also for the non-Adventist comparison study (American Cancer Society Study). Clearly there were proportionately many more elderly Adventists enrolled, but disease rate comparisons adjust for this difference in age structure between the two studies.

DESIGN OF THE LATER ADVENTIST HEALTH STUDY

During 1973 to 1976, two questionnaires were developed for use in an upcoming new prospective cohort study (Beeson et al, 1989). The first questionnaire was designed primarily as a census instrument to be completed by the head of the household; it documented basic demographic variables, along with a brief history of church membership and education for all householders. The second, the lifestyle questionnaire, was much longer and was designed to be completed by each individual in the household, documenting his or her own medical history, use of selected medications, diet, exercise, psychosocial variables, and certain religious activities.

This second cohort of Adventists was identified in 1974 with the goal of enrolling all Adventists over the age of 25 years living at that time in California. Current directories from all Adventist churches in California were computerized, and a census questionnaire was sent to all 63,530 identified households. The 36,805 replies from heads of households identified 59,081 individuals more than 25 years old.

In 1976, a lifestyle questionnaire was sent to all of these individuals who still survived. Of the 45,537 non-Hispanic white subjects, 34,192 re-

Table A–2. Adventist Health Study: Non-Hispanic White Participants Who Completed Both Census and Lifestyle Questionnaires

Sex	Age at Census Return	Incidence Population[a]	
		No. of Adventists	No. of Non-Adventists
Male	25–34	2,431	409
	35–44	1,925	416
	45–54	2,381	462
	55–64	2,201	497
	65–74	1,651	322
	75–84	842	112
	85–94	188	15
	95+	3	2
	All ages	11,622	2,235
Female	25–34	3,662	178
	35–44	3,008	142
	45–54	3,566	131
	55–64	3,821	127
	65–74	3,289	100
	75–84	1,811	58
	85–94	412	16
	95+	17	3
	All Ages	19,586	755
Total, all ages		31,208	2,990

[a]Incidence population consists of all non-Hispanic whites in the study population who completed both the census and the lifestyle questionnaires and who lived in a home with at least one Adventist. Thus about 10% were non-Adventists

turned lifestyle questionnaires; of the 3475 black subjects 1739 returned these questionnaires. Table A–2 shows the numbers of non-Hispanic white subjects, enrolled by age and sex, who completed both census and lifestyle questionnaires. The roughly 10% of non-Adventists were enrolled because they lived in households containing at least one Adventist member who was also enrolled.

As the number of black subjects was much smaller, certain analyses took advantage of the larger number who completed the census questionnaire only, while other analyses require data from the lifestyle questionnaire and relate to the smaller group who completed both questionnaires. Table A–3 shows the person-years at risk (as well as the deaths) in these two overlapping cohorts of black subjects in the Adventist Health Study. The person-years concept used in this table is often used to represent the effective size of the population, rather than simply the number of persons who began the study.

The evaluation of diet was by 55 food-frequency questions and a dozen other qualitative dietary questions. The food-frequency method is usually considered the only practical way to assess diet by questionnaire in thousands of subjects. In the Adventist Health Study, questions simply required

Table A–3. Adventist Health Study: Person-Years in the Black Population by Age and Gender, also Divided into Those Completing Only the Census Questionnaire or Both Questionnaires

| | Census Questionnaire Population[a] (n = 3475) | | | | Lifestyle Questionnaire Population[b] (n = 1739) | | | |
| | Males | | Females | | Males | | Females | |
Age	Deaths	P-Y	Deaths	P-Y	Deaths	P-Y	Deaths	P-Y
25–34	4	1,656	0	2,061	0	414	0	606
35–44	7	3,252	7	4,403	2	1,062	3	1,886
45–54	17	3,218	12	4,619	7	1,241	4	2,160
55–64	35	2,836	27	4,404	13	1,222	6	2,257
65–74	43	1,993	53	3,552	17	886	19	1,964
75–84	37	879	64	2,228	19	427	29	1,194
85–94	36	343	58	750	14	197	17	350
95+	5	39	11	82	1	8	2	19
Totals	184	14,216	232	22,099	73	5,457	80	10,436

P-Y, person-years between study baseline and fatal event or removal from study.

[a]Follow-up 1974–1985.

[b]Follow-up 1977–1985. These subjects also completed the census questionnaire

Table A–4. Example of Dietary Questions from the AHS Lifestyle Questionnaire

1. What ONE type of bread do you use most of the time? *Mark only the one type used most frequently.*

White (*enriched or unenriched*) .... □
100% whole wheat or whole grain .... □
Sprouted wheat or wheatberry .... □
Other (*rye, cracked wheat, pumpernickel, soy, etc.*) .... □

2. Mark the box which comes closest to how often you use each food when you are following your usual routine. <u>*Be sure*</u> *to mark in the correct column and mark "never" if never used.*

a. Eggs (*except those used in recipes*)   (a)
b. Cheese (*except cottage cheese*)   (b)
c. Meat, poultry, or fish   (c)
d. Sweets and desserts   (d)

		d	c	b	a
Current use:	Never	□	□	□	□
	Less than one/MONTH	□	□	□	□
	1–2 times per MONTH	□	□	□	□
	1–2 times per WEEK	□	□	□	□
	3–4 times per WEEK	□	□	□	□
	5–6 times per WEEK	□	□	□	□
	Once per DAY	□	□	□	□
	More than once/DAY	□	□	□	□

3. Mark the box which comes closest to how frequently you NOW use each food or beverage when following your usual routine. <u>*Be sure*</u> *to mark in the correct column and mark "never" for foods you never use.*

a. Low fat (2%) milk   (a)
b. Nonfat (skim) milk   (b)
c. Soymilk   (c)

		c	b	a
Current use:	Never or almost never	□	□	□
	Less than once/WEEK	□	□	□
	Several times per WEEK	□	□	□
	Once per DAY	□	□	□
	2–3 times per DAY	□	□	□
	4–5 times per DAY	□	□	□
	Over 5 times per DAY	□	□	□

subjects to nominate one of eight frequencies of consumption for each of the 55 foods. The frequencies ranged from "rarely or never" to "more than six times daily" (see Table A–4).

For most variables in the census and lifestyle questionnaires, the rate of missing data was between 4% and 7%. There did not appear to be any excess for "sensitive" variables among Adventists, such as pork consumption, cigarette smoking, or use of alcohol (Beeson et al., 1989). Thus, investigators believe that the population responded as accurately to these variables as any others. Nevertheless, with this potential sensitivity in mind, the investigators gave much effort to assuring study subjects of the anonymity of their responses.

Upon completion of the lifestyle questionnaire, the non-Hispanic white population was followed for six years, until December 1982, to collect all new or incident events of cancer and coronary heart disease. The same population was again followed, until 1988, to document fatalities only and to obtain death certificates for those deceased. Black Adventists were followed through 1985, collecting fatalities only, but as death certificates were not obtained, the causes of death are unknown.

The follow-up of the non-Hispanic white subjects between 1976 and 1982 required documentation of subsequent fatal and nonfatal events. This was accomplished using several methods, but first by the use of an annual mailed contact, when subjects indicated on a simple questionnaire whether they had been hospitalized since they completed the last such questionnaire, and if so where and when. The response rates to those annual questionnaires always exceeded 90%, and in the most important final contact early in 1993, the response was 99.5%.

Investigators used this information to guide study field representatives who collected details of these hospitalizations. They visited each California hospital named by any subject and reviewed the individual's medical chart. If there was any mention of cancer, tumor, neoplasm, or malignancy, selected contents of the chart were microfilmed. Similarly, if there was any mention of myocardial infarction, coronary thrombosis, cardiac arrest, myocardial ischemia, coronary insufficiency, coronary angiography, or heart catheterization, the medical and nursing history and electrocardiographs were microfilmed, and cardiac enzymes results were abstracted to coding forms.

In this way, field representatives visited 698 hospitals within California. Study participants also were hospitalized outside of California, if they had moved or were on vacation. The same data was obtained from 960 out-of-state hospitals by mail. These contacts concerned 32,451 hospitalizations for 18,053 individuals.

Fatal events in non-Hispanic white subjects, many of which occurred out of the hospital, were also found by the use of church records, by responses to our annual mailed questionnaires by next of kin, and by computerized matching to the California State Death Tapes (Beeson et al., 1990). As 15% or so of our population moved out of state, computerized matching with the National Death Index was also used to find deaths out of state beginning in 1979 when this service became available.

The copied materials were used to establish a diagnosis of cancer, which required histologic confirmation. The diagnosis of definite coronary heart disease used published international diagnostic criteria (Gillum et al.,

1984), following detailed coding (known as Minnesota coding) of the electrocardiographs (Prineas et al., 1982), and contact with friends or next of kin to establish the circumstances of a death. Cardiac enzyme results were also used as required by the criteria.

As a result of the study design, 8.7% of the individuals who completed both questionnaires were non-Adventist members of Adventist households. This varied little by age; however, 3.9% of females—but 19.2% of males—were non-Adventist. Non-Adventists were usually excluded from coronary heart disease analyses, but not from cancer analyses, where statistical power was a greater problem due to smaller numbers of a particular cancer. Non-Adventist husbands could be considered an intermediate group, who often ate quite similarly to their wives.

Follow-up of total mortality in Black Adventists was less formal, based on intensive tracing using church records, friends, and fellow parishioners. In addition, computerized matching with the California State Death Tapes was performed. The status of about 7% of these individuals could not be determined by these means, and as investigators had had no contact since completing the baseline data, these subjects were excluded from survival analyses.

During the development phase of the Adventist Health Study, a number of substudies were conducted to assess the likely accuracy of the questionnaire information to be obtained and to help with selection of the best questions for the questionnaire. The most significant of these is the Special Nutrition Substudy (SNSS). This study, perhaps the first validation study of a food-frequency questionnaire, allowed us to assess the accuracy of the dietary component of the lifestyle questionnaire. From the area close to Loma Linda, California, 147 subjects—41 men and 106 women—were randomly selected from church directories. Over a period of three months, these subjects completed five 24-hour recalls by telephone, documenting what they had eaten on three weekdays, one Saturday, and one Sunday. During this period, they also completed an extensive food-frequency questionnaire, from which dietary questions were subsequently selected for the lifestyle questionnaire. Correlations between food-frequency questions and important nutrients, calculated from the 24-hour recalls, were used to select the best food-frequency questions.

More recent analyses of the SNSS data have allowed us to estimate the amount of random error that is incorporated into our food-frequency estimates of dietary habits. For some foods and nutrients, this is considerable but very similar to that found in other studies (Willett, 1998b). Understanding the nature and magnitude of dietary measurement errors is extremely important, as investigators can then use newly developed statistical techniques to correct for such errors, although this is at the expense of requiring longer and larger studies (Fraser and Stram, 2001; Rosner et al,

1990). These errors are one reason why it is difficult to establish reliable links between diet and disease and, if appropriate corrections are not made, why some studies find quite different estimates of associations than others. The lay person should place more emphasis on stronger associations (relative risk greater than 1.50, or a protective relative risk of less than 0.67) that are highly statistically significant ($p < 0.01$) and that are found in at least two or three well-analyzed studies. This would avoid much confusion.

STUDY DESIGNS FOR ADVENTISTS IN NORWAY, THE NETHERLANDS, DENMARK, AND JAPAN

Norway

The first published comparison of mortality between Adventists and non-Adventists outside California came from Norway (Waaler and Hjort, 1981). Doctors Waaler and Hjort used a church membership question in the 1960 population census to identify 5292 Adventists. The Central Office of Statistics registered deaths and emigration for the whole population, including the Adventists. However, members of the cohort leaving the church during follow-up could not be identified and were not removed. The investigators followed 4044 of these individuals between ages 35 and 90, during the observation period from January 1961 through December 1977. There was a relative excess of older women and fewer younger men in the study group than in the general population. The endpoints were deaths and cause of death, found from the national data bank. During the 48,175 person-years of follow-up, 1173 observed deaths were then compared to expected deaths, the latter also based on national mortality statistics, to form age-standardized mortality ratios.

An extension of this design and improvement on it underlies three reports by Dr. V. Fønnebø (Fønnebø, 1992, 1994; Fønnebø and Helseth, 1991). He identified Adventists in January 1961 by using official church records, but he also constructed this as a dynamic cohort whereby persons entered, remained, or left the group between 1961 and 1986 as they joined, retained membership, left the church, or died. This study included 7253 individuals.

The follow-up for all-cause mortality and cancer incidence used two sources of information. Norwegians have an 11-digit personal identification number, which can be linked to national mortality files. Vital status follow-up by this means was possible in 98% of the individuals. In addition, linkage was possible to the Norwegian Cancer Registry, which is a virtually complete register for solid tumors. During the 26 years of follow-up, 712 cancers were observed from 121,448 person-years, and 2476

Table A–5. The Population Studied for Mortality in Norway, 1962–1986

| Age group | Person-Years | |
	Men ($n = 2476$)	Women ($n = 4697$)
<45	17,656	23,385
45–54	5,412	10,539
55–64	6,021	13,982
65–74	5,940	15,377
75–84	3,939	10,866
85–94	1,020	2,944
95+	78	130
Total	40,066	77,223

Source: Adapted and reprinted from Fonnebo V, Mortality in Norwegian Seventh-day Adventists 1962–1986, *J Clin Epidemiol* 45:157–167, 1992. Copyright 1992, with permission from Elsevier Science.

deaths from 117,289 person-years of Adventist follow-up. The age and gender structure of the mortality population is shown in Table A–5 (the population for the cancer incidence differed to a minor extent). Observed cases were compared to expected cases using rates from the Norwegian National Cancer Registry or national mortality statistics, to form standardized cancer incidence or mortality ratios.

Denmark

Dr. O. M. Jensen (Jensen, 1983) identified a group of Adventist men by virtue of their membership in the Danish Temperance Union, the great majority of whom had been lifelong teetotalers. All such Adventists who had Temperance Union membership between 1939 and 1963 were included and followed through December 1977. This represented 16,748 person-years of observation.

As with the first Norwegian Study, subjects leaving the Adventist church during follow-up were apparently neither noted nor excluded. Nearly 96% of the potentially eligible subjects were identified on various municipal and national registries and could be followed until death or emigration using national data bases. Follow-up included 781 individuals, and during this period, 61 incident cancers were identified by linkage with the Danish Cancer Registry. Cases observed in Adventists were compared to those expected, using Copenhagen age- and gender-specific incidence rates to form standardized incidence ratios.

Netherlands

Doctors J. Berkel and F. de Waard (Berkel, 1979; Berkel and deWaard, 1983) used church records to identify all Adventist church members in the

Table A–6. The Population Studied in the Netherlands, 1968–1977

	Person-Years	
Age group	Men	Women
10–24	1,540	2,286
25–34	2,212	3,140
35–44	2,087	2,929
45–54	1,820	3,355
55–64	1,744	3,729
65–74	1,364	3,980
75–84	655	2,162
85+	79	514
Total	11,501	22,095

Source: Adapted from Berkel J, *The Clean Life* (Amsterdam: Drukkerij Insulinde, 1979). Reprinted by permission.

Netherlands from 1968 to 1977. During this period, church membership in the Netherlands was between 3500 and 4000 persons. Individuals were eliminated from the study by death, but not for leaving the Adventist church. New church members were added to the study group. In this way 11,501 male and 22,095 female person-years were accumulated with an age distribution as shown in Table A–6 (Berkel and deWaard, 1983).

Church records were used for mortality follow-up, as was linkage with the Central Bureau of Statistics, which allowed determination of the cause of death. A total of 522 individuals died during the follow-up period, and the cause of death was identified for 92.3%.

Japan

Doctor M. Kuratsune and colleagues (Kuratsune et al., 1986) used church records to identify church members in January 1975 and then used the updates of these same records to confirm vital status during follow-up from January 1975 to January 1981. Individuals needed to have been Adventists at least five years before the study began and to have complete records regarding age, gender, and date of baptism from church record offices. These latter requirements excluded approximately 20% of the potential cohort. A further 951 individuals were excluded due to inadequate addresses, which interfered with follow-up. Thus the cohort finally consisted of 6742 individuals, about 30% male. In addition to church records, the "koseki" system of national records was also used to determine vital status where necessary.

During follow-up, 95 men and 197 women died. Observed deaths were compared to expected deaths using rates from the Japanese population in 1975, to produce standardized mortality ratios.

Table A-7. Number of Common Site-Specific Cancers and Coronary Heart Disease (CHD) Events in the Various Studies of Adventists[a]

		AMS[b] (1960-1976)	AHS[c] (1976-1982)	AHS[b] (1976-1988)	Norway[d]	Netherlands	Denmark (Males)	Japan
Total fatalities	M	2,400	1,030	2,130	815	149	—	86
	F	3,804	1,446	3,422	1661	333	—	197
Fatal cardiovascular events	M	—	—	—	443	—	—	—
	F	—	—	—	902	—	—	—
Fatal CHD	M	901	136	358	—	—	—	18
	F	1,252	166	536	—	—	—	29
	M & F	—	—	—	197	99	—	—
Incident CHD events	M	—	411	—	—	—	—	—
	F	—	355	—	—	—	—	—
Fatal cerebrovascular disease	M	—	—	—	122	—	—	12
	F	—	—	—	—	—	—	32
	M & F	—	—	—	—	83	—	—
All fatal cancer	M	388	—	—	167	—	—	7
	F	661	—	—	297	—	—	36
	M & F	—	—	—	—	115	—	—
All incident cancer	M	—	598	—	247	—	61	—
	F	—	862	—	465	—	—	—
	M & F	—	—	—	—	—	—	—
Colon cancer[e]	M	59	62	—	—	—	1	1
	F	91	95	—	—	—	—	1
	M & F	—	—	—	58	—	—	—
Lung cancer[e]	M	24	—	—	—	—	3	0
	F	18	—	—	—	—	—	4
	M & F	—	37	—	64	15	—	—
Breast cancer[e]	F	160	15	—	32	12	—	2
Prostate cancer[e]	M	78	180	—	92	18	10	—

—, not available.

[a] Incident cases include fatal and nonfatal cases having no history of the disease at study baseline. Incident cases are reported from AHS, Norway, and Denmark, else fatal cases only.

[b] Fatal CHD cases were diagnosed as ICD9 codes 410–414 on the death certificate. Nonincident fatalities for both cancer and CHD are included.

[c] Reported here is follow-up 1976–1982 for non-Hispanic white subjects. Deaths for black AHS subjects are shown in Table A-3. Only incident cancers and CHD are reported. Total fatalities and coronary disease events include only Adventists. Cancer cases include non-Adventists living in Adventist households.

[d] Norwegian data are that of Fønnebø, which overlaps that of Waaler and Hjort (1960–1977). See page 287.

[e] Incident where available, else fatal only.

EVENT NUMBERS IN THE DIFFERENT STUDIES

Finally, Table A–7 shows numbers of deaths or disease events in the various studies described (see Table A–3 for deaths observed in the Black Adventist Health Study cohorts). Note the distinction between incident and fatal cases of both ischemic heart disease and cancer that needs to be made when comparing these studies. Incident cases refer to all new cases, whether or not the subject survived, whereas fatal cases are only those in which death resulted. These two categories may be numerically quite different for the same disease. For instance, in the Adventist Health Study only about 18% of breast cancer cases become fatal breast cancers within five years of diagnosis. It is seen that the studies in California and Norway have provided the greatest numbers of disease events, although the other smaller studies are valuable by demonstrating a broad consistency of findings across several geographical locations.

Glossary

Acetylcholine: A chemical produced normally by nerve endings to transmit an impulse from one nerve cell to the next. In addition, this chemical will dilate arteries by stimulating the release of certain chemicals from the normal endothelium.

Adenocarcinoma: Adeno is a prefix that refers to glandular or secretory epithelial cells that are found in many organs of the body (e.g., lung, bowel, pancreas, prostate). An adenocarcinoma is a cancer that mainly involves such glandular cells.

Adipose: Fat beneath the skin.

Ancel Keys: Dr. Ancel Keys first convincingly linked dietary fat with blood cholesterol. This discovery spurred the American Heart Association to assume a leading role in urging Americans to change their eating habits.

Angiotensin: *See* Renin

Antemortem: Before death.

Antibody: *See* comment under Cellular immune response.

Antioxidant: A substance that suppresses chemical reactions characterized by the loss of an electron (a particle in an atom carrying negative charge). Oxidation reactions can seriously interfere with cellular chemistry.

Antiproliferative and Differentiating: Forces that reduce the rate of multiplication and division of cells, and lead them to express all the features of mature cells in that particular tissue.

Arrhythmia: Each heartbeat is stimulated in a regular pattern by a natural pacemaker within the heart called the sinus node. A variety of abnormalities, either of the sinus node or other parts of the heart, can produce irregular, very rapid, or very slow heart beats, all of which are called arrhythmias.

Baseline Data: That information gathered at the beginning of a cohort study against which later disease experience will be compared.

Bias: A technical term for playing favorites in choosing individuals for the study or in assessing their exposure or disease status. *Selection bias* can occur when not everyone eligible to be in a study can be selected, and when those selected are different in some way from those excluded. *Recall bias* occurs when the individual's ability to report past experiences may be affected by his or her preconceived ideas about what the answer should be. These and other problems can systematically lead to wrong estimates of effect measures such as the relative risk. Then the relative risk is biased.

Bias-Correction Techniques: Errors in measuring either risk factors (exposure variables) or disease outcome will often lead to an incorrect assessment of the effect of that risk factor on risk of disease. Bias-correction techniques are statistical methods that may at least partially correct these problems. *See* Regression calibration.

Biochemical Risk Factor: Chemicals found in living organisms that relate to risk of disease.

Biological Mechanism: The bodily chemistry or cellular interactions that result in a particular health outcome.

Blood Clotting Factors: The clotting of blood is a remarkably complicated process. Several chains of chemical reactions, along with the clumping of platelets, are necessary to form fibrin, the main chemical in the clot, from fibrinogen. The major chemicals that contribute to these chains of reactions are called clotting factors. Examples include factor VII, factor VIII, and thrombin.

Body Mass Index (BMI): A common measure of obesity that adjusts body weight for height. In fact, BMI = body weight/height^2. In the U.S. it is commonly in the range of 22 to 27 kg/m^2.

California State Lifetables: Publically available statistics that tabulate mortality rates and use them in lifetable analyses to predict life expectancy and related variables for the whole state of California.

Calorie-Dense: A food that contains more calories than the average food per gram of weight.

Carcinogen: A chemicals that can cause cancer, accelerate its growth, or both.

Cardiac Enzymes: Chemicals that are released to the bloodstream from damaged heart cells. Thus abnormally high blood levels will help diagnose a heart attack.

Carotenoids: A class of chemicals that are widespread among vegetables and fruits. They often give these foods their yellow, orange, or red colors. Beta-carotene is a particularly common member of this group, giving carrots their orange color, for instance. Lycopene is another, responsible for the red color of tomatoes. Several carotenoids have strong antioxidant properties.

Carotid Artery Wall Thickness: Over recent years advances in ultrasound technology have allowed researchers to image the wall of the carotid arteries (the main arteries in the neck supplying the head and brain with blood). A thicker wall is generally due to atherosclerosis (see Chapter 2) and seems to correlate moderately well with a higher risk of heart attack or stroke.

Case-Control Studies: *See* Retrospective studies.

Catecholamines: *See* Epinephrine.

Cellular Immune Response: The body's immune system is its defense against foreign chemicals, bacteria, viruses, and other microorganisms that may enter the body. Part of this system involves cells that accumulate around the foreign agent, may absorb and digest it, or secrete chemicals that immobilize or kill microorganisms. Another immunologic defense, the humoral immune system, comes from cells located in the spleen and lymph nodes that release chemicals (antibodies) into the bloodstream to attach to and disable specific foreign agents wherever they are located in the body.

Cellular Immunocompetence: The state of the cellular immune system. *See* Cellular immune response.

Cerebrospinal Fluid Levels of Corticotrophin-Releasing Factor: Corticotrophin-releasing factor is produced by the hypothalamus (a portion of the brain), that then causes the release of a hormone from the pituitary gland, which in turn stimulates the adrenal gland to release cortisone to the bloodstream. Levels of the releasing factor can be measured in cerebrospinal fluid, a clear fluid that surrounds the brain and spinal cord.

Chronic Obstructive Pulmonary Disease (COPD): A common disorder, particularly in smokers, where the lungs having been subject to chronic inflammation and bronchitis lose their elasticity and many of the alveoli (oxygen exchange sacs) are destroyed. Common clinical variants of COPD are chronic bronchitis and emphysema.

Cluster Analysis: The statistical analysis of a population and (in this case) their dietary habits so as to find groups of people who have similar preferences for many foods or nutrients. The clusters are groups of people whose diets, in a broad sense, show many similarities.

Cohort Effects: Usually refers to a birth cohort, who are a group of individuals born in about the same calendar year. There may be differences in the risk of different birth cohorts, even when they pass through the same ages (obviously, at different calendar years). Different risks at the same age are known as birth cohort effects and are due to the cumulative effects of different conditions experienced during aging in a different set of calendar years.

Cohort Studies: Also known as "what will happen to me" studies. They follow a group of people with different levels of exposure to the risk factors under study and assess what happens to their health over time. The risk factor status is measured <u>before</u> there is evidence of disease.

Collaborative Analysis: *See* Meta-analysis.

Collagen: A fibrous protein that is a prominent part of the connective tissues that hold structures together within the body. Collagen is also an important component of scar tissue, or fibrosis, at any bodily site.

Colonic Crypt: A glandular indentation in the wall of the large bowel (colon); it contains rapidly dividing cells that spread to continuously replace the lining of the colon.

Competing Causes of Death: When lifetime risk or age at death from a particular cause are of interest, life table analyses must also take into account other (competing) causes of death. Subjects dying of a competing cause are of course no longer at risk from the cause of interest. Life tables that account for competing causes of death are called multiple-decrement life tables.

Compression of Mortality: Occurs if an average increase in life expectancy is accomplished mainly by avoiding deaths at younger ages. Then a greater proportion of the population survive to older ages, but have a higher mortality at these ages.

Confounding: The effect of one variable to change risk is confused or mixed with that of another closely related variable. For instance, heavy meat-eaters may have a greater risk for a certain disease, but as a group they also eat less fiber. Is it meat or the associated lower fiber intake, or both, that actually causes the change in disease risk? Meat-eating and fiber consumption are closely associated potentially causal variables in this example. Statistical techniques are available that can help prevent the intermingling of effects, as long as both meat consumption and fiber are measured in the study.

Coronary Arteries: Arteries that supply the heart muscle with blood.

Correlated Nutrients: This means that those who eat more or less than average of one particular nutrient tend to be the same people who have systematically higher or lower intakes of a second nutrient. Then knowing the intake of the first nutrient allows some prediction of the level of intake of the second nutrient.

Cortisol: *See* Cortisone

Cortisone: A hormone produced by the cortex of the adrenal gland that helps the body cope with stress.

Current Life Table: A method of predicting the mortality experience at different ages, the average age at death, and other similar characteristics of a whole population. This method starts with a hypothetical newborn population, then applies age-specific mortality rates to predict deaths and survivors at different ages in sequence, till all hypothetical subjects have died.

Death Certificate: In most countries, a legal document that must be signed by a medical practitioner. It details the time and likely causes of death for a deceased individual. Usually only a minority of these diagnoses are supported by an autopsy, and they are thus less than perfectly accurate.

Death Rate: *See* Mortality rate.

Demographic Studies: Demographics is the study of the characteristics of human populations, such as size, growth, density, distribution, predicted longevity, and other vital statistics.

Detoxifying Enzyme: Toxic substances are poisons and, interpreted broadly, this will also include carcinogens. Detoxifying enzymes speed up chemical interactions in the body that neutralize the toxin.

Diagnostic Bias: Results when some characteristic of an individual gives them an atypical probability of having their disease diagnosed. For instance, economically disadvantaged subjects may be less likely to be diagnosed as they visit doctors less often.

Disease Rate: A measure of disease frequency that is usually standardized for the number of people at risk and also the time period of observation. Typically such a rate is the number of new cases of disease per 100,000 people at risk during a one-year period.

DNA: Acronym for deoxyribonucleic acid, a long helical (spiral) molecule consisting of a sequence of pairs of chemicals called nucleotides. DNA contains the genetic information of a cell and is located in the cell nucleus.

Double-Blind Crossover Study: An experimental study in which neither the subjects in the study nor the researchers having contact with the subjects know whether particular subjects have been assigned to the experimental treatment or to placebo. In theory, that the subjects do not know keeps balance between the treatment groups for any psychological effects they may experience from simply being in a study. Moreover, any unconscious tendency for researchers to treat or measure subjects in the experimental treatment group differently from those in the placebo group is removed, as the researchers who contact the subjects also do not know who is on which treatment.

Ecologic Study: Looks for associations between the disease rates of whole communities or countries and the average risk factor levels in those communities (e.g., average intake of fat). Contrasted with usual epidemiologic work that deals with risk factor values of individuals. Ecologic studies have a major weakness that any chosen risk factor will almost certainly be a good marker for a number of other cultural or social differences between communities or countries. Then it is unclear which risk factor is responsible for differences in disease experience—the usual confounding problem is exacerbated.

Effect Modification: If the effect of one variable on risk of disease differs according to the value of a second risk factor, the effect of the first variable is said to be modified by the second. For instance, if the effect of meat-eating on CHD risk differs at different ages, the effect of meat-eating is said to be modified by age. The term *interaction* is sometimes used to describe this situation.

Eicosanoids: A diverse group of biologically active substances based on 20-carbon chains. These include the prostaglandins, thromboxanes, and leukotrienes that mediate the balance of platelet and endothelial function, as well as the inflammatory response.

Endothelial Function: The endothelium is the layer of cells that line the interior of blood vessels; however, they are much more than a passive structural feature. The cells release potent chemicals in response to various stimuli that can cause constriction of vessels and clumping of platelets, for instance. Endothelial function in atherosclerotic vessels is abnormal and may cause further narrowing by stimulating constrictor muscles in the walls of arteries.

Energy-Adjusted: A method of scoring intake of a nutrient in such a way that there is adjustment, or compensation, for differences in total energy intake. For instance, a big man may eat twice as much saturated fat as a small woman, but more importantly, as a proportion of total calories there may be no difference.

Enzymatic Abnormalities: Enzymes are very highly specialized proteins, whose three-dimensional folding is critical to their proper function. Genes provide the coding for the manufacture of these enzymes. Alterations in genes (mutations) may alter the shape of the enzymes. If this alteration is in a critical region, the enzyme's chemical activity may be impaired.

Enzyme: A body protein that has the unique ability to facilitate and markedly accelerate either the combination of two other chemicals or the splitting of another chemical. Many bodily functions depend on enzymes.

Epidemiology: The scientific study of widely prevalent diseases and the factors that influence their onset, development, and outcome.

Epinephrine (Adrenaline): A "fight and flight" hormone produced by the medulla of the adrenal gland (and by certain nerves) that increases blood pressure and heart rate among other effects. Another similar hormone is norepinephrine (noradrenaline).

Epithelial: An adjective describing cells that form internal and external surfaces of the organs and tubes (e.g., bowel, ureter) of the body. An exception is the cells lining blood vessels, which are known as *endothelial*.

Estrogens, Estriol, and Plasma Prolactin: Chemicals in the steroid family that stimulate the human organism to express female secondary sexual characteristics. Secreted by ovaries in women or produced in smaller quantities by fatty tissue, particularly in postmenopausal women. Estrogens also tend to promote a healthy endothelium and raise HDL cholesterol levels in women. Prolactin is a hormone associated with milk production during normal breast-feeding. High levels of prolactin may modestly increase risk of pre-menopausal breast cancer.

Exponential in Exposures: A mathematical model often used in epidemiology, whereby changing the risk factor by a fixed increment changes the relative risk by a fixed multiplier (e.g. 2-fold). *See* Nonparametric for further discussion.

Factor Analysis: A multivariate statistical technique that finds groups of variables such that those within a particular group (or factor) are statistically related to each other. It provides these related variables with a high weighting coefficient for that factor. One variable may be an important contributor to several factors. The factors are considered to measure underlying constructs such that each important variable in the factor contributes some additional information. Researchers often give each factor a label that describes the common features of the important variables for that factor, in an attempt to identify the underlying construct.

False "Positive" and "Negative" Results: Where test results are in terms of positive (say, disease present) or negative (say, disease absent), a false positive is where the test result is "Yes" but, due to imperfections in the test, the truth is "No." The equivalent but opposite situation is a false negative. These situations are real as no clinical test is perfect. A false negative may miss a disease diagnosis. A false positive creates unnecessary anxiety, as in fact disease was never present.

Fatal and Nonfatal Events: Fatal events are occurrences of the particular disease in question that resulted in death. Nonfatal events are occurrences of the particular disease in question that did not result in death.

Fiber (Dietary): Complex carbohydrates found only in plant foods that are not digested, but nevertheless lower blood cholesterol, probably by affecting its absorption in the small bowel.

Fibrinogen, Factor VII: *See* Blood clotting factors

Fibrinolytic Activity: A group of chemicals in the blood that act to reduce blood clotting and may even dissolve clot.

Flavonoids: A large class of polyphenolic chemicals found in many fruits and vegetables. Many flavonoids have antioxidant properties. One group, the isoflavones, also have weak estrogenic activity and are thus one category of phytoestrogens.

Follow-Up: In the context of this book, this usually refers to a period of some years after obtaining baseline dietary and other information in a prospective study. During this follow-up period, there is an attempt to gather information about all new cases of the disease of interest that develop.

Food-Frequency Questions: A method that is often used to measure diet in large numbers of people. A question for a particular food simply asks how often (each week or day), on average, the subject eats this food. Typically, 50 to 130 foods are covered in such a questionnaire. There may be a comparative portion size listed also.

Framingham Heart Study: Since 1948 the federal government has followed 5209 adult residents in Framingham, Massachusetts, to learn the circumstances under which cardiovascular diseases arise, evolve, and terminate fatally in the general population. The Framingham study is designed to find out how those who develop cardiovascular diseases differ from those who remain free of the diseases over a long period of time.

Genitals: Sex organs—e.g., prostate in men and uterus, cervix, and ovaries in women.

Hazard: A technical term describing a quantity closely related to a disease rate, but often considered a little more accurate. It describes disease experience during a short time period and diminishes the denominator over follow-up time to take account of subjects who die or drop out of the study for other reasons which preclude them from subsequently contributing to disease events.

HDL Cholesterol: The cholesterol content of high density lipoprotein (HDL) particles. This is thought to be largely cholesterol moving from the artery walls to the liver, some of which will be excreted. Subjects with higher HDL (good) cholesterol levels are at lower risk of CHD.

Healthy-Volunteer Effect: People who are unwell are less likely to volunteer for research. Thus volunteer research populations may have lower mortality than average for the early period of follow-up. This distortion can usually be minimized by eliminating the first two to three years of follow-up from the analysis.

Heterocyclic Amine: A carcinogenic chemical that can be produced when frying, grilling, or barbecuing meats at high temperatures. These amines are formed from amino acids in protein, creatine in muscle, and sugars, in combination.

Heterogeneity Between Studies: When several studies are combined to one analysis, the usual assumption is that the true effect of the variable of interest on disease is the same in all studies (although the observed values in different studies will vary by chance). A heterogeneity test evaluates whether the data are compatible with this assumption of uniform effect. If the test is statistically significant, this suggests that the individual studies have disparate effects and perhaps should not be combined in a single analysis.

Histology: The microscopic structure of normal and abnormal cells and tissues. An assessment of histology is necessary for the detailed diagnosis of cancer.

HMGCoA Reductase Inhibitor: HMGCoA reductase is an important chemical (an enzyme) in liver cells and is essential for their manufacture of cholesterol. Most cholesterol in the body is made in the liver. Common drugs, known as statins, inhibit this enzyme and so reduce blood cholesterol levels.

Homocysteine: A sulfur-containing amino acid formed during the metabolism of methionine. The breakdown of homocysteine is slower in some individuals because of genetic factors, or because of a lack of the vitamins folate, B_{12}, or pyridoxine, all necessary to its breakdown. A good deal of evidence suggests that high levels of blood homocysteine are associated with increased risk of CHD, but it is not yet clear if this association is causal.

Hyperlipidemic: High levels of total blood cholesterol or triglycerides.

Hypothesis: An idea about cause and effect that is usually proposed for further data-based evaluation.

ICD9: International Classification of Diseases, Revision 9. A system whereby any particular disease is assigned a number, according to a careful definition of the disease. This coding scheme allows an efficient summary of death statistics from whole populations.

Immune System: A complicated system of defense cells called lymphocytes and macrophages, and chemicals, such as antibodies and cytokines, that deactivate or kill harmful foreign chemicals, bacteria, viruses, and other microorganisms that may enter the body.

Incident Event: Refers to the first diagnosis of the disease—for instance, the first heart attack or the first manifestation of arthritis.

Indoles and Isothiocyanates: Pungent (smelly) substances formed when the cells of brassica vegetables (the cabbage and broccoli family) are ruptured. Enzymes are released that transform glucosinolates in the intact cells to isothiocyanates and indoles. These chemicals stimulate detoxifying enzymes in the liver that neutralize carcinogens and may inhibit other enzymes that convert procarcinogens to carcinogens. Both of these changes in theory reduce risk of cancer. Indoles and isothiocyanates are found elsewhere in nature and also have some antioxidant capacity.

Independent Contribution: An effect ascribed to a single variable. Conceptually this is the effect observed on health status when this variable changes but all other variables are held constant.

Inflammatory Cell: A white blood cell—especially neutrophils, lymphocytes, and monocytes—that repairs damage to the body tissues.

Insulin-Like Growth Factors (IGF) and Binding Proteins: A family of proteins normally produced by a wide variety of tissues and necessary for growth and differentiation (maturing) of these tissues. These have some chemical similarities to insulin. Proteins on the cell surface that capture and bind these IGFs are the binding proteins.

Interaction: *See* Effect modification.

Intervening Variable: The way in which a variable X causes disease D is often complex. In particular, there may be a causal chain. Variable X changes variable Y, which, in turn, affects risk of D. Then Y is an intervening variable. Adjusting for differences in Y in a multivariate analysis will completely negate the apparent effect of X. In such a situation, Y should not usually be included as a covariate. Often the effect of X through Y may be only partial, and then there is still some direct effect of X on D.

Inverse Association: As one of a pair of variables gets larger, the other tends to get smaller. For instance, an inverse association between polyunsaturated fat intake and risk of CHD implies that when much polyunsaturated fat is eaten, the risk of disease is smaller, and vice versa.

Isoflavones: *See* Flavonoids; Phytoestrogens.

Keys' Score: Keys' score is a mathematical combination of dietary cholesterol and fats that predicts average blood cholesterol in men (and probably approximately in women).

Korotkoff Sounds: These are the thudding noises heard through the stethoscope in time with the heartbeat by the doctor or nurse taking the blood pressure. The sounds fade or disappear when cuff pressure equals diastolic pressure. The "fade" point is the fourth Korotkoff sound (K4) and disappearance of sound is K5, both possible measures of diastolic blood pressure, although K4 is usually preferred.

Lacto-Ovo Vegetarian: A person who does not eat meat, poultry, fish, or seafood but does consume milk, milk products, and eggs. This is the most common type of vegetarianism in the United States.

LDL Cholesterol: An acronym for low-density lipoprotein cholesterol. Cholesterol is carried in the blood within small "packages" called lipoprotein particles. Higher levels of the LDL "packages" increase the risk of coronary heart disease. Moreover, it appears to be the smaller LDL particles that are particularly dangerous.

LDL Particle Size: *See* LDL cholesterol.

Life Expectancy at a Specified Age: A prediction of the number of years of life remaining on average, starting at this age.

Life Span: The genetically endowed upper limit to age for an individual free of other environmental or lifestyle risk factors. It is a theoretical quantity that cannot be directly observed.

Lignans: *See* Phytoestrogens.

Logistic Regression: A mathematical model that allows the prediction of risk of disease, for instance, by some combination of risk factors. In the analysis of a cohort study, it will give results very similar to the generally more accurate proportional hazards method of analysis as long as the subjects who develop disease and those who drop out during follow-up form only a small percentage (5% to 10%) of those starting the study.

Lp(a) (Lipoprotein a): A special class of lipid particles like LDL, except that the proteins in the particle are joined to a molecule very similar to plasminogen, one of the fibrinolytic factors, and interferes with normal plasminogen action, thus promoting blood clotting. Higher blood levels of Lp(a) have been associated with increased risk of CHD in many, but not all, well-designed studies.

Lumbar Arteries: Medium-sized arteries that arise from the aorta and feed the vertebrae and spine with blood, oxygen, and nutrients.

Mean: Another name for average, calculated as the sum of values to be averaged, divided by their number.

Measurement Error: Occurs when investigators do not measure exactly what they wish to measure. This may be because their questions are poorly constructed or because subjects are not careful with their responses, or perhaps cannot remember accurately. If about equal numbers of people provide erroneously high as low answers, on average, the errors may cancel out. Then the errors do not cause bias as the average value is correct. However, this will often not be the case, if most responses are erroneously high, for instance. Further, even if errors are balanced they continue to cause problems when such measurements are used in regression analyses to predict risk of disease (see bias correction techniques).

Meat Analogue: Meat substitute containing vegetable protein. Typically contains soy, nut, or wheat gluten as protein sources.

Mediterranean Diet: A loosely defined dietary pattern somewhat typical of Mediterranean countries. Traditionally there is an emphasis on fruits, vegetables, legumes, nuts, olives, olive oil, moderate wine, and smaller servings of red meats.

Meta-Analysis: An analysis that combines the results of several studies that address the same question in order to increase statistical power. A disadvantage may be the need to take account of different definitions of variables in different studies, the use of different diagnostic methods, or even the possibility that the association being investigated is actually different in the different populations of the studies (suggested by a statistically significant test of heterogeneity).

Metabolic Rate: The amount of energy produced by the body per minute as it metabolizes foods or burns stored fats, carbohydrates, and proteins. This energy supports cellular activity, bodily functions such as digestion, and movement.

Metabolite: A "daughter" chemical that results when the "parent" chemical is changed within the body. A common site for these chemical changes (metabolism) is the liver.

Methylation: The addition of a methyl group ($-CH_3$) to some other molecule.

Mid-Luteal Phase: The luteal phase is approximately the second half of the normal menstrual cycle, when the developing egg and the ovary secrete increasing quantities of progesterone and estrogens. An investigation of the effect of diet or other factors on sex-hormone levels in women needs to specify the part of the menstrual cycle during which these levels are measured.

Millerites and the Great Disappointment: Between 1831 and 1844, William Miller—a Baptist preacher—launched the "great second advent awakening" which eventually spread throughout much of Christianity in the United States. Based on his study of biblical prophecy, Miller calculated that Jesus would return to earth on October 22, 1844. When Jesus did not appear, Miller's followers experienced what came to be called "the Great Disappointment."

Model: Scientific research involves the repetition of four steps: (*1*) observation, (*2*) explaining the observation with a model, (*3*) using the model to predict, and (*4*) testing whether future observations agree with the prediction. Thus a model may be a precise mathematical representation of postulated relationships, or it may make allowance for random errors (stochastic). Alternatively, it may take less precise qualitative rather than quantitative form.

Monounsaturated Fats: *See* Unsaturated fats.

Morbidity: Nonfatal illness.

Mortality Rate: Same idea as disease rate (see above), except that the disease of interest is "death", hence, the term *mortality*.

Mortality Ratio: The ratio of mortality rates from two groups to be compared.

Multiple Decrement Life Table: *See* Competing causes of death.

Multivariate: An analysis that includes more than just one exposure (risk factor) or one outcome (disease) variable in the model.

Mutation: A change or disorganization of specific portions of the DNA. This changes the genes and thus may change the development of an organism or its metabolic functions.

Myocardial Infarction: A "heart attack," often due to the total blockage of a coronary artery, results in the death of a portion of the heart muscle. In time this is converted to a scar.

N-Acetyl Transferase: An enzyme (with "slow" and "fast" genetic variants), especially found in the liver, that can add acetyl segments to many molecules. In so doing, it may convert procarcinogens (e.g., heterocyclic amines) to carcinogens or by contrast may detoxify other carcinogens.

National Death Index: A computerized system that covers the whole United States and has tabulated basic demographic information and the causes of death for all deceased persons since 1978. For a fee, this information can be matched to the data files of a research study and thus provides a mechanism to identify most deaths in the research group without the need for attempted personal contacts.

Nitrosamines: Well-known carcinogens that are formed by chemical actions in the stomach and bowel on nitrates and nitrites. These nitrates and nitrites may come from foods, or in the past, from preservatives added to foods. Higher levels of nitrosamines are formed in the bowel of meat-eaters.

Nocebo: Anything that creates an expectation of illness and may, through this expectation, actually cause the experience of illness.

Nonparametric: Parametric methods of analysis force the data to conform to a mathematical pattern or model. Most commonly, this is a linear pattern, where irrespective of the starting value, changing the value of a risk factor by some quantity X, always changes the value of the outcome variable by a quantity Y. In epidemiology, the most common kind of modeling is when the risk factor is linearly related to log [relative risk] of a disease. A nonparametric method (e.g., Kaplan-Meier product-limit survival analysis) is more flexible as it does not impose these mathematical patterns on the relationships. Although the analysis is often more complicated, it may describe the relationship more accurately.

Noradrenaline, Adrenaline: See Epinephrine

Nutrients: Chemicals found in foods that provide energy when they are metabolized ("burned") within the body.

Odds Ratio: The measure of relative risk that naturally results from logistic regression.

Omega-3 Fatty Acids: A family of polyunsaturated fatty acids found particularly in fatty fish. However, modest quantities of linolenic acid, which is in the omega-3 family, are found in some plant foods, such as walnuts, rapeseed (canola oil), and flaxseed (linseed oil).

Osteoarthritis: The most common arthritis, due to degeneration of the cartilage, a cushioning material between the bones of the joint. One cause is "wear-and-tear," but there are clearly also other less well identified causes.

Oxidizing: A chemical reaction characterized by the loss of an electron (a particle in an atom carrying a negative charge). Oxidation occurs naturally in the body and if not suppressed (see antioxidants) will damage tissues.

p Value: A statistical measure that attempts to quantify uncertainty about whether an outcome is due to chance or whether it actually reflects a true difference. Using a formula that considers the number of subjects or events, epidemiologists calculate a probability of the observed result happening by chance, if in fact there is no real difference. Then the p value is an index such that a very small value (5%, 1%, or less) gives more confidence that there is a true difference, and in that case the result is called statistically significant. The 5% and 1% values are usually expressed as decimals, .05 and .01.

Pathologic Risk Factors: A pathologic condition (disease) that increases the risk of a second disease. For instance, diabetes mellitus predicts a higher risk of stroke or coronary heart disease.

Person-Years at Risk: Obtained by finding the numbers of people in the cohort, still alive and contactible during each year of the follow-up period, and then totaling this for all years. So each person contributes one person-year for each year he or she remains alive and in the study.

Physiologic Risk Factors: A physical characteristic or measure of bodily function that relates to risk of disease. Examples are physical fitness, endothelial function, and blood pressure (even within the usually accepted normal range).

Phytochemicals: The many special chemicals found in vegetables and fruits, many of which can have effects on human physiology and chemistry when eaten. Little is known about most phytochemicals, but it is an area of very active research.

Phytoestrogens: Chemicals in plants that have weak estrogenic activity. These are mainly isoflavones, found especially in soybeans, and, to a lesser extent garbanzos; they also include lignans, which are formed in the bowel from substances present in many fruits, cereals, and vegetables, especially linseed. The major isoflavones are genistein and daidzein. The major lignans are enterolactone and enterodiol.

Phytosterols: Sterols are a class of chemicals of which cholesterol is the best known member. Phytosterols are members of this family found in plants. In contrast to cholesterol, eating certain phytosterols (e.g., sitosterol, sitostanol) lowers blood cholesterol, as they interfere with the absorption of dietary cholesterol.

Placebo: Usually a fake medicine or intervention that cannot easily be distinguished from the true medicine or intervention. This is used in some experiments where subjects randomly allocated not to receive the medicine of interest are instead given the placebo. Thus, by prior agreement, subjects do not know whether they are taking the medicine or the placebo. This compensates for any expectation of better health through "pill-taking" (placebo effects) in the experimental comparison, as it would now affect both groups equally.

Platelet Aggregability: See platelet clumping.

Platelet Clumping: Platelets are tiny membrane-covered packages of chemicals in the bloodstream which, if stimulated by damaged blood vessels or certain chemicals, become "sticky" and clump together. They then release many chemicals, some of which are clotting factors, and their clumps become the "scaffolding" on which a clot can form.

Polycyclic Hydrocarbon: A chemical often formed when plant or animal materials are burned. A widely known example is the chemical benzopyrene found in tobacco smoke, which is a well-known carcinogen in animals. Somewhat similar chemicals may be formed when meat is very well done, or burned.

Polyunsaturated Fats: See Unsaturated fats.

Positively Related: A term that describes an association between two variables such that as one variable takes greater values, on average, the other variable also takes greater values. When variables are negatively related, as one takes greater values, on average, the other takes smaller values.

Postmortem Angiographic Examination: A test in which the arteries are filled with a fluid that shows up white on an X-ray. If performed after death it is called postmortem. Narrowings of the arteries are seen as constrictions of the white arterial images on the X-ray.

Primary Prevention: Attention to lifestyle and risk factors where the goal is to prevent the first episode of a disease.

Product Term: When a disease regression model contains both a main term for risk factor X, and a product-term with age, for instance $X^\star$Age, each with its β coefficient, the effect of X on disease risk is estimated by $\exp(\beta_1 X + \beta_2 X^\star \text{Age}) = \exp[(\beta_1 + \beta_2^\star \text{Age})X]$. In other words, changing X by one unit changes risk by a factor $\exp(\beta_1 + \beta_2^\star \text{Age})$, and this is clearly different at different values of age. Hence the effect of X is modeled to change with age, and this will be so if the coefficient of the product term, β_2, is different from zero, an example of effect modification.

Proportional Hazard: An assumption that often seems justified in health-related analyses and markedly simplifies the calculations—hence, the popularity of proportional hazards regression analysis. Essentially, the assumption is that whatever a subject's baseline risk of disease due to other risk factors, changing the factor of special interest by a fixed amount always changes risk by a fixed multiplying factor (e.g., doubles risk). That this assumption is reasonable should always be checked in the data being used.

Prospective: *See* Cohort study.

Prostaglandins: A family of tissue hormones produced by many tissues. Among other effects, they influence the size of blood vessels, blood pressure, and platelet function. Many are excreted in the urine. Thromboxane B_2 is one prostaglandin that stimulates clumping of platelets, formation of clots, and constriction of blood vessels.

Protease Inhibitor: Proteases are enzymes secreted by the pancreas into the bowel to break down proteins that are eaten. Protease inhibitors, found particularly in legumes (including peanuts), allow additional undigested protein to enter the colon. It has been hypothesized that this may reduce risk of colon cancer.

Proto-Oncogene: A normal human gene that when altered, or mutated, promotes the formation or growth of cancers.

P/S Ratio: Amount of polyunsaturated divided by the saturated fat in the diet.

Psychosocial Factors: Include personality attributes such as anxiety, depression, and hostility, as well as measures of social interaction, such as social support.

Quality of Life: This has also become a technical term and is typically measured by a series of questions that include an assessment of levels of physical, mental, social, and role functioning, along with the ability to perform certain common tasks, an evaluation of significant personal relationships, and satisfaction with life.

Quantile: If the values of a variable are ordered from smallest to largest, then the quantile of a particular value is the percentage of all values that lies below or equal to it.

Quartile: If the values of a variable are ordered from smallest to largest, then sequential quarters of this list are each called quartiles.

Quintile: If the values of a variable are ordered from smallest to largest, then sequential fifths of this list are each called quintiles.

Random Error: Errors that are due to undetermined factors. In most statistical applications, they are thought of being balanced in that an equal number are "upside" as "downside" errors. Hence, they cancel each other when averages are calculated.

Randomized Trial: An attempt to prevent the confounding that is always at least a theoretical problem in observational studies (cohort studies, case-control studies). Randomized trials are experiments in which an intervention is imposed on a representative subgroup of the study subjects. Confounding is prevented by controlling the intervention so that it is present in one group of subjects (the intervention group) and absent in another group (the controls) who do not differ systematically from the first group in any other way. In theory, this can be achieved by a random assignment of subjects to one group or the other. While randomized trials are often considered the most rigorous study design to test an idea about cause and effect, they often have problems when applied to diet. Most people will not agree to, or comply with, a request to change their diet for years at a time, or those who do agree may be a quite atypical group.

Rates of Disease: *See* Disease rates.

Regression Calibration: A statistical procedure whereby instead of using a crude or food-frequency estimate of diet (that incorporates measurement errors) in a regression predicting the risk of disease, the predicted (or average) value of the true diet given the crude estimate, is used instead. This procedure will provide unbiased estimates of the association of disease with the true diet. The average value of the true diet in those with a particular crude value is found by a separate regression analysis in a smaller calibration study where ideally subjects provide both crude and true data. In practice, a true dietary value is usually never available for use in a calibration study, but data from a more detailed so-called reference method may be considered "close enough" to the true intake.

Relative Risk: The measure of risk for those exposed compared to those who are not exposed. For instance, those counted as exposed by having a particular risk factor, or behaving in a particular way, may have 1.5 times the risk of those not so exposed.

Renin, Angiotensin: Tissue hormones that exert important effects on blood pressure. Renin is produced in the kidney and chemically transforms angiotensin (a chemical produced by the liver) to an active form that constricts blood vessels and increases blood pressure.

Retrospective *or* Case-Control Studies: Studies in which the risk factor (often called an exposure) is measured after the disease has developed. The frequency of the risk factor in diseased subjects (cases) identified at the beginning of the study is compared with its frequency in a control, nondiseased group. This allows the calculation of a relative risk measure called the odds ratio. There is no follow-up aspect to these studies. One weakness is that the retrospective (looking backward) measurement of diet, for instance, depends on memory and may be influenced by the fact that disease is already present in the case group but not in the controls.

Rheumatoid Arthritis: Arthritis is the inflammation of joints. Rheumatoid arthritis results when the immune system attacks the lining of the joints (synovium) and causes pain, swelling, and often (in time) destruction of the whole joint. Sometimes other bodily tissues are also involved.

Risk-Factor Profile: Risk factors are elements that have been proven to contribute to the development of a particular disease. A risk-factor profile is a compilation of all risk factors involved for an individual or a group.

Saponins: Chemicals found especially in soy and other legumes. They have a chemical structure somewhat similar to cholesterol but do, however, lower blood cholesterol when eaten. They also have antioxidant properties.

Saturated Fats: Fats that chemically have no unsaturated bonds in the carbon chain. They come mainly from animal sources (coconut is an exception) and raise blood LDL cholesterol levels.

Secondary Prevention: Attention to lifestyle, risk factors, and medications where the goal is to prevent further episodes or death in subjects who already have diagnosed disease.

Sex-Hormone-Binding Globulin: A protein in the blood that binds estrogens and so reduces their activity on target organs (e.g., sexual organs) and in so doing may affect the risk of certain cancers.

Sex-Specific: Calculated separately for men and women.

Site-Specific Cancers: Cancers can occur in any organ, or site, within the body. A site-specific cancer is a cancer of a particular named organ— for example, breast cancer.

SMR: *See* Standardized mortality ratio.

Social Support: The physical assistance and psychological benefits derived from contact with supportive family and friends. Some studies evaluate the effects of social networks, which are groups of socially connected individuals.

Spondylosis: A form of arthritis of the spine where rough projections or spurs develop on the margins of the bony vertebrae, and the soft intervertebral disks may rupture.

Squamous Cell: A flattened type of epithelial cell that is stacked in layers to form the surface of several organs, particularly those that experience abrasive forces. Thus this is the type of epithelial cell found in the skin and the esophagus.

Stages of Progression of Cancer: Different systems of classification of the stages of cancer have been used. A more advanced stage indicates that the cancer is larger or has spread further within the body. A common progression would be (*1*) cancer-in-situ, (*2*) microinvasive, (*3*) locally invasive, and (*4*) metastatic (spread to other parts of the body).

Standard Deviation (SD): A measure of variation among a group of values. It is the square root of the mean of squared deviations about the mean of the values.

Standardized Mortality Ratios (SMR): A method to allow fair comparisons of disease rates between study groups that have different proportions of older and younger subjects. In the context of our discussion, assume that the age-specific national mortality rates (number of deaths per year in 1000 persons of a particular age) are applied to the corresponding ages of the study population. Then add up the total deaths that would be expected under this assumption, across all ages in the study population. Express the total deaths actually observed in the study population as a percentage of this expected number. This is a standardized mortality ratio.

Statistical Power: Statistical power is the probability that one will detect the effect or risk being studied if there really is one. Well-designed studies have a greater statistical power than poorly designed ones.

Statistical Significance: *See p* value.

Stool Transit Time: The time for food to traverse the alimentary system from mouth to anus. This time is quite variable, but typically around 18 to 36 hours in Western cultures.

Sulfotransferase *1A1* Genotype: One member of a large family of enzymes that combine various chemicals in the body with sulfur-containing molecules. By doing so, they may detoxify certain carcinogens. However, their reactions with isothiocyanates (*see* Indoles and isothiocyanates) may also inactivate these chemicals and prevent their potentially helpful actions. Sulfotransferases may also activate certain procarcinogens directly.

Survival Curve: The curve that charts survival as 100% at some beginning age and then plots the proportion of these subjects who survive to subsequent ages.

Sympatho-Adrenal Hyperactivity: High levels of sympathetic nervous system activity or adrenergic hormone (e.g., epinephrine) levels. These are the typical "fight or flight" response mechanisms characterized by increased alertness and higher heart rates, blood pressure, and sweating.

Systolic and Diastolic Blood Pressures: Systolic blood pressure is the higher blood pressure that coincides with a heartbeat. Diastolic blood pressure is that between heartbeats. These are usually expressed as systolic/diastolic (e.g., 120/80).

Tertiles: If the values of a variable are ordered from smallest to largest, then sequential thirds of this list are each called tertiles.

Thromboxane: *See* Prostaglandins.

Tissue Culture: Tissues grown on special plates in the laboratory. These cultures can be used to study the effects of various chemicals on living cells.

Tissues: The fabric of bodily organs. A particular tissue commonly describes a portion of an organ composed mainly of one or a few cell types.

***Trans*-Fatty Acids:** These are fatty acids with at least one double bond in the carbon chain, but this double bond forms a different angle to the rest of the molecule than the usual (natural) version of this unsaturated fat. The usual version is called a *cis*-fatty acid. *Trans*-acids especially result from commercial hydrogenation of polyunsaturated fats, which makes them less liquid at room temperature (e.g., in some harder margarines). *Trans*-fatty acids in the diet raise blood cholesterol.

Triglycerides: These are the traditional fats. They are combinations of three fatty acid molecules with one glycerol molecule. Cholesterol, by contrast, is actually not a fat, but a sterol. However, it does have a somewhat fatty appearance when seen in the lining of arteries.

Triglyceride-Rich Remnant Particles: Some of the fat and cholesterol-laden particles in the blood stream are rich in triglycerides. Remnant particles are derived from these triglyceride-rich chylomicrons and VLDL that have been partly broken down, lost some of their triglycerides, and are enriched with cholesterol. These are then often called intermediate-density lipoproteins and smaller VLDL particles. Such remnant particles particularly promote atherosclerotic artery disease.

Type A Behavior Pattern: Has been defined by Jenkins et al. (1974) as a style of living characterized by excesses of competitiveness, striving for achievement, aggressiveness (sometimes stringently repressed), time urgency, acceleration of common activities, restlessness, hostility, hyper-alertness, explosiveness of speech amplitude, tenseness of facial musculature, and feelings of struggle against the limitations of time and the insensitivity of the environment.

Twenty-Four Hour Dietary Recall: A detailed listing from memory of all food and drink consumed in the preceding 24 hours.

Unsaturated Fats: Fatty acids with one (monounsaturated) or more (polyunsaturated) unsaturated (double) bonds in the carbon chain. Polyunsaturated fats are largely obtained from vegetable sources (mainly omega-6) or fatty fish (mainly omega-3). Monounsaturates are also common in foods of vegetable origin, but there are significant animal sources. Eating unsaturated fats tends to lower blood cholesterol, and polyunsaturated fats have more effect than do monounsaturated fats.

Validation Study: A small substudy of subjects that properly represent those in the main study and allows an independent assessment of the accuracy of dietary measurement by the main study's food-frequency questionnaire. This is compared to a more accurate, but usually time-intensive, method of dietary assessment, such as diet diaries or repeated 24-hour recalls. Understanding the nature of the inaccuracies in the food-frequency data may allow at least partial correction of the effects of these errors when trying to relate diet to risk of disease in the main study. See Regression calibration.

Values: The thoughts, feelings, and behaviors that are important and pervasive in a person's life. Values are not merely "held"; rather, people care passionately and deeply about them. They help direct the decisions a person makes in their life.

Vegan: A person who avoids eating all animal products, including dairy, eggs, and possibly honey.

Ventricular Arrhythmia: One type of "skipped heart beats." These abnormal beats that often precede a pause are initiated by cells in the ventricle of the heart rather than the usual natural pacemaker in the upper portion of the heart. Rarely such ventricular beats come in rapid runs called ventricular tachycardia, but when this occurs it can be fatal.

Vitamin D Receptor: A specific chemical on the surface of many cells that binds to vitamin D and then transfers it to the interior of these cells.

VLDL Cholesterol: The cholesterol content of very low density lipoprotein (VLDL) particles.

VLDL Particles: One of several lipid-carrying particles in the bloodstream. VLDL is secreted by the liver and is very rich in triglycerides. These particles are only weakly associated with the risk of CHD, but when there are high blood levels of partly broken down VLDL particles that are less rich in triglyceride and enriched with cholesterol, such remnant particles do increase risk.

Water Hardness: In some localities the water contains relatively high concentrations of calcium and magnesium salts and is termed "hard."

References

Abbey M, Noakes M, Belling GB, Nestel PJ. Partial replacement of saturated fatty acids with almonds or walnuts lowers total plasma cholesterol and low-density-lipoprotein cholesterol. *Am J Clin Nutr* 59:995–999, 1994.

Abrass IB. The biology and physiology of aging. *West J Med* 153:641–645, 1990.

ADA Reports. Position of the American Dietetic Association: vegetarian diets. *J Am Diet Assoc* 97:1317–1321, 1997.

Adler CM, Hillhouse JJ. Stress, health, and immunity: a review of the literature. In: T. W. Miller (ed.), *Theory and Assessment of Stressful Life Events.* International Universities Press Stress and Health Series. Madison, CT. International Universities Press, 1996, pp. 109–138.

Adlercreutz H, Fotsis T, Bannwart C, Wahala K, Makela T, Brunow G, Hase T. Determination of urinary lignans and phytoestrogen metabolites, potential antiestrogens and anticarcinogens in urine of women on various habitual diets. *J Steroid Biochem* 25:791–797, 1986.

Adorno T. *The Authoritarian Personality.* New York: Harper and Row, 1950.

Agren JJ, Tormala M-L, Nenonen MT, Hanninen OO. Fatty acid composition of erythrocyte, platelet, and serum lipids in strict vegans. *Lipids* 30:365–369, 1995.

Ahern DK, Gorkin L, Anderson JL, Tierney C, Hallstrom A, Ewart C, Capone RJ, Schron E, Kornfeld D, Herd JA, et al. Behavioral variables and mortality or cardiac arrest in the Cardiac Arrhythmia Pilot Study (CAPS). *Am J Cardiol* 66:59–62, 1990.

Ajzen I, Fishbein M. *Understanding Attitudes and Predicting Social Behavior.* Englewood Cliffs, NJ: Prentice Hall, 1980.

Ajzen I. The theory of planned behavior. *Organizational Behaviour and Human Decision Processes* 50:179–211, 1991.

Albert CM, Hennekens CH, O'Donnell CJ, Ajani UA, Carey VJ, Willett WC, Ruskin JN, Manson JE. Fish consumption and risk of sudden cardiac death. *JAMA* 279:23–28, 1998a.

Albert CM, Willett WC, Manson JE, Hennekens CH. Nut consumption and the risk of sudden and total cardiac death in the Physicians' Health Study (Abstract). *Circulation* 98(Suppl. I):582, 1998b.

Albrink MJ, Ullrich IH. Interaction of dietary sucrose and fiber on serum lipids in healthy young men fed high carbohydrate diets. *Am J Clin Nutr* 43:419–428, 1986.

Alfthan G, Pekkanen J, Jauhiainen M, Pitkaniemi J, Karvonen M, Tuomilehto J, Salonen JT, Ehnholm C. Relation of serum homocysteine and lipoprotein (a) concentrations to atherosclerotic disease in a prospective Finnish population based study. *Atherosclerosis* 106:9–19, 1994.

Allen NE, Appleby PN, Davey GK, Key TJ. Hormones and diet: low insulin-like growth factor-I, but normal bioavailable androgens in vegan men. *Br J Cancer* 83:95–97, 2000.

Allport GW, Ross JM. Personal religious orientation and prejudice. *J Per Soc Psychol* 5, 432–443, 1967.

Alpha-Tocopherol, Beta Carotene Cancer Prevention Study Group. The effect of vitamin E and beta carotene on the incidence of lung cancer and other cancers in male smokers. *N Engl J Med* 330:1029–1035, 1994.

Anda R, Williamson D, Jones D, Macera C, Eaker E, Glassman A, Marks J. Depressed affect hopelessness, and the risk of ischemic heart disease in a cohort of U.S. adults. *Epidemiology* 4:285–294, 1993.

Anderson F, Cowan NR. Survival of healthy older people. *Br J Prev Soc Med* 30:231–232, 1976.

Anson O, Antonovsky A, Sagy S. Religiosity and well-being among retirees: a question of causality. *Behav Health Aging* 1(2):85–97, 1990a.

Anson O, Carmel S, Bonneh DY, Levenson A, Maoz B. Recent life events, religiosity, and health: an individual or collective effect. *Hum Relations* 43(11): 1051–1066, 1990b.

Antonovsky, A. Can attitudes contribute to health? *Advances* 8(4):33–49, 1992.

Appel LJ. Non-pharmacologic therapies that reduce blood pressure: a fresh perspective. *Clin Cardiol* 22(Suppl. III):1–5, 1999.

Appel LJ, Miller ER, Jee SH, Stolzenberg-Solomon R, Lin P-H, Erlinger T, Nadeau MR, Selhub J. Effect of dietary patterns on serum homocysteine. *Circulation* 102:852–857, 2000.

Appleby PN, Thorogood M, McPherson K, Mann JI. Associations between plasma lipid concentrations and dietary, lifestyle and physical factors in the Oxford Vegetarian Study. *J Hum Nutr Diet* 8:305–314, 1995.

Appleby PN, Thorogood M, Mann JI, Key TJ. Low body mass index in non-meat eaters: the possible roles of animal fat, dietary fibre and alcohol. *Int J Obes Relat Metab Disord* 22:454–460, 1998.

Appleby PN, Thorogood M, Mann JI, Key TJA. The Oxford Vegetarian Study: an overview. *Am J Clin Nutr* 70(Suppl.):525S–531S, 1999.

Appleby PN, Key TJ, Thorogood M, Burr ML, Mann J. Mortality in British vegetarians. *Public Health Nutr* 5:29–36, 2002

Armstrong B, Clarke H, Martin C, Ward W, Norman N, Masarei J. Urinary sodium and blood pressure in vegetarians. *Am J Clin Nutr* 32:2472–2476, 1979.

Armstrong BK, Brown JB, Clarke HT, Crooke DK, Hahnel R, Masarei JR, Ratajczak T. Diet and reproductive hormones: a study of vegetarian and non-vegetarian postmenopausal women. *J Natl Cancer Inst* 67:761–767, 1981.

Arnesen E, Refsum H, Bonaa KH, Ueland PM, Forde OH, Nordrehang JE. Serum total homocysteine and coronary heart disease. *Int J Epidemiol* 24:704–709, 1995.

Aro A, Kardinaal AFM, Salminen I, Kark JD, Riemersma RA, Delgardo-Rodriguez M, Gomez-Aracena J, Huttunen JK, Kohlmeier L, Martin BC, et al. Adipose tissue isomeric trans fatty acids and risk of myocardial infarction in nine countries: the EURAMIC Study. *Lancet* 345:273–278, 1995.

Arroll B, Beaglehole R. Exercise for hypertension (Editorial). *Lancet* 341:1248–1249, 1993.

Ascherio A, Rimm EB, Giovannucci EL, Colditz GA, Rosner B, Willett WC, Sacks F, Stampfer MJ. A prospective study of nutritional factors and hypertension among U.S. men. *Circulation* 86:1475–1484, 1992.

Ascherio A, Rimm EB, Stampfer MJ, Giovannucci EL, Willett WC. Dietary intake of marine *n*-3 fatty acids, fish intake, and the risk of coronary disease among men. *N Engl J Med* 332:977–982, 1995.

Ascherio A, Rimm EB, Giovannucci EL, Spiegelman D, Stampfer M, Willett WC. Dietary fat and risk of coronary artery disease in men: cohort follow-up study in the United States. *Br Med J* 313:84–90, 1996.

Baldwin D, Naco G, Petersen F, Fraser G, Song B, Ruckle H. The effect of nutritional and clinical factors on prostate specific antigen and prostate cancer in a population of elderly California men (Abstract). *J Urology* 157(4) Supplement:54, 1997.

Bandura A. *Social Learning Theory*. Englewood Cliffs, NJ: Prentice Hall, 1977. Bandura, A. *Self-efficacy: The Exercise of Control*. New York: W.H. Freeman, 1997.

Banks DA, Fossel M. Telomeres, cancer and aging. *JAMA* 278:1345–1348, 1997.

Barefoot JC, Dahlstrom WG, Williams RB. Hostility, CHD incidence, and total mortality: a 25 year follow-up study of 255 physicians. *Psychosom Med* 45:59–63, 1983.

Barefoot JC, Larsen S, von der Lieth L, Schroll M. Hostility, incidence of acute myocardial infarction, and mortality in a sample of older Danish men and women. *Am J Epidemiol* 142:477–484, 1995.

Barefoot JC, Schroll M. Symptoms of depression, acute myocardial infarction, and total mortality in a community sample. *Circulation* 93:1976–1980, 1996.

Barkas, Jane. *The Vegetable Passion*. London: Routledge and Kegan Paul, 1975.

Barnes S. Effect of genistein on in vitro and in vivo models of cancer. *J Nutr* 125:777S–783S, 1995.

Barnhouse R. Changing mortality patterns among California's older population: 1960–1986. In: *Data Matters*. Sacramento: Department of Health Services, State of California, 1988.

Barrett-Connor E. Epidemiology, obesity, and non-insulin-dependent diabetes mellitus. *Epidemiol Rev* 11:172–181, 1989.

Battie MC, Videman T, Gill K, Moneta GB, Nyman R, Kaprio J, Koskenvuo M. Smoking and lumbar intervertebral disc degeneration: an MRI study of identical twins. *Spine* 16:1015–1021, 1991.

Bazzano LA, Jiang H, Ogden LG, Loria C, Vupputuri S, Myers L, Whelton PK. Legume consumption and risk of coronary heart disease in U.S. men and women. *Arch Int Med* 161:2573–2578, 2001.

Beckmann MW, Niederacher D, Bender HG. Mechanisms of steroid hormone action and resistance in endometrial and breast cancer. *Eur J Cancer Prev* 7(Suppl 1):S25–S28, 1998.

Beeson WL, Mills PK, Phillips RL, Andress M, Fraser GE. Chronic disease among Seventh-day Adventists, a low risk group. *Cancer* 64:557–581, 1989.

Beeson WL, Fraser GE, Mills. PK Validation of record linkage to two California population-based tumor registries in a cohort study. In: *Proceedings of the 1989 Public Health Conference on Records and Statistics*. Publication No. (PHS) 90–1214. Washington, D.C.: Department of Health and Human Services, 1990, pp. 196–201.

Beilin LJ. Lifestyle and hypertension: an overview. *Clin Exp Hypertens* 21:749–762, 1999.

Belfrage P, Borg B, Cronholm T, Elmqvist D, Hagerstrand I, Johansson B, Nilsson-Ehle P, Norden G, Sjovall J, Wiebe T. Prolonged administration of ethanol to young, healthy volunteers: effects on biochemical, morphological and neurophysiological parameters. *Acta Med Scand* (Suppl.)552:1–44, 1973.

Bell MR, Holmes DR, Berger PB, Garratt KN, Bailey KR, Gersh BJ. The changing in-hospital mortality of women undergoing percutaneous transluminal coronary angioplasty. *JAMA* 269:2091–2095, 1993.

Benfante RJ, Reed DM, MacLean CJ, Yano K. Risk factors in middle age that predict early and late onset of coronary heart disease. *J Clin Epidemiol* 42:95–104, 1989.

Beral V, Hermon C, Key T, Hannaford P, Darby S, Reeves G. Mortality associated with oral contraceptive use: 25 year followup of a cohort of 46,000 women from Royal College of General Practitioners' Oral Contraceptive Study. *Br Med J* 318:96–100, 1999.

Bergin AE, Masters KS, Richards PS. Religiousness and mental health reconsidered: a study of an intrinsically religious sample. *J Couns Psychol* 34(2):197–204, 1987.

Bergstrom A, Pisani P, Tenet V, Wolk A, Adami H-O. Overweight as an avoidable cause of cancer in Europe. *Int J Cancer* 91:421–430, 2001.

Berkel J. *The Clean Life: Some Aspects of Nutritional and Health Status of Seventh-day Adventists in the Netherlands.* Amsterdam: Drukkerij Insulinde, 1979.

Berkel J, deWaard F. Mortality pattern and life expectancy of Seventh-day Adventists in the Netherlands. *Int J Epidemiol* 12:455–459, 1983.

Berkman L, Syme SL. Social contacts, host resistance, and mortality: a nine-year follow-up study of Alameda County residents. *Am J Epidemiol* 109:186, 1979.

Berkman LF, Breslow L. *Health and Ways of Living. The Alameda County Study.* New York: Oxford University Press, 1983, chap. 1.

Berkman LF, Glass T. Social integration, social network, social support and health. In: L. F. Berkman and I. Kawachi (eds.), *Social Epidemiology.* New York: Oxford University Press, 2000, pp. 137–173.

Bernstein L, Henderson BE, Hanisch R, Sullivan-Halley J, Ross RK. Physical exercise and reduced risk of breast cancer in young women. *J Natl Cancer Inst* 86:1403–1408, 1994.

Berry EM, Eisenberg S, Haratz D, Fredlander Y, Norman Y, Kaufmann NA, Stein Y. Effects of diets rich in monounsaturated fatty acids on plasma lipoprotein—the Jerusalem Nutrition Study: high MUFAs vs. high PUFAs. *Am J Clin Nutr* 53:899–907, 1991.

Berry EM, Eisenberg S, Fredlander Y, Haratz D, Kaufmann NA, Norman Y, Stein Y. Effects of diets rich in monounsaturated fatty acids on plasma lipoproteins—the Jerusalem Nutrition Study: II. Monounsaturated fatty acids vs. carbohydrates. *Am J Clin Nutr* 56:394–403, 1992.

Berscheid E, Reis HT. Attraction and close relationships. In: D. T. Gilbert and S. T. Fiske (eds.), *The Handbook of Social Psychology*, vol. 2 (4th ed.) Boston: McGraw-Hill, 1998, pp.193–281.

Bertone ER, Hankinson SE, Newcomb PA, Rosner B, Willett WC, Stampfer MJ, Egan KM. A population-based case-control study of carotenoid and vitamin A intake and ovarian cancer (United States). *Cancer Causes Control* 12:83–90, 2001.

Bingham S. Meat, starch and non-starch polysaccharides: are epidemiological and experimental findings consistent with acquired genetic alterations in sporadic colorectal cancer? *Cancer Lett* 114:25–34, 1997.

Bingham SA. High meat diets and cancer risk. *Proc Nutr Soc* 58:243–248, 1999.

Blutt SE, Weigel NL. Vitamin D and prostate cancer. *Proc Soc Exp Biol Med* 221:89–98, 1999.

Boffa LC, Luptian JR, Mariani MR, Coppi M, Newmark H, Scalmati A, Lipkin M. Modulation of caloric cell proliferation, histone, acetylation and luminal short chain fatty acids by variation of dietary fibers (wheat bran) in rats. *Cancer Res* 52:5906–5912, 1992.

Bogardus C, Lillioja S, Mott DM, Hollenbeck C, Reaven G. Relationship between degree of obesity and in vivo insulin action in man. *Am J Physiol* 248:E286–E291, 1985.

Bolton-Smith C, Woodward M, Tunstall-Pedoe H. The Scottish Heart Health Study—dietary intake by food frequency questionnaire and odds ratios for coronary heart disease risk: II. The antioxidant vitamins and fibre. *Eur J Clin Nutr* 46:85–93, 1992.

Bortner RW. A short rating scale as a potential measure of pattern A behavior. *J Chron Dis* 22:87–91, 1969.

Bostick RM, Potter JD, Sellers TA, McKenzie DR, Kushi LH, Folsom AR. Relation of calcium, vitamin D, and dairy foods to incidence of colon cancer in older women: the Iowa Women's Health Study. *Am J Epidemiol* 137:1302–1317, 1993.

Bostick RM, Potter JD, Kushi LH, Sellers TA, Steinmetz KA, McKenzie DR, Gapstur SM, Folsom AR. Sugar, meat, and fat intake, and non-dietary risk factors for colon cancer incidence in Iowa women (United States). *Cancer Causes Control* 5:38–52, 1994.

Bostick RM, Fosdick L, Wood JR, Grambsch P, Grandits GA, Lillemoe TJ, Louis TA, Potter JD. Calcium and colorectal epithelial cell proliferation in sporadic adenoma patients: a randomized, double-blinded, placebo controlled clinical trial. *J Natl Cancer Inst* 87:1307–1315, 1995.

Bostom AG, Selhub J. Homocysteine and arteriosclerosis (Editorial). *Circulation* 99:2361–2363, 1999.

Bracht, N. (ed.). *Health Promotion at the Community Level.* Newbury Park, CA: Sage, 1990.

Bray GA, Popkin BM. Dietary fat intake does affect obesity! *Am J Clin Nutr* 68:1157–1173, 1998.

Brezinka V, Kittel L. Psychosocial factors of coronary heart disease in women: a review. *Soc Sci Med* 42:1351–1365, 1996.

Brown L, Rosner B, Willett WC, Sacks FM. Cholesterol-lowering effects of dietary fiber: a meta-analysis. *Am J Clin Nutr* 69:30–42, 1999a.

Brown L, Rosner B, Willett WC, Sacks FM. Nut consumption and risk of recurrent coronary heart disease (Abstract). *FASEB J Abstracts* 13(4):A538, 1999b.

Brown M. Do vitamin E and fish oil protect against ischaemic heart disease? (Editorial). *Lancet* 354:441–442, 1999.

Brussaard JH, van Raaij JMA, Stasse-Wolthuis M, Katan MB, Hautvost JGAJ. Blood pressure and diet in normotensive volunteers: absence of an effect of dietary fiber, protein or fat. *Am J Clin Nutr* 34:2023–2029, 1981.

Bryant S, Rakowski W. Predictors of mortality among elderly African-Americans. *Res Aging* 14(1):50–67, 1992.

Bucher HC, Cook RJ, Guyatt GH, Lang JD, Cook DJ, Hatala R, Hunt DL. Effects of dietary calcium supplementation on blood pressure. *JAMA* 275:1016–1022, 1996.

Burchfiel CM, Sharp DS, Curb JD, Rodriguez BL, Hwang L-J, Marcus EB, Yano K. Physical activity and incidence of diabetes: the Honolulu Heart Program. *Am J Epidemiol* 141:360–368, 1995.

Burr ML, Bates CJ, Fehily AM, St. Leger AS. Plasma cholesterol and blood pressure in vegetarians. *J Hum Nutr* 35:437–441, 1981.

Burr ML, Sweetnam PM. Vegetarianism, dietary fiber, and mortality. *Am J Clin Nutr* 36:873–877, 1982.

Burr ML, Butland BK. Heart disease in British vegetarians. *Am J Clin Nutr* 48 (Suppl.):830–832, 1988.

Burr ML, Gilbert JF, Holliday RM, Elwood PC, Fehily AM, Rogers S, Sweetnam PM, Deadman NM. Effects of changes in fat, fish, and fibre intakes on death and myocardial reinfarction: diet and reinfarction trial (DART). *Lancet* 2:757–761, 1989.

Burslem J, Schonfeld G, Howald MA, Weidman SW, Miller JP. Plasma apoprotein and lipoprotein lipid levels in vegetarians. *Metabolism* 27:711–719, 1978.

Byers T, Perry G. Dietary carotenes, vitamin C and vitamin E as protective antioxidants in human cancers. *Annu Rev Nutr* 12:139–159, 1992.

Byrd RC. Positive therapeutic effects of intercessory prayer in a coronary care unit population. *South Med J* 81(7):826–829, 1998.

Calkins BM, Whittaker DJ, Rider AA, Turjman N. Diet, nutrition, and metabolism in populations at high and low risk for colon cancer. Population: demographic and anthropometric characteristics. *Am J Clin Nutr* 40:887–895, 1984.

Callegari PE, Zurier RB. Botanical lipids: potential role in modulation of immunological responses and inflammatory reactions. *Rheum Dis Clin North Am* 17:415–426, 1991.

Cappuccio FP. The epidemiology of diet and blood pressure (Editorial). *Circulation* 86:1651–1653, 1992.

Carroll RJ, Ruppert D, Stefanski LA. Measurement error in non-linear models. New York: Chapman and Hall, 1995, p. 34.

Case RB, Heller SS, Case NB, Moss AJ. Type A behaviour and survival after acute myocardial infarction. *New England J Med* 312:737–741, 1985.

Casscells W. Magnesium and myocardial infarction (Editorial). *Lancet* 343:807–809, 1994.

Cassel J. Incidence of coronary heart disease by ethnic group, social class, and sex. *Arch Int Med* 128:901–906, 1971.

Cauley JA, Lucas FL, Kuller LH, Stone K, Browner W, Cummings SR. Elevated serum estradiol and testosterone concentrations are associated with a high risk for breast cancer. *Ann Int Med* 130:270–277, 1999.

Center for Health Statistics. Department of Health Services, Sacramento, CA. (Electronic data sent to G. Fraser, 1999).

Cha MC, Jones PJH. Dietary fat type and energy restriction interactively influence plasma leptin concentration in rats. *J Lipid Res* 39:1655–1660, 1998.

Chadwick BA, Top BL. Religiosity and delinquency among LDS adolescents. *J Sci Study Religion* 32(1):51–67, 1993.

Chan J, Knutsen SMF, Blix GG, Lee JW, Fraser GE. Water, other fluids and fatal coronary heart disease: the Adventist Health Study. *Am J Epidemiol* 155:827–833, 2002.

Chan JM, Giovannucci E, Andersson S-D, Yuen J, Adami H-O, Wolk A. Dairy products, calcium, phosphorus, vitamin D, and risk of prostate cancer (Sweden). *Cancer Causes Control* 9:559–566, 1998a.

Chan JM, Stampfer MJ, Giovannucci E, Gann PH, Ma J, Wilkinson P, Hennekens CH, Pollak M. Plasma insulin-like growth factor-I and prostate cancer risk: a prospective study. *Science* 279:563–566, 1998b.

Chan JM, Stampfer MJ, Ma J, Gann PH, Gaziano JM, Giovannucci EL. Dairy products, calcium, and prostate cancer risk in the Physicians' Health Study. *Am J Clin Nutr* 74:549–554, 2001.

Chang-Claude J, Frentzel-Beyme R, Eilber U. Mortality pattern of German vegetarians after 11 years of follow-up. *Epidemiology* 3:395–401, 1992.

Chang-Claude J, Frentzel-Beyme R. Dietary and lifestyle determinants of mortality among German vegetarians. *Int J Epidemiol* 22:228–236, 1993.

Chason-Taber L, Selhub J, Rosenberg IH, Malinow R, Terry P, Tishler PV, Willett WC, Hennekens CH, Stampfer MJ. A prospective study of folate and vitamin B6 and risk of myocardial infarction in U.S. physicians. *J Am Coll Nutr* 15:136–143, 1996.

Chipperfield B, Chipperfield JR. Heart-muscle magnesium, potassium, and zinc concentrations after sudden death from heart-disease. *Lancet* 2:293–295, 1973.

Chyou PH, Nomura AMY, Stemmermann GN. A prospective study of diet, smoking, and lower urinary tract cancer. *Ann Epidemiol* 3:211–216, 1993.

Clarkson P, Montgomery HE, Mullen MJ, Donald AE, Powe AJ, Bull T, Jubb M, World M, Deanfield JE. Exercise training enhances endothelial function in young men. *J Am Coll Cardiol* 33:1379–1385, 1999.

Cleland LG, James MJ. Rheumatoid arthritis and the balance of dietary *n*-6 and *n*-3 essential fatty acids (Editorial). *Br J Rheumatol* 36:513–515, 1997.

Coe RM, Romeis JC, Hall MM. Sense of coherence and survival in the chronically ill elderly: a five-year follow-up. In: H. I. McCubbin and E. A. Thompson (eds.), *Stress, Coping, and Health in Families: Sense of Coherence and Resiliency*. Resiliency in Families Series, 1. Thousand Oaks, CA: Sage, 1998, pp.265–275.

Coggon D, Kellingray S, Inskip H, Croft P, Campbell L, Cooper C. Osteoarthritis of the hip and occupational lifting. *Am J Epidemiol* 147:523–528, 1998.

Cohen S, Herbert TB. Health psychology: psychological factors and physical disease from the perspective of human psychoneuroimmunology. *Annu Rev Psychol* 47:113–142, 1996.

Cohen S, Doyle WJ, Skoner DP, Rabin BS, Gualtney JM. Social ties and susceptibility to the common cold. *JAMA* 277:1940–1944, 1997.

Colditz GA, Manson JE, Stampfer MJ, Rosner B, Willett WC, Speizer FE. Diet and risk of clinical diabetes in women. *Am J Clin Nutr* 55:1018–1023, 1992.

Colditz GA, Cannuscio CC, Frazier AL. Physical activity and reduced risk of colon cancer: implications for prevention. *Cancer Causes Control* 8:649–667, 1997.

Collaborative Group on Hormonal Factors in Breast Cancer. Breast cancer and hormonal contraceptives: collaborative reanalysis of individual data on 53,297 women with breast cancer and 100,239 women without breast cancer from 54 epidemiologic studies. *Lancet* 347:1713–1728, 1996.

Collaborative Group on Hormonal Factors in Breast Cancer. Breast cancer and hormone replacement therapy: collaborative reanalysis of data from 51 epidemiologic studies of 52,705 women with breast cancer and 108,411 women without breast cancer. *Lancet* 350:1047–1059, 1997.

Colquhoun DM, Humphries JA, Moores D, Somerset SM. Effects of a macadamia nut enriched diet on serum lipids and lipoproteins compared to a low fat diet. *Food Australia* 48:216–222, 1996.

Comstock GW, Partridge KB. Church attendance and health. *J Chron Dis* 25:665–672, 1972.

Cooper C, Inskip H, Croft P, Campbell L, Smith G, McLaren M, Coggon D. Individual risk factors for hip osteoarthritis: obesity, hip injury, and physical activity. *Am J Epidemiol* 147:516–522, 1998.

Cooper RS, Goldberg RB, Trevisan M, Tsong Y, Liu K, Stamler J, Rubenstein A, Scanu AM. The selective lipid-lowering effect of vegetarianism on low density lipoproteins in a cross-over experiment. *Atherosclerosis* 44:293–305, 1982.

Cooper RS, Ford E. Comparability of risk factors for coronary heart disease among blacks and whites in the NHANES-I epidemiologic follow-up study. *Ann Epidemiol* 2:637–645, 1992.

Cooper RS. Health and social status of blacks in the United States. *Ann Epidemiol* 3:137–144, 1993.

Cowley MJ, Kelsey SF, Costigan TM, Detre KM. Percutaneous coronary transluminal angioplasty in women: gender differences in outcome. In: E. D. Eaker, B. Packard, N. K. Wenger, T. B. Clarkson, and H. A. Tyroler (eds.), *Coronary Heart Disease in Women*. New York: Haymarket Doyma, 1987, pp. 251–256.

Criqui MH, Wallace RB, Heiss G, Mishkel M, Schonfeld G, Jones GTL. Cigarette smoking and plasma high-density lipoprotein cholesterol. *Circulation* 62(Suppl. 4):70–76, 1980.

Cummings JH. Fermentation in the human large intestine: evidence and implications for health. *Lancet* 1:1206–1209, 1983.

Curb JD, Reed DM. Fish consumption and mortality from coronary heart disease. *N Engl J Med* 313:821–822, 1985.

Curb JD, Wergowske G, Dobbs JC, Abbott RD, Huang B. Serum lipid effects of a high-monounsaturated fat diet based on macadamia nuts. *Arch Int Med* 160:1154–1159, 2000.

Davidson MH, Hunninghake D, Maki KC, Kwiterovich PO, Kafonek S. Comparison of the effects of lean red meat vs lean white meat on serum lipid levels among free-living persons with hypercholesterolemia. *Arch Int Med* 159:1331–1338, 1999.

Daviglus ML, Stamler J, Orencia AJ, Dyer AR, Liu K, Greenland P, Walsh MK, Morris D, Shekelle RB. Fish consumption and the 30-year risk of fatal myocardial infarction. *N Engl J Med* 336:1046–1053, 1997.

Davis KB. Coronary artery bypass graft surgery in women. In E. D. Eaker, B. Packard, N. K. Wenger, T. B. Clarkson, and H. A. Tyroler (eds.), *Coronary Heart Disease in Women*. New York: Haymarket Doyma, 1987, pp. 247–250.

Dayton S, Pearce ML, Hashimoto S, Dixon WJ, Tomiyasu U. A controlled clinical trial of a diet high in unsaturated fat in preventing complications of atherosclerosis. *Circulation* 40(Suppl. 2):1–63, 1969.

Deighton CM, Gray JW, Bint AJ, Walker DJ. Anti-proteus antibodies in rheumatoid arthritis same-sexed sibships. *Br J Rheumatol* 31:241–245, 1992.

Deitz AC, Zheng W, Leff MA, Gross M, Wen WQ, Doll MA, Xizo GH, Folsom AR, Hein DW. N-acetyl transferase-2 genetic polymorphism, well-done meat intake, and breast cancer risk among postmenopausal women. *Cancer Epidemiol Biomarkers Prev* 9:905–910, 2000.

De Lorgeril M, Renaud S, Mamelle N, Salen P, Martin J-M, Monjaud I, Guidollet J, Touboul P, Delaye J. Mediterranean α-linoleic rich diet in the secondary prevention of coronary heart disease. *Lancet* 343:1454–1459, 1994.

DeLuca P, Rothman D, Zurier RB. Marine and botanical lipids as immunomodulatory agents in the treatment of rheumatoid arthritis. *Rheum Dis Clin North Am* 21:759–777, 1995.

Der Simonian R, Laird N. Meta-analysis in clinical trials. *Control Clin Trials* 7:177–188, 1986.

Di Pietro L. Physical activity in the prevention of obesity: current evidence and research issues. *Med Sci Sports Exerc* 31(Suppl.):S542–S546, 1999.

Dizik M, Christman JK, Wainfan E. Alterations in expression and methylation of specific genes in livers of rats fed a cancer promoting methyl-deficient diet. *Carcinogenesis* 12:1307–1312, 1991.

Dolocek TA, Grandits G. Dietary polyunsaturated fatty acids and mortality in the Multiple Risk Factor Intervention Trial (MRFIT). In: A. P. Simopoulos, R. R. Kifer, R. E. Martin, and S. M. Barlow (eds.), *Health Effects of Polyunsaturated Fatty Acids in Seafoods. World Rev Nutr Diet* (Basel: Karger) 66:205–216, 1991.

Dolecek TA. Epidemiologic evidence of relationships between dietary polyunsaturated fatty acids and mortality in the Multiple Risk Factor Intervention Trial. *Proc Soc Exp Biol* 200:177–182, 1992.

Doll R, Peto R. The causes of cancer. *J Nat Cancer Inst* 66:1191–1308, 1981.

Donaldson AN. The relation of protein foods to hypertension. *Calif West Med* 24:328–331, 1926.

Dudley R, Gillespie V. *Valuegenesis: Faith in the Balance.* Riverside, CA: La Sierra University Press, 1992.

Dudley RL, Mutch PB, Cruise RJ. Religious factors and drug usage among Seventh-day Adventist youth in North America. *J Sci Study Religion* 26(2):218–233, 1987.

Durak I, Koksal I, Kacmaz M, Buyukkocak S, Cimen B, Ozturk H. Hazelnut supplementation enhances plasma antioxidant potential and lowers plasma cholesterol levels. *Clinica Chimica Acta* 284:113–115, 1999.

Durazo-Arvizu R, Cooper RS, Luke A, Previtt TE, Liao Y, McGee DL. Relative weight and mortality in U.S. blacks and whites: findings from representative national samples. *Ann Epidemiol* 7:383–395, 1997.

Durlach J, Rayssiguier Y. Fatty acid profile, fibre content and high magnesium density of nuts may protect against risk of coronary heart disease events (Editorial). *Magnesium Res* 6:191–192, 1993.

Dvilansky A, Bar-Am J, Nathan I. Hematologic values in healthy older people in the Negev area. *Isr J Med Sci* 15:821–825, 1979.

Dysinger PW, Lemon FR, Crenshaw GL, Walden RT. Pulmonary emphysema in a non-smoking population. *Dis Chest* 43:17–26, 1963.

Ebringer A, Ptaszynska T, Corbett M, Wilson C, Macafee Y, Avakian H, Baron P, James DC. Antibodies to proteus in rheumatoid arthritis. *Lancet* 2:305–307, 1985.

Editorial. Folate, alcohol, methionine, and colon cancer risk: is there a unifying theme? *Nutr Rev* 52:18–28, 1994.

Ellison CG, Gay DA. Religion, religious commitment, and life satisfaction among black Americans. *Sociol Q* 31(1):123–147, 1990.

Ellison CG. Religious involvement and subjective well-being. *J Health Soc Behav* 32(1):80–99, 1991.

Ellison CG, Levin JS. The religion–health connection: evidence, theory, and future directions. *Health Educ Behav* 25(6):700–720, 1998.

Elwood PC, Beasley WH. Myocardial magnesium and ischaemic heart disease. *Artery* 9:200–204, 1981.

Enstrom JE, Kanim LE, Klein MA. Vitamin C intake and mortality among a sample of the United States population. *Epidemiology* 3:194–202, 1992.

Erdman JW for the AHA Nutrition Committee. Soy protein and cardiovascular disease. *Circulation* 102:2555–2559, 2000.

Ernst E, Pietsch L, Matrai A, Eisenberg J. Blood rheology in vegetarians. *Br J Nutr* 45:555–560, 1986.

Ernst E. Hematocrit and cardiovascular risk. *J Int Med* 237:527–528, 1995.

Esrey KL, Joseph L, Grover SA. Relationship between dietary intake and coronary heart disease mortality: Lipid Research Clinics Prevalence Followup Study. *J Clin Epidemiol* 49:211–216, 1996.

Evans RW, Shaten BJ, Hempel JD, Cutler JA, Kuller LH for MRFIT Research Group. Homocyst(e)ine and risk of cardiovascular disease in the Multiple Risk Factor Intervention Trial. *Arterioscler Thromb Vasc Biol* 17:1947–1953, 1997.

Everson SA, Kauhanen J, Kaplan GA, Goldberg DE, Julkunen J, Tuomilehto J, Salonen JT. Hostility and increased risk of mortality and acute myocardial infarction: the mediating role of behavioral risk factors. *Am J Epidemiol* 146:142–152, 1997.

Eysenck HJ. Psychosocial factors, cancer, and ischemic heart disease. *Br Med J* 305:457–459, 1992.

Fairfield KM, Hankinson SE, Rosner BA, Hunter DJ, Colditz GA, Willett WC. Risk of ovarian carcinoma and consumption of vitamins A, C, and E and specific carotenoids. *Cancer* 92:2318–2326, 2001.

Famodu AA, Osilesi O, Makinde YO, Osonuga OA. Blood pressure and blood lipid levels among vegetarian, semi-vegetarian, and non-vegetarian native Africans. *Clin Biochem* 31:545–549, 1998.

Famodu AA, Osilesi O, Makinde YO, Osonuga OA, Fakoya TA, Ogunyemi EO, Egbenehkhuere IE. The influence of a vegetarian diet on haemostatic risk factors for cardiovascular disease in Africans. *Thromb Res* 95:31–36, 1999.

Farchi G, Mariotti S, Menotti A, Seccareccia F, Torsello S, Fidanza F. Diet and 20-year mortality in two rural population groups of middle-aged men in Italy. *Am J Clin Nutr* 50:1095–1103, 1989.

Fehily AM, Burr ML, Butland BK, Eastham RD. A randomised controlled trial to investigate the effect of a high fibre diet on blood pressure and plasma fibrinogen. *J Epidemiol Community Health* 40:334–337, 1986.

Fisher M, Levine PH, Weiner B, Ockene IS, Johnson B, Johnson MH, Natale AM, Vaudreuil CH, Hoogasian J. The effect of vegetarian diets on plasma lipids and platelet levels. *Arch Int Med* 146:1193–1197, 1986.

Fisher S, Greenberg RP. The curse of the placebo: fanciful pursuit of a pure biological therapy. In: S. Fisher and R. P. Greenberg (eds.), *From Placebo to Panacea: Putting Psychiatric Drugs to the Test*. New York: Wiley, 1997, pp. 3–56.

Fitchett G, Rybarczyk BD, DeMarco GA, Nicholas JJ. The role of religion in medical rehabilitation outcomes: a longitudinal study. *Rehabil Psychol* 44(4):333–353, 1999.

Fleming SE, O'Donnell AU, Perman JA. Influence of frequent and long-term bean consumption on colonic function and fermentation. *Am J Clin Nutr* 41:909–918, 1985.

Folkman, S. Personal control and stress and coping processes: a theoretical analysis. *J Pers Soc Psychol* 46(4):839–852, 1984.

Folsom AR, Burke GL, Ballew C, Jacobs DR Jr, Haskell WL, Donahue RP, Liu KA, Hilner JE. Relation of body fatness and its distribution to cardiovascular risk factors in young blacks and whites: the role of insulin. *Am J Epidemiol* 130:911–924, 1989.

Folsom AR, Nieto FJ, McGovern P, Tsai MY, Malinow MR, Eckfeldt JH, Hess DL, Davis CE. Prospective study of coronary heart disease incidence in relation to fasting total homocysteine, related genetic polymorphisms and B vitamins: the Atherosclerosis Risk in Communities (ARIC) Study. *Circulation* 98:204–210, 1998a.

Folsom AR, Stevens J, Schreiner PJ, McGovern PG. Body mass index, waist/hip ratio, and coronary heart disease incidence in African Americans and whites. *Am J Epidemiol* 148:1187–1194, 1998b.

Folsom AR, Kushi LH, Anderson KE, Mirk PJ, Olson JE, Hong C-P, Sellers TA, Lazowich D, Prineas RJ. Associations of general and abdominal obesity with multiple health outcomes in older women. *Arch Int Med* 160:2117–2128, 2000.

Fønnebø V. The Tromsø Heart Study: coronary risk factors in Seventh-day Adventists. *Am J Epidemiol* 122:789–793, 1985.

Fønnebø V. The Tromsø Heart Study: diet, religion, and risk factors for coronary heart disease. *Am J Clin Nutr* 48:826–829, 1988.

Fønnebø V, Helseth A. Cancer incidence in Norwegian Seventh-day Adventists 1961 to 1986. *Cancer* 68:666–671, 1991.

Fønnebø V. Mortality in Norwegian Seventh-day Adventists 1962–1986. *J Clin Epidemiol* 45:157–167, 1992.

Fønnebø V. The healthy Seventh-day Adventists lifestyle: what is the Norwegian experience? *Am J Clin Nutr* 59:1124S–1192S, 1994.

Ford DE, Mead LA, Chang PP, Cooper-Patrick L, Wang N-Y, Klag MJ. Depression is a risk factor for coronary artery disease in men. *Arch Int Med* 158:1422–1426, 1998.

Ford ES, Byers TE, Giles WH. Serum folate and chronic disease risk: findings from a cohort of United States adults. *Int J Epidemiol* 27:592–598, 1998.

Ford ES. Serum magnesium and ischaemic heart disease: findings from a national sample of US adults. *Int J Epidemiol* 28:645–651, 1999.

Fortes C, Forastiere F, Farchi S, Rapiti E, Pastori G, Perucci CA. Diet and overall survival in a cohort of very elderly people. *Epidemiology* 11:440–445, 2000.

Fortmann SP, Flora JA, Winkleby MA, Schooler C, Taylor CB, Farquhar JW. Community intervention trials: reflection on the Stanford Five-City Project experience. *Am J Epidemiol* 142:576–586, 1995.

Fortmann SP, Marcovina SM. Lipoprotein (a), a clinically elusive lipoprotein particle. *Circulation* 95:295–296, 1997.

Fraser GE. Sudden death in Auckland. *Aust N Z J Med* 8:490–499, 1978.

Fraser GE, Swannell RJ. Diet and serum cholesterol in Seventh-day Adventists: a cross-sectional study showing significant relationships. *J Chronic Dis* 34:487–501, 1981.

Fraser GE, Dysinger PW, Best C, Chan R: IHD risk factors in middle-aged Seventh-day Adventist men and their neighbors. *Am J Epidemiol* 126:638–646, 1987.

Fraser GE, Phillips RL, Beeson WL. Hypertension, antihypertensive medication, and risk of renal carcinoma in California Seventh-day Adventists. *Int J Epidemiol* 19:832–838, 1990.

Fraser GE, Beeson WL, Phillips RL. Diet and lung cancer in California Seventh-day Adventists. *Am J Epidemiol* 133:683–693, 1991.

Fraser GE, Strahan TM, Sabaté J, Beeson WL. Effects of traditional coronary risk factors on rates of incident coronary events in a low risk population. *Circulation* 86:406–413, 1992a.

Fraser GE, Sabaté J, Beeson WL, Strahan TM. A possible protective effect of nut consumption on risk of coronary heart disease. *Arch Int Med* 152:1416–1424, 1992b.

Fraser GE. Diet and coronary heart disease: beyond dietary fats and low-density-lipoprotein cholesterol. *Am J Clin Nutr* 59(Suppl.):1117S–1123S, 1994.

Fraser GE, Lindsted KD, Beeson WL. Effect of risk factor values on lifetime risk of and age at first coronary event. *Am J Epidemiol.* 142:746–758, 1995.

Fraser GE, Shavlik DJ. Risk factors for all-cause and coronary heart disease mortality in the oldest-old. *Arch Int Med* 157:2249–2258, 1997a.

Fraser GE, Shavlik D. Risk factors, lifetime risk, and age at onset of breast cancer. *Ann Epidemiol* 7:375–382, 1997b.

Fraser GE, Haller-Wade TM, Morrow S. Selected social support variables in middle-aged Seventh-day Adventist men and their neighbors. *J Religion Health* 36:231–239, 1997a.

Fraser GE, Sumbureru D, Pribis P, Neil RL, Frankson MAC. Association among health habits, risk factors, and all-cause mortality in a black California population. *Epidemiology* 8:168–174, 1997b.

Fraser GE, Shavlik DJ. The estimation of lifetime risk and average age at onset of a disease using a multivariate exponential hazard rate model. *Stat Med* 18:397–410, 1999.

Fraser GE, Butler J, Myint T. Marked differences in effects of CHD risk factors by age: Adventist Health Study. (Abstract). In *Epidemiology for Sustainable Health*. The XV International Scientific Meeting of the International Epidemiologic Association, Florence, Italy, September 1999. Abstract Book II:7.

Fraser GE. Associations between diet and cancer, ischemic heart disease, and all-cause mortality in non-Hispanic white California Seventh-day Adventists. *Am J Clin Nutr* 70(Suppl.):532S–538S, 1999a.

Fraser GE. Nut consumption, lipids, and risk of a coronary event. *Clin Cardiol* 22(Suppl. 3):11–15, 1999b.

Fraser GE. Diet as primordial prevention in Seventh-day Adventists. *Prev Med* 29(Suppl.):S18–S23, 1999c.

Fraser GE, Welch A, Luben R, Bingham SA, Day NE. The effect of age, sex, and education on food consumption of a middle-aged English cohort: EPIC in East Anglia. *Prev Med* 30:26–34, 2000.

Fraser GE, Shavlik DJ. Ten years of life: is it a matter of choice? *Arch Int Med* 161:1645–1652, 2001.

Fraser GE, Stram D. An illustration of the effect of calibration study size, power loss, and bias correction in regression calibration models containing two correlated dietary variables. *Am J Epidemiol* 154:836–844, 2001.

Fraser GE, Bennett HW, Sabaté J, Jaceldo KB. Effect of a free 320 calorie daily supplement of almonds on body weight. *J Am Coll Nutr* 21:275–283, 2002.

Frasure-Smith N, Lespérance F, Talajic M. Depression following myocardial infarction: impact on 6-month survival. *JAMA* 270:1819–1825, 1993.

Frasure-Smith N, Lespérance F, Granel G, Masson A, Juneau M, Talajic M, Bourassa MG. Social support, depression, and mortality during the first year after myocardial infarction. *Circulation* 101:1919–1924, 2000.

Frentzel-Beyme R, Claude J, Eilber U. Mortality among German vegetarians: first results after five years of follow-up. *Nutr Cancer* 11:117–126, 1988.

Frentzel-Beyme R, Chang-Claude J. Vegetarian diets and colon cancer: the German experience. *Am J Clin Nutr* 59(Suppl.):1143S–1152S, 1994.

Freud S. *Die Zukunft einer Illusion.* Leipzig: Internationaler Psychoanalytischer Verlag, 1927.

Friedman M, Rosenman RH. Association of specific overt behavior pattern with blood and cardiovascular findings: blood cholesterol level, blood clotting time, incidence of arcus senilis and clinical coronary artery disease. *JAMA* 169:1286–1296, 1959.

Friedman M, Thoresen CE, Gill JJ, Powell JH, Ulmer D, Thompson L, Price VA, Rabin DD, Breall WS, Dixon T et al. Alteration of type A behavior and reduction in cardiac recurrences in postmyocardial infarction patients. *Am Heart J* 108:237–48, 1984.

Fukushima S, Takada N, Hori T, Wanibuchi T. Cancer prevention by organosulfur compounds from garlic and onions. *J Cell Biochem Suppl* 27:100–105, 1997.

Fulton-Kehoe DL, Eckel RH, Shetterly SM, Hamman RF. Determinants of total high density lipoprotein and high density lipoprotein subfraction levels among Hispanic and nonHispanic white persons with normal glucose tolerance: the San Luis Valley Diabetes Study. *J Clin Epidemiol* 45:1191–1200, 1992.

Gaard M, Tretli S, Loken EB. Dietary fat and the risk of breast cancer: a prospective study of 25,892 Norwegian women. *Int J Cancer* 63:13–17, 1995.

Gammon MD, John EM, Britton JA. Recreational and occupational physical activities and risk of breast cancer. *J Natl Cancer Inst* 90:100–117, 1998.

Gann PH, Hennekens CH, Sacks FM, Grodstein F, Giovannucci EL, Stampfer MJ. Prospective study of plasma fatty acids and risk of prostate cancer. *J Natl Cancer Inst* 86:281–286, 1994.

Gann PH, Ma J, Giovannucci E, Willett W, Sacks FM, Hennekens CH, Stampfer MJ. Lower prostate cancer risk in men with elevated plasma lycopene levels: results of a prospective analysis. *Cancer Res* 15:1225–1230, 1999.

Garg A. High-monounsaturated-fat diets for patients with diabetes mellitus: a meta-analysis. *Am J Clin Nutr* 67(Suppl.):577S–582S, 1998.

Garland C, Shekelle RB, Barrett-Connor E, Criqui MH, Rossof AH, Paul O. Dietary vitamin D and calcium and risk of colorectal cancer: a 19-year prospective study in men. *Lancet* 1:307–309, 1985.

Gartner J, Larson DB, Allen GD. Religious commitment and mental health: a review of the empirical literature. Special Issue: Spirituality: Perspectives in theory and research. *J Psychol Theol* 19(1):6–25, 1991.

Gear JS, Mann JI, Thorogood M, Carter R, Jelfs R. Biochemical and haematological variables in vegetarians. *Br Med J* 1:1415, 1980.

Genia, V. Intrinsic, extrinsic, quest, and fundamentalism as predictors of psychological and spiritual well-being. *J Sci Study Religion* 35(1):56–64, 1996.

Geronimus AT, Bound J, Waidmann TA, Hillmeier MM, Burns PB. Excess mortality among blacks and whites in the United States. *N Engl J Med* 335:1552–1558, 1996.

Giacosa A, Franceschi S, La Vecchia C, Favero A, Andreatta R. Energy intake, overweight, physical exercise and colorectal cancer risk. *Eur J Cancer Prev* 8(Suppl 1):S53–S60, 1999.

Giles WH, Kittner SJ, Croft JB, Anda RF, Casper ML, Ford ES. Serum folate and risk for coronary heart disease: results from cohort of US adults. *Ann Epidemiol* 8:490–496, 1998.

Gilligan DM, Sack MN, Guetta V, Casino PR, Quyyumi AA, Rader DJ, Panza JA, Cannon RO. Effect of antioxidant vitamins on low density lipoprotein oxidation and impaired endothelium dependent vasodilation in patients with hypercholesterolemia. *J Am Coll Cardiol* 24:1611–1617, 1994.

Gillum, RF, Fortman, SP, Prineas, RJ, Kottke, TE. International diagnostic criteria for acute myocardial infarction and stroke. *Am Heart J* 108:150–158, 1984.

Gillum RF. Trends in acute myocardial infarction and coronary heart disease death in the United States. *J Am Coll Cardiol* 23:1273–1277, 1993.

Gillum RF, Mussolino ME, Madans JH. The relationship between fish consumption and stroke incidence: the NHANES I Epidemiologic Follow-up Study. *Arch Int Med* 156:537–542, 1996.

Gillum RF, Mussolino ME, Madaus JH. Coronary heart disease risk factors and attributable risks in African-American women and men: NHANES I Epidemiology Follow-up Study. *Am J Public Health* 88:913–917, 1998.

Giovannucci E, Stampfer MJ, Colditz GA, Rimm EG, Trichopoulos D, Rosner BA, Speizer FE, Willett WC. Folate, methionine, and alcohol intake and risk of colorectal adenoma. *J Natl Cancer Inst* 85:875–884, 1993a.

Giovannucci E, Rimm EG, Colditz GA, Stampfer MJ, Ascherio A, Chute CC, Willett WC. A prospective study of dietary fat and risk of prostate cancer. *J Natl Cancer Inst* 85:1571–1579, 1993b.

Giovannucci E, Rimm EB, Stampfer MJ, Colditz GA, Ascherio A, Willett WC. Intake of fat, meat and fiber in relation to risk of colon cancer in men. *Cancer Res* 54:2390–2397, 1994.

Giovannucci E. Insulin and colon cancer. *Cancer Causes Control* 6:164–179, 1995.

Giovannucci E, Ascherio A, Rimm EG, Stampfer MJ, Colditz GA, Willett WC. Intake of carotenoids and retinol in relation to risk of prostate cancer. *J Natl Cancer Inst* 87:1767–1776, 1995.

Giovannucci E, Rimm EG, Wolk A, Ascherio A, Stampfer MJ, Colditz GA, Willett WC. Calcium and fructose intake in relation to risk of prostate cancer. *Cancer Res* 58:442–447, 1998.

Giovannucci E. Dietary influences of 1,25 $(OH)_2$ vitamin D in relation to prostate cancer: a hypothesis. *Cancer Causes Control* 9:567–582, 1998.

GISSI-Prevenzione Investigators. Dietary supplementation with n-3 polyunsaturated fatty acids and vitamin E after myocardial infarction: results of the GISSI-Prevenzione trial. *Lancet* 354:447–455, 1999.

Glyn SA, Albanes D. Folate and cancer: a review of the literature. *Nutr Cancer* 22:101–119, 1994.

Godin G, Kok G. The theory of planned behavior: a review of its applications to health-related behaviors. *Am J Health Promot* 11:87–98, 1996.

Goen GC. In: E. James, JW James, PS Boyer (eds.), *Notable American Women, 1607–1950*. Vol. 3. Boston: Belknap Press, Harvard University, 1971, pp. 585–588.

Goldberg AD. The Sabbath as dialectic: implications for mental health. *J Religion Health* 25(3):237–244, 1986.

Goldberg AD. The Sabbath: implications for mental health. *Couns Values* 31(2):147–156, 1987.

Goldbohm RA, Van den Brandt PA, Van't Veer P, Brants HAM, Dorant E, Sturman SF, Hermus RJJ. A prospective cohort study on the relation between red meat consumption and the risk of colon cancer. *Cancer Res* 54:718–723, 1994.

Goldin BR, Gorbach SL. Effect of diet on the plasma levels, metabolism, and excretion of estrogens. *Am J Clin Nutr* 48(Supplement):787–790, 1988.

Golner JH. The Sabbath and mental health intervention: some parallels. *J Religion Health* 21(2):132–144, 1982.

Gordon T, Kagan A, Garcia-Palmieri M, Kannel WB, Zukel WJ, Tillotson J, Sorlie P, Hjortland M. Diet and its relation to coronary heart disease and death in three populations. *Circulation* 63:500–515, 1981.

Gould AL, Rossouw JE, Santanello NC, Heyse JF, Furberg CD. Cholesterol reduction yields clinical benefit. *Circulation* 97:946–952, 1998.

Graham S, Haughey B, Marshall J, Priore R, Byers T, Rzepka T, Mettlin C, Pontes JE. Diet in the epidemiology of carcinoma of the prostate gland. *J Natl Cancer Inst* 70:687–692, 1983.

Grant WB. The role of meat in the expression of rheumatoid arthritis. *Br J Nutr* 84:589–595, 2000.

Gray GE, Williams P, Gerkins V, Brown JB, Armstrong B, Phillips R, Casagrande JT, Pike MC, Henderson BE. Diet and hormone levels in Seventh-day Adventist teenage girls. *Prev Med* 11:103–107, 1982.

Greenberg MA, Mueller HS. Why the excess mortality in women after PTCA? *Circulation* 87:1030–1032, 1993.

Gregoire RC, Stern HS, Yeung KS, Sadler J, Langley S, Furrer R, Bruce WR. Effect of calcium supplementation on mucosal cell proliferation in high risk patients for colon cancer. *Gut* 30:376–382, 1989.

Groen JJ, Tijong KB, Koster M, Willebrands AF, Verdonck G, Pierloot M. The influence of nutrition and ways of life on blood cholesterol and the prevalence of hypertension and coronary heart disease among Trappist and Benedictine monks. *Am J Clin Nutr* 10:456–470, 1962.

Grover SA, Paquet S, Levinton C, Coupal L, Zowall H. Estimating the benefits of modifying risk factors of cardiovascular disease. *Arch Int Med* 158:655–662, 1998.

Grundy SM. Small LDL, atherogenic dyslipidemia and the metabolic syndrome. *Circulation* 95:1–4, 1997.

Grusec J, Kuczynski L, Marshall S, Schell K. Historical overview of parental influence and bidirectionality. In: J. Grusec and L. Kuczynski (eds.), *Parenting and Children's Internalization of Values: A Handbook of Contemporary Theory*. New York: Wiley, 1997, pp. 3–50.

Gussow JD. Ecology and vegetarian considerations: does environmental responsibility demand the elimination of livestock? *Am J Clin Nutr* 59(Suppl.):1110S–1116S, 1994.

Haddad EH. Development of a vegetarian food guide. *Am J Clin Nutr* 59(Suppl.):1248S–1254S, 1994.

Haddad EH, Berk LS, Kettering JD, Hubbard RW, Peters WR. Dietary intake and biochemical, hematologic, and immune status of vegans compared to nonvegetarians. *Am J Clin Nutr* 70(Suppl.):586S–593S, 1999a.

Haddad EH, Sabaté J, Whitten CG. Vegetarian food guide pyramid: a conceptual framework. *Am J Clin Nutr* 70(Suppl.):615S–619S, 1999b.

Haddad EH, Sabaté J. Effect of pecan consumption on stool fat. *FASEB J (Abstracts)* 14(4):A294, 2000.

Hahn RA. Expectations of sickness: concept and evidence of the nocebo phenomenon. In: I. Kirsch (ed.), *How Expectancies Shape Experience*. Washington, DC: American Psychological Association, 1999, pp. 333–356.

Haines AP, Chakrabarti R, Fisher D, Meade TW, North WRS, Stirling Y. Haemostatic variables in vegetarians and non-vegetarians. *Thromb Res* 19:139–148, 1980.

Hammond, EC. Smoking in relation to the death rates of one million men and women. *Natl Cancer Inst Monogr* 19:127–204, 1966.

Hankinson SE, Colditz GA, Hunter DJ, Willett WC, Stampfer MJ, Rosner B, Hennekens CH, Speizer FE. A prospective study of reproductive factors and risk of epithelial ovarian cancer. *Cancer* 76:284–290, 1995.

Hankinson SE, Willett WC, Colditz GA, Hunter DJ, Michand DS, Deroo B, Rosner B, Speizer FE, Pollak M. Circulatory concentrations of insulin-like growth factor-I and risk of breast cancer. *Lancet* 351:1393–1396, 1998a.

Hankinson SE, Willett WC, Manson JE, Colditz GA, Hunter DJ, Spiegelman D, Barbieri RL, Speizer FE. Plasma sex steroid hormone levels and risk of breast cancer in postmenopausal women. *J Natl Cancer Inst* 90:1292–1299, 1998b.

Hansen RK, Bissell MJ. Tissue architecture and breast cancer: the role of extracellular matrix and steroid hormones. *Endocr Relat Cancer* 7:95–113, 2000.

Hanson BS, Mattisson I, Steen B. Dietary intake and psychosocial factors in 68-year old men. *Compr Gerontol* 1:62–67, 1987.

Hanson NR. *Perception and Discovery*. Freeman Cooper, 1969, Chapter 9.

Hardinge MG, Stare FJ. Nutritional studies of vegetarians: I. Nutritional, physical, and laboratory studies. *J Clin Nutr* 2:73–82, 1954a.

Hardinge MG, Stare FJ. Nutritional studies of vegetarians: II. Dietary and serum levels of cholesterol. *J Clin Nutr* 2:83–88, 1954b.

Hardinge MG, Crooks H, Stare FJ. Nutritional studies of vegetarians: IV. Dietary fatty acids and serum cholesterol levels. *Am J Clin Nutr* 10:516–524, 1962.

Harmon RL, Myers MA. Prayer and meditation as medical therapies. *Phys Med Rehabil Clin North Am* 10(3):651–662, 1999.

Harris RD, Phillips RL, Williams PM, Kuzma JW, Fraser GE. The child-adolescent blood pressure study: I. Distribution of blood pressure levels in Seventh-day Adventist (SDA) and non-SDA children. *Am J Public Health* 71:1342–1349, 1981.

Harris WS, Gowda M, Kolb JW, Strychacz CP, Vacek JL, Jones PG, Forker A, O'Keefe JH, McCallister BD. A randomized, controlled trial of the effects of remote, intercessory prayer on outcomes in patients admitted to the coronary care unit. *Arch Int Med* 159(19):2273–2278, 1999.

Harsha DW, Lin P-H, Obarzanek E, Karanja NM, Moore TM, Caballero B. Dietary Approaches to Stop Hypertension: a summary of study results. *J Am Diet Assoc* 99:S35–S39, 1999.

Haskell WL, Camargo C, Williams PT, Vranizan KM, Krauss RM, Lindgren FT, Wood PD. The effect of cessation and resumption of moderate alcohol intake on serum high-density lipoprotein subfractions. *N Engl J Med* 310:805–810, 1984.

Haugen MA, Kjeldsen-Kragh J, Bjerve KS, Hostmark AT, Forre O. Changes in plasma phospholipid fatty acids, and their relationship to disease activity in rheumatoid arthritis patients treated with a vegetarian diet. *Br J Nutr* 72:555–566, 1994.

Havlik RJ, Feinleib M (eds.). *Proceedings of the Conference on the Decline in Coronary Heart Disease Mortality.* NIH Publication No. 79-1610. Bethesda, MD: Department of Health, Education and Welfare, 1979.

Heart Outcomes Prevention Evaluation Study Investigators. Vitamin E supplementation and cardiovascular events in high risk patients. *N Engl J Med* 342:154–160, 2000.

Heath GW, Macera CA, Croft JB, Mace ML, Gillette T, Wheeler FC. Correlates of high-density lipoprotein cholesterol in black and white women. *Am J Public Health* 84:98–101, 1994.

Heilbrun LK, Nomura A, Hankin JH, Stemmerman GN. Diet and colorectal cancer with special reference to fiber intake. *Int J Cancer* 44:1–6, 1989.

Heitzer T, Yla-Herttuala S, Luoma J, Kurz S, Munzel T, Just H, Olschewski M, Drexler H. Cigarette smoking potentiates endothelial dysfunction of forearm resistance vessels in patients with hypercholesterolemia. *Circulation* 93:1346–1353, 1996.

Helmrich SP, Ragland DR, Leung RW, Paffenbarger RS. Physical activity and reduced occurrence of non-insulin-dependent diabetes mellitus. *N Engl J Med* 325:147–152, 1991.

Henderson BE, Pike MC, Bernstein L, Ross RK. Breast cancer. In: D. Schottenfeld and J. F. Fraumeni (eds.), *Cancer Epidemiology and Prevention*, 2nd ed. New York: Oxford University Press, 1996, pp. 1022–1039.

Henderson CJ, Panush RS. Diets, dietary supplements, and nutritional therapies in rheumatic diseases. *Rheumatoid Dis Clin North Am* 25:937–968, 1999.

Henderson JB, Dunnigan MG, McIntosh WB, Abdul-Motaal AA, Gettinby G, Glekin BM. The importance of limited exposure to ultraviolet radiation and dietary factors in the aetiology of Asian rickets: a risk factor model. *Q J Med* 63:413–425, 1987.

Hennekens CH, Buring JE, Manson JE, Stampfer M, Rosner B, Cook NR, Belanger C, LaMotte F, Gaziano JM, Ridker PM, et al. Lack of effect of longterm supplementation with beta carotene on the incidence of malignant neoplasms and cardiovascular disease. *N Engl J Med* 334:1145–1149, 1996.

Henry, M. *Concise Commentary on the Whole Bible.* Chicago: Moody Press, 1983.

Herman C, Adlercreutz T, Goldin BR, Gorbach SL, Hockerstedt KAV, Watanabe S, Hamalainen EK, Markkanen MH, Makela TH, Wahala KT, et al. Soybean phytoestrogen intake and cancer risk. *J Nutr* 125:757S–770S, 1995.

Hertog MGL, Feskens EJM, Hollman PCH, Katan MB, Kromhout D. Dietary antioxidant flavonols and risk of coronary heart disease: the Zutphen Elderly Study. *Lancet* 342:1007–1011, 1993.

Hertog MGL, Feskens EJM, Kromhout D. Antioxidant flavonols and coronary heart disease risk. *Lancet* 349:699, 1997a.

Hertog MGL, Sweetnam PM, Fehily AM, Elwood PC, Kromhout D. Antioxidant flavonols and ischaemic heart disease in a Welsh population of men: the Caerphilly Study. *Am J Clin Nutr* 65:1489–1494, 1997b.

Heymsfield SB, Darby PC, Muhlheim LS, Gallagher D, Wolper C, Allison DB. The calorie: myth, measurement, and reality. *Am J Clin Nutr* 62(Suppl.): 1034S–1041S, 1995.

Hill PC, Butter EM. The role of religion in promoting physical health. *J Psychol Christianity* 14(2):141–155, 1995.

Hill PB, Wynder EL. Effect of a vegetarian diet and dexamethasone on plasma prolactin, testosterone and dehydroepiandrosterone in men and women. *Cancer Letters* 7:273–282, 1979.

Hirayama T. An analytical epidemiology of ovarian cancer and possible environmental carcinogenesis (In Japanese and quoted by Kushi et al., 1999). *Med Chugai* 34:282–286, 1981.

Hirayama T. A large-scale study on cancer risks by diet, with special reference to the risk reducing effects of green-yellow vegetable consumption. In: Y. Hayaishi (ed.), *Diet, Nutrition and Cancer.* Tokyo: Japan Scientific Societies Press, 1986, pp. 41–53.

Hirayama T. Epidemiology of pancreatic cancer in Japan. *Jpn J Clin Oncol* 19:208–215, 1989.

Hirokawa K. Understanding the mechanism of the age-related decline in immune function. *Nutr Rev* 50:361–366, 1992.

Hjermann I, Holme I, Velve Byre K, Leren P. Effect of diet and smoking intervention on the incidence of coronary heart disease. *Lancet* 2:1303–1210, 1981.

Hodis HN. Triglyceride-rich lipoprotein remnant particles and risk of atherosclerosis. *Circulation* 99:2852–2854, 1999.

Hokin BD, Butler T. Cyanocobalamin (vitamin B-12) status in Seventh-day Adventist ministers in Australia. *Am J Clin Nutr* 70(Suppl.):576S–578S, 1999.

Hollenbeck CB. Dietary fructose effects on lipoprotein metabolism and risk for coronary artery disease. *Am J Clin Nutr* 58(Suppl.):800S–809S, 1993.

Hopkin K. Caloric restriction may put the brakes on aging. *J NIH Res* 7:47–50, 1995.

Horton ES. Exercise and physical training: effects on insulin sensitivity and glucose metabolism. *Diabetes Metab Rev* 2:1–17, 1986.

Howard BV, Kritchevsky D. Phyto chemicals and cardiovascular disease. *Circulation* 95:2591–2593, 1997.

Howell WH, McNamara DJ, Tosca MA, Smith BT, Gaines JA. Plasma lipid and lipoprotein responses to dietary fat and cholesterol: a meta-analysis. *Am J Clin Nutr* 65:1747–1764, 1997.

Hu FB, Stampfer MJ, Manson JE, Rimm E, Colditz GA, Rosner BA, Hennekens CH, Willett WC. Dietary fat intake and the risk of coronary heart disease in women. *N Engl J Med* 337:1491–1499, 1997.

Hu FB, Stampfer MJ, Manson JE, Rimm EB, Colditz GA, Rosner BA, Speizer FE, Hennekens CH, Willett WC. Frequent nut consumption and risk of coronary heart disease in women: prospective cohort study. *Br Med J* 317:1341–1345, 1998.

Hu FB, Stampfer MJ, Manson JE, Rimm EB, Wolk A, Colditz GA, Hennekens CH, Willett WC. Dietary intake of α-linoleic acid and risk of fatal ischemic heart disease among women. *Am J Clin Nutr* 69:890–897, 1999.

Hu FB, Rimm EB, Stampfer MJ, Ascherio A, Spiegelman D, Willett WC. Prospective study of major dietary patterns and risk of coronary heart disease in men. *Am J Clin Nutr* 72:912–921, 2000.

Hu FB, Leitzmann MF, Stampfer MJ, Colditz GA, Willett WC, Rimm EB. Physical activity and television watching in relation to risk for type 2 diabetes mellitus in men. *Arch Int Med* 161:1542–1548, 2001.

Hua NW, Stoohs RA, Facchini FS. Low iron status and enhanced insulin sensitivity in lacto-ovo vegetarians. *Br J Nutr* 86:515–519, 2001.

Hughes K, Aw TC, Kuperan P, Choo M. Central obesity, insulin resistance, syndrome X, lipoprotein (a), and cardiovascular risk in Indians, Malays and Chinese in Singapore. *J Epidemiol Community Health* 51:394–399, 1997.

Humble CG, Malarcher AM, Tyroler HA. Dietary fiber and coronary heart disease in middle-aged hypercholesterolemic men. *Am J Prev Med* 9:197–202, 1993.

Hummer RA, Rogers RG, Nam CB, Ellison CG. Religious involvement and U.S. adult mortality. *Demography* 36(2):273–285, 1999.

Hunink MGM, Goldman L, Tosteson ANA, Mittleman MA, Goldman PA, Williams LW, Tsevat J, Weinstein MC. The recent decline in mortality from coronary heart disease, 1980–1990. *JAMA* 277:535–542, 1997.

Hunter D. Biochemical indicators of dietary intake. In: W. Willet (ed.), *Nutritional Epidemiology*, 2nd ed. New York: Oxford University Press, 1998, pp. 174–243.

Hunter DJ, Stampfer MJ, Colditz GA, Stampfer MJ, Rosner B, Hennekens CH, Speizer FE, Willett WC. A prospective study of intake of vitamin C, E, and A and the risk of breast cancer. *N Engl J Med* 329:234–240, 1993.

Hunter DJ, Spiegelman D, Adami HO, Beeson L, van den Brandt PA, Folsom AR, Fraser GE, Goldbohm RA, Graham S, Howe GR, et al. Cohort studies of fat intake and the risk of breast cancer: a pooled analysis. *N Engl J Med* 334:356–361, 1996.

Idler EL, Kasl SV. Religion, disability, depression, and the timing of death. *Am J Sociol* 97(4):1052–1079, 1992.

Idler EL, Kasl SV. Religion among disabled and nondisabled persons: II. Attendance at religious services as a predictor of the course of disability. *J Gerontol B Psychol Sci Soc Sci* 56(6):S306–S316, 1997.

Ingles SA, Coetzee GA, Ross RK, Henderson BA, Kolonel LN, Crocitto L, Wang W, Haile RW. Association of prostate cancer with vitamin D receptor haplotypes in African-Americans. *Cancer Res* 58(8):1620–1623, 1998.

Iso H, Rexrode KM, Stampfer MJ, Manson JE, Colditz GA, Speizer FE, Hennekens CH, Willett WC. Intake of fish and omega-3 fatty acids and risk of stroke in women. *JAMA* 285:304–312, 2001.

Jacobs DR, Anderson JT, Blackburn H. Diet and serum cholesterol: do zero correlations negate the relationship? *Am J Epidemiol* 110:77–87, 1979.

Jacobs DR, Meyer KA, Kushi LH, Folsom AR. Whole-grain intake may reduce the risk of ischemic heart disease in post-menopausal women: the Iowa Women's Health Study. *Am J Clin Nutr* 68:248–257, 1998.

Jacobsen B, Knutsen SF, Fraser GE. Does high soy milk intake reduce prostate cancer incidence? The Adventist Health Study (United States). *Cancer Causes Control* 9:553–557, 1998.

Jagerstad M, Skog K, Grivas S, Olsson K. Formation of heterocyclic amines using model systems. *Mutat Res* 259:219–233, 1991.

Jarvis GK, Northcott HC. Religion and differences in morbidity and mortality. *Soc Sci Med* 25(7):813–824, 1987.

Jebb SA, Moore MS. Contribution of a sedentary lifestyle and inactivity to the etiology of overweight and obesity: current evidence and research issues. *Med Sci Sports Exerc* 31(Suppl.):S534–S541, 1999.

Jekel JF, Elmore JG, Katz DL. *Epidemiology, Biostatistics and Preventive Medicine*. Philadelphia: W. B. Saunders, 1996, pp.66–67.

Jemal A, Thomas A, Murray T, Thun M. Cancer statistics, 2002. *CA: Cancer J Clin* 52:23–47, 2002.

Jenkins CD. Risk of new myocardial infarction in middle-aged men with manifest coronary heart disease. *Circulation* 53:342–347, 1976.

Jenkins DJ, Josse RG, Jenkins AL, Wolever TM, Vuksan V. Implications of altering the rate of carbohydrate absorption from the gastrointestinal tract. *Clin Invest Med* 18:296–302, 1995.

Jenkins DJA, Wolever TM, Kalmusky J, Giudici S, Giordano C, Wong GS, Bird JN, Patten R, Hall M, Buckley G et al. Low glycemic index carbohydrate foods in the management of hyperlipidemia. *Am J Clin Nutr* 42:604–617, 1985.

Jenkins DJA, Wolever TMS, Collier GR, Ocana A, Rao V, Buckley G, Lam Y, Mayer A, Thompson LU. Metabolic effects of a low glycemic index diet. *Am J Clin Nutr* 46:968–975, 1987.

Jenkins DJ, Kendall CW, Marchie A, Parker Tl, Connelly PW, Qian W, Haight JS, Faulkner D, Vidgen E, Lapsley KG, Spiller GA. Dose response of almonds on coronary heart disease risk factors: blood lipids, oxidized low-density lipoproteins, lipoprotein (a), homocysteine and pulmonary nitric oxide: a randomized, controlled, crossover trial. *Circulation* 106:1327–1332, 2002.

Jensen OM. Cancer risk among Danish male Seventh-day Adventists and other temperance society members. *J Natl Cancer Inst* 70:1011–1014, 1983.

Jernstrom H, Barrett-Connor E. Obesity, weight change, fasting insulin, proinsulin, C-peptide, and insulin-like growth factor-1 levels in women with and without breast cancer: the Rancho Bernardo Study. *J Womens Health Gend Based Med* 8:1265–1272, 1999.

Johnson CJ, Peterson DR, Smith EK. Myocardial tissue concentrations of magnesium and potassium in men dying suddenly from ischemic heart disease. *Am J Clin Nutr* 32:967–979, 1979.

Jongen WMF. Glucosinolates in brassica: occurrence and significance as cancer modulating agents. *Proc Nutr Soc* 55:433–446, 1996.

Kamarck TW, Everson SA, Kaplan GA, Manuck SB, Jennings JR, Salonen R, Salonen JT. Exaggerated blood pressure responses during mental stress are associated with enhanced carotid atherosclerosis in middle-aged Finnish men. *Circulation* 96:3842–3848, 1997.

Kannel WB, Thomas HE. Sudden coronary death: the Framingham Study. *Ann N Y Acad Sci.* 382:3–20, 1982.

Kant AK, Schatzkin A, Graubard BI, Schairer C. A prospective study of diet quality and mortality in women. *JAMA* 283:2109–2115, 2000.

Kaplan GA, Seeman TE, Cohen RD, Knudsen LP, Guralnik J. Mortality among the elderly in the Alameda County Study: behavioral and demographic risk factors. *Am J Public Health* 77:307–312, 1987.

Kaplan GA, Keil JE. Socioeconomic factors and cardiovascular disease: a review of the literature. *Circulation* 88:1973–1998, 1993.

Kaplan JR, Pettersson K, Manuck SB, Olsson G. Role of sympathoadrenal medullary activation in the initiation and progression of atherosclerosis. *Circulation* 84(Suppl 6):VI-23–VI-32, 1991.

Kardinaal AFM, Aro A, Kark JE, Riemersma RA, van't Veer P, Gomez-Aracena J, Kohlmeier L, Ringstad J, Martin BC, Mazaev VP, et al. Association between â-carotene and acute myocardial infarction depends on polyunsaturated fatty acid status. *Arterioscler Thromb Vasc Biol* 15:726–732, 1995.

Karpe F, Hellenius ML, Hamsten A. Differences in postprandial concentrations of very low density lipoprotein and chylomicron remnants between normotriglyceridemic and hypertriglyceridemic men with and without coronary disease. *Metabolism* 48:301–307, 1999.

Kasper H, Thiel H, Ehl M. Response of body weight to a low carbohydrate, high fat diet in normal and obese subjects. *Am J Clin Nutr* 26:197–204, 1973.

Kato I, Akhmedkhanov A, Koenig K, Toniolo PG, Share RE, Riboli E. Prospective study of diet and female colorectal cancer: the New York University Women's Health Study. *Nutr Cancer* 28:276–2817, 1997.

Katzel LI, Bleecker ER, Colman EG, Rogus EM, Sorkin JD, Goldberg AP. Effects of weight loss vs. aerobic exercise training on risk factors for coronary heart disease in healthy, obese, middle-aged and older men: a randomized controlled trial. *JAMA* 274:1915–1921, 1995.

Kaufman JS, Long AE, Liao Y, Cooper RS, McGee DL. The relation between income and mortality in U.S. blacks and whites. *Epidemiology* 9:147–155, 1998.

Kauppila LI, Tallroth K. Post mortem angiographic findings for arteries supplying the lumbar spine: their relationship to low-back symptoms. *J Spinal Disord* 6:124–129, 1993.

Kauppila LI, Penttila A, Karhunen PJ, Lalu K, Hannikainen P. Lumbar disc degeneration and atherosclerosis of the abdominal aorta. *Spine* 19:923–929, 1994.

Kearney J, Giovannucci E, Rimm EB, Ascherio A, Stampfer MJ, Colditz GA, Wing A, Kampman E, Willett WC. Calcium vitamin D, dairy foods, and the occurrence of colon cancer in men. *Am J Epidemiol* 143:907–917, 1996.

Kennedy AR. The Bowman–Birk inhibitor from soy beans as an anticarcinogenic agent. *Am J Clin Nutr* 68(Suppl.):1394S–1399S, 1998.

Keri SO, Feskens EJM, Kromhout D. Fish consumption and the risk of stroke: the Zutphen Study. *Stroke* 25:328–332, 1994.

Key TJ, Davey GK. Prevalence of obesity is low in people who do not eat meat (Letter). *Br Med J* 313:816–817, 1996.

Key TJ, Roe L, Thorogood M, Moore JW, Clark GM, Wang DY. Testosterone, sex hormone-binding globulin, calculated free testosterone, and oestradiol in male vegans and omnivores. *Br J Nutr* 64:111–119, 1990.

Key TJ, Thorogood M, Appleby PN, Burr ML. Dietary habits and mortality in 11,000 vegetarians and health-conscious people: result of a 17-year follow-up. *Br Med J* 313:775–779, 1996.

Key TJ, Fraser GE, Thorogood M, Appleby PN, Beral V, Reeves G, Burr ML, Chang-Claude J, Frentzel-Beyme R, Kuzma JW, et al. Mortality in vegetarians and non-vegetarians: a collaborative analysis of 8,300 deaths among 76,000 men and women in five prospective studies. *Public Health Nutr* 1:33–41, 1998.

Key TJ. Serum oestradiol and breast cancer risk. *Endocr Relat Cancer* 6:175–180, 1999.

Key TJ, Fraser GE, Thorogood M, Appleby PN, Beral V, Reeves G, Burr ML, Chang-Claude J, Frentzel-Beyme R, Kuzma JW, et al. Mortality in vegetarians and non-vegetarians: detailed findings from a collaborative analysis of 5 prospective studies. *Am J Clin Nutr* 70(Suppl.):516–524, 1999a

Key TJ, Davey GK, Appleby PN. Health benefits of a vegetarian diet. *Proc Nutr Soc* 58:271–275, 1999b.

Keys A. *Seven Countries: A Multivariate Analysis of Death and Coronary Heart Disease*. Cambridge, MA: Harvard University Press, 1980.

Keys A, Menotti A, Karvonen MJ, Aravanis C, Blackburn H, Buzina R, Djordje-vic BS, Dontas AS, Fidanza F, Keys MH, et al. The diet and 15-year death rate in the Seven Countries Study. *Am J Epidemiol* 124:903–915, 1986.

Khaw KT, Barrett-Connor E. Dietary fiber and reduced ischemic heart disease mortality rates in men and women: a 12-year prospective study. *Am J Epidemiol* 126:1093–1102, 1987.

Khaw KT, Bingham S, Welch A, Luben R, Wareham N, Oakes S, Day N. Rela-tion between plasma ascorbic acid and mortality in men and women in EPIC-Norfolk prospective study: a prospective population study. *Lancet* 357:657–663, 2001.

Kiani F, Knutsen S, Fraser G. Diet and risk of fatal ovarian cancer among Sev-enth-day Adventist women. The Adventist Health Study (Abstract). *Am J Epidemiol* 153(11):S197, 2001.

Kiecolt-Glaser JK, Malarkey WB, Cacioppo JT, Glaser R. Stressful personal rela-tionships: immune and endocrine function. In: R. Glaser and J. K. Kiecolt-Glaser (eds.), *Handbook of Human Stress and Immunity*. San Diego: Acade-mic Press, 1994, pp. 321–339.

Kim Y-I. Methylenetetrahydrofolate reductase polymorphisms, folate, and cancer risk: a paradigm of gene–nutrient interactions in carcinogenesis. *Nutr Rev* 58:205–209, 2000.

King KB. Psychologic and social aspects of cardiovascular disease. *Ann Behav Med* 19(3):264–270, 1997.

King M, Speck P, Thomas A. The effect of spiritual beliefs on outcome from ill-ness. *Soc Sci Med* 48(9):1291–1299, 1999.

Kinlen LJ. Meat and fat consumption and cancer mortality: a study of strict reli-gious orders in Britain. *Lancet* 1:946–949, 1982.

Kissinger DG, Sanchez A. The association of dietary factors with age of menar-che. *Nutr Res* 7:471–479, 1987.

Kjeldsen-Kragh J, Haugen M, Borchgrevink CF, Laerum E, Eek M, Mowinkel P, Hovi K, Forre O. Controlled trial of fasting and one year vegetarian diet in rheumatoid arthritis. *Lancet* 338:899–902, 1991.

Kjeldsen-Kragh J, Mellbye OJ, Haugen M, Mollnes TE, Hammer HB, Sioud M, Forre O. Changes in laboratory variables in rheumatoid arthritis patients during a trial of fasting and one-year vegetarian diet. *Scand J Rheumatol* 24:85–93, 1995.

Kjeldsen-Kragh J. Rheumatoid arthritis treated with vegetarian diets. *Am J Clin Nutr* 70(Suppl.):594S–5600S, 1999.

Knekt P, Reunanen A, Jarvinen R, Seppanen R, Heliovaara M, Aromaa A. Anti-oxidant vitamin intake and coronary mortality in a longitudinal population study. *Am J Epidemiol* 12:1180–1189, 1994a.

Knekt P, Steineck G, Jaervinen R, HakulinenT, Aromaa A. Intake of red meat and risk of cancer: a followup study in Finland. *Int J Cancer* 59:756–760, 1994b.

Knekt P, Jarvinen R, Reunanen A, Maatela J. Flavonoid intake and coronary mor-tality in Finland: a cohort study. *Br Med J* 312:478–481, 1996.

Knox SS, Uvnas-Moberg K. Social isolation and cardiovascular disease: an ather-osclerotic pathway? *Psychoneuroendocrinology* 23:877–890, 1998.

Knutsen SF. Lifestyle and the use of health services. *Am J Clin Nutr* 59(Suppl.):1171S–1175S, 1994.

Koenig HG, Cohen HJ, Blazer DG, Pieper C, Meador KG, Shelp F, Goli V, Di-Pasquale R. Religious coping and depression among elderly, hospitalized mentally ill men. *Am J Psychiatry* 149:1693–1700, 1992.

Koenig HG, George LK, Peterson BL. Religiosity and remission of depression in medically ill older patients. *Am J Psychiatry* 155(4):536–542, 1998a.

Koenig W, Sund M, Filipak B, Doring A, Lowel H, Ernst E. Plasma viscosity and the risk of coronary heart disease: results from the MONICA–Augsburg cohort study, 1984 to 1992. *Arterioscler Thromb Vasc Biol* 18:768–772, 1998b.

Krauss RM, Dreon DM. Low-density-lipoprotein subclasses and response to a low-fat diet in healthy men. *Am J Clin Nutr* 62(Suppl.):478S–487S, 1995.

Kris-Etherton PM (ed.). Expert Panel on Trans Fatty Acids and Coronary Heart Disease: trans fatty acids and coronary heart disease risk. *Am J Clin Nutr* 62(Suppl.):655S–708S, 1995.

Kristal-Boneh E, Glusman JG, Chaemovitz C. Improved thermoregulation caused by forced water intake in desert dwellers. *Eur J Appl Physiol* 57:220–224, 1988.

Kromhout D, Bosschieter EB, Coulander C de L. Dietary fiber and 10-year mortality from coronary heart disease, cancer, and all causes. *Lancet* 2:518–522, 1982.

Kromhout D, Bosschieter EB, Coulander C de L. The inverse relationship between fish consumption and 20-year mortality from coronary heart disease. *N Engl J Med* 312:1205–1209, 1985.

Kromhout D, Feskens EJ, Bowles CH. The protective effect of a small amount of fish on coronary heart disease mortality in an elderly population. *Int J Epidemiol* 24:340–345, 1995.

Kuller LH, Evans RW. Homocysteine, vitamins, and cardiovascular disease. *Circulation* 98:196–199, 1998.

Kuratsune M, Ikeda M, Hayashi T. Epidemiologic studies on possible health effects of intake of pyrolysates of foods, with reference to mortality among Japanese Seventh-day Adventists. *Environ Health Perspect* 67:143–146, 1986.

Kurowska EM, Spence JD, Jordan J. HDL-cholesterol-raising effect of orange juice in subjects with hypercholesterolemia. *Am J Clin Nutr* 72:1095–1100, 2000.

Kushi LH, Lew RA, Stare FJ, Ellison CR, el Lozy M, Bourke G, Daly L, Graham I, Hickey N, Mulcahy R, et al. Diet and 20-year mortality from coronary heart disease. *N Engl J Med* 312:811–818, 1985.

Kushi LH, Samonds KW, Lacey JM, Brown PT, Bergan JG, Sacks FM. The association of dietary fat with serum cholesterol in vegetarians: the effect of dietary assessment on the correlation coefficient. *Am J Epidemiol* 128:1054–1064, 1988.

Kushi LH, Folsom AR, Prineas RJ, Mink PJ, Wu Y, Bostick RM. Dietary antioxidant vitamins and death from coronary heart disease in postmenopausal women. *N Engl J Med* 334:1156–1162, 1996.

Kushi LH, Mink PJ, Folsom AR, Anderson KE, Zhang W, Lazovich DA, Sellers TA. Prospective study of diet and ovarian cancer. *Am J Epidemiol* 149:21–31, 1999.

Kuzma JW, Beeson WL. The relationship of lifestyle characteristics to mortality among California Seventh-day Adventists. In: *Proceedings of the 18th National Meeting of the Public Health Conference on Records and Statistics*. Publication No. (PHS) 81-1214. Washington, DC: Department of Health and Human Services, 1981, pp. 195–200.

Kuczmarski RJ, Anderson JJB, Koch GG. Correlates of blood pressure in Seventh-day Adventist (SDA) and non-SDA adolescents. *J Am Coll Nutr* 13:165–173, 1994.

Ladwig KH, Kieser M, Konig J, Breithardt G, Borggrefe M. Affective disorders and survival after myocardial infarction: results from the postinfarction late potential study. *Eur Heart J* 12:959–964, 1991.

Langer RD, Klauber MR, Criqui MH, Barrett-Connor EL. Exercise and survival in the very old. *Am J Geriatr Cardiol* 3:24–34, 1994.

Lantz PM, House JS, Lepkowski JM, Williams DR, Mero RP, Chen J. Socioeconomic factors, health behaviors, and mortality. *JAMA* 279:1703–1708, 1998.

Lapidus L, Andersson H, Bengtsson C, Bosaeus I. Dietary habits in relation to incidence of cardiovascular disease and death in women: a 12-year followup of participants in a population study of women in Gothenburg, Sweden. *Am J Clin Nutr* 44:444–448, 1986.

Larson DB, Sherrill KA, Lyons JS, Craigie FC Jr., Thielman SB, Greenwold MA, Larson SS. Associations between dimensions of religious commitment and mental health reported in the *American Journal of Psychiatry* and *Archives of General Psychiatry*: 1978–1989. *Am J Psychiatry* 149(4):557–559, 1992.

Lassere B, Spoerri M, Moullet V, Theubet MP. Should magnesium therapy be considered for the treatment of coronary heart disease? Epidemiologic evidence in outpatients with and without coronary heart disease. *Magnesium Res* 7:145–153, 1994.

La Vecchia C, Decarli A, Pagano R. Vegetable consumption and risk of chronic disease. *Epidemiology* 9:208–210, 1998.

La Vecchia C, Gallus S, Talamini R, Decarly A, Negri E, Franceschi S. Interaction between selected environmental factors and familial propensity for colon cancer. *Eur J Cancer Prev* 8:147–150, 1999.

Layton DW, Bogen KT, Knize MG, Hatch FT, Johnson VM, Felton JS. Cancer risk of heterocyclic amines in cooked foods: an analysis and implications for research. *Carcinogenesis* 16:39–52, 1995.

Lazarus RS, Launier R. Stress-related transactions between person and environment. In: L. A. Pervin and M. Lewis (eds.), *Perspectives in International Psychology*. New York: Plenum Press, 1978, pp. 1287–1327.

Lazarus RS, Folkman S. *Stress, Appraisal, and Coping*. New York: Springer, 1984.

Leaf A. Cardiovascular effects of fish oils. *Circulation* 82:624–628, 1990.

Lee HP, Gowley L, Duffy SW, Esteve J, Lee J, Day NE. Dietary effects on breast cancer risk in Singapore. *Lancet* 337:1197–1200, 1991.

Lee IM, Manson JE, Ajani U, Paffenbarger RS, Hennekens CH. Physical activity and risk of colon cancer: the Physicians' Health Study (United States). *Cancer Causes Control* 8:568–574, 1997.

Lee JW, Rice GT, Gillespie VB. Family worship patterns and their correlation with adolescent behavior and beliefs. *J Sci Study Religion* 36(3):372–381, 1997.

Le Marchand L, Kolonel LN, Wilkens LR, Myers BC, Hirohata T. Animal fat consumption and prostate cancer: a prospective study in Hawaii. *Epidemiology* 5:276–282, 1994.

Lemon FR, Walden RT, Woods RW. Cancer of the lung and mouth in Seventh-day Adventists: a preliminary report on a population study. *Cancer* 17:486–497, 1964.

Lemon FR, Walden RT. Death from respiratory system disease among Seventh-day Adventist men. *JAMA* 198:117–126, 1966.

Lemon FR, Kuzma JW. A biologic cost of smoking: decreased life expectancy. *Arch Environ Health* 18:950–955, 1969.

Leon A, Connett J. Physical activity and 10.5 year mortality in the Multiple Risk Factor Intervention Trial (MRFIT). *Int J Epidemiol* 20:690–697, 1991.

Leon GR, Finn SE, Murray D, Bailey JM. Inability to predict cardiovascular disease from hostility scores or MMPI items related to type A behavior. *J Consult Clin Psych* 56:597–600, 1988.

Levin JS, Schiller PL. Is there a religious factor in health? *J Religion Health* 26:9–36, 1987.

Levin JS, Vanderpool HY. Is frequent religious attendance really conducive to better health? Toward an epidemiology of religion. *Soc Sci Med* 24(7):589–600, 1987.

Levin JS, Vanderpool HY. Is religion therapeutically significant for hypertension? *Soc Sci Med* 29(1):69–78, 1989.

Levin JS, Vanderpool HY. Religious factors in physical health and the prevention of illness. *Prev Human Serv* 9(2):41–64, 1991.

Levin JS. Religion and health: is there an association, is it valid, and is it causal? *Soc Scie Med* 38(11):1475–1482, 1994.

Levin JS. How prayer heals: a theoretical model. *Altern Ther Health Med* 2(1):66–73, 1996.

Levin JS, Chatters LM. Religion, health, and psychological well-being in older adults: findings from three national surveys. *J Aging Health* 10(4):504–531, 1998a.

Levin JS, Chatters LM. Research on religion and mental health: an overview of empirical findings and theoretical issues. In: H. G. Koenig (ed.), *Handbook of Religion and Mental Health*. San Diego: Academic Press, 1998b, pp. 33–50.

Levin JS, Taylor RJ. Panel analyses of religious involvement and well-being in African Americans: contemporaneous vs. longitudinal effects. *J Sci Study Religion* 37(4):695–709, 1998c.

Levine AS, Silvis SE. Absorption of whole peanuts, peanut oil and peanut butter. *N Engl J Med* 303:917–918, 1980.

Lewis S. An opinion on the global impact of meat consumption. *Am J Clin Nutr* 59(Suppl.):1099S–1102S, 1994.

Li D, Sinclair A, Mann N, Turner A, Ball M, Kelly F, Abedin L, Wilson A. The association of diet and thrombotic risk factors in healthy male vegetarians and meat-eaters. *Eur J Clin Nutr* 53:612–619, 1999.

Liao F, Folsom AR, Brancati FL. Is low magnesium concentration a risk factor of coronary heart disease? The Atherosclerosis Risk in Communities (ARIC) Study. *Am Heart J* 136:480–490, 1998.

Lichtman SW, Pisarska K, Berman ER, Pestone M, Dowling H, Offenbacher E, Weisel H, Heshka S, Matthews DE, Heymsfield SB. Discrepancy between self-reported and actual caloric intake and exercise in obese subjects. *N Engl J Med* 327:1893–1898, 1992.

Lin HJ, Probst-Hensch NM, Louie AD, Kau IH, Witte JS, Ingles SA, Frankl HD, Lee ER, Haile RW. Glutathione *S*-transferase null genotype, broccoli, and lower prevalence of colorectal adenomas. *Cancer Epidemiol Biomarkers Prev* 7:647–652, 1998.

Lindahl O, Lindwall L, Spangberg A, Stenram A, Ockerman PA. A vegan regime with reduced medication in the treatment of hypertension. *Br J Nutr* 52:11–20, 1984.

Lindsted KD, Fraser GE, Steinkohl M, Beeson WL. Healthy volunteer effect in a cohort study: temporal resolution in the Adventist Health Study. *J Clin Epidemiol* 49:783–790, 1996.

Linos A, Kaklamani VG, Kaklamani E, Koumantaki Y, Giziaki E, Papazoglou S, Mantzoros CS. Dietary factors in relation to rheumatoid arthritis: a role for olive oil and cooked vegetables? *Am J Clin Nutr* 70:1077–1082, 1999.

Lipkin M, Uehara K, Winawer S, Sanchez A, Bauer C, Phillips R, Lynch HT, Blattner WA, Fraumeni JF. Seventh-day Adventists have a quiescent proliferative activity in colonic mucosa. *Cancer Lett* 26:139–144, 1985.

Lipkin M, Newmark HL. Vitamin D, calcium and prevention of breast cancer: a review. *J Am Coll Nutr* 18:392S–397S, 1999.

Liu S, Stampfer MJ, Hu FB, Giovannucci E, Rimm E, Manson JE, Hennekens CH, Willett WC. Whole-grain consumption and risk of coronary heart disease: results from the Nurses' Health Study. *Am J Clin Nutr* 70:412–419, 1999.

Liu S, Manson JE, Lee IM, Cole SR, Hennekens CH, Willett WC, Buring JE. Fruit and vegetable intake and risk of cardiovascular disease: the Women's Health Study. *Am J Clin Nutr* 72:922–928, 2000a.

Liu S, Manson JE, Stampfer MJ, Rexrode KM, Hu FB, Rimm EB, Willett WC. Whole grain consumption and risk of ischemic stroke in women: a prospective study. *JAMA* 284:1534–1540, 2000b.

Loh MY, Flatt WP, Martin RJ, Hausman DB. Dietary fat type and level influence adiposity development in obese but not lean Zucker rats. *Proc Soc Exp Biol Med* 218:38–44, 1998.

London SJ, Yuan J-M, Chung F-L, Gao Y-T, Coetzee GA, Ross RK, Yu MC. Isothiocyanates, glutathione-*S*-transferase M1 and T1 polymorphisms, and lung cancer risk: a prospective study of men in Shanghai, China. *Lancet* 356:724–729, 2000.

Loria CM, Ingram DD, Feldman JJ, Wright JD, Madans JH. Serum folate and cardiovascular disease mortality among U.S. men and women. *Arch Int Med* 160:3258–3262, 2000.

Losonczy KG, Harris TB, Havlik RJ. Vitamin E and vitamin C supplement use and risk of all-cause and coronary mortality in older persons: the Established Populations for Epidemiologic Studies of the Elderly. *Am J Clin Nutr* 64:190–196, 1996.

Lu LJ, Anderson KE, Grady JJ, Kohen F, Nagamani M. Decreased ovarian hormones during a soya diet: implications for breast cancer prevention. *Cancer Res* 60:4112–4121, 2000.

Lundgren H, Bengtsson C, Blohmé G, Isaksson B, Lapidus L, Lenner RA, Soaek A, Winther E. Dietary habits and incidence of noninsulin-dependent diabetes mellitus in a population of women in Gothenburg, Sweden. *Am J Clin Nutr* 49:708–712, 1989.

Ma J, Folsom A, Melnick SL, Eckfeldt JH, Sharrett AR, Nabulsi AA, Hutchinson RG, Metcalf PA. Associations of serum and dietary magnesium with cardiovascular disease, hypertension, diabetes, insulin, and carotid arterial wall thickness: the ARIC study. *J Clin Epidemiol* 48:927–940, 1995.

Ma J, Pollak M, Giovannucci E, Chan JM, Tao Y, Hennekens C, Stampfer MJ. A prospective study of plasma levels of insulin-like growth factor 1 (IGF-1) and IGF-binding protein-3, and colorectal cancer risk among men. *Growth Horm IGF Res* (Suppl. A):S28–S29, 2000.

Mack TM. Cancer surveillance program of Los Angeles County. *Natl Cancer Inst Monogr* 47:99–101, 1977.

Maltby J, Lewis CA, Day L. Religious orientation and psychological well-being:

the role of the frequency of personal prayer. *Br J Health Psychol* 4(Part 4):363–378, 1999.

Mangge H, Herman J, Schauenstein K. Diet and rheumatoid arthritis: a review. *Scand J Rheumatol* 28:201–209, 1999.

Mann JI, Appleby PN, Key TJ, Thorogood M. Dietary determinants of ischaemic heart disease in health-conscious individuals. *Heart* 78:450–455, 1997.

Manson JE, Colditz GA, Stampfer MJ, Willett WC, Rosner B, Monson RR, Speizer FE, Hennekens CH. A prospective study of obesity and risk of coronary heart disease in women. *N Engl J Med* 322:882–889, 1990.

Manson JE, Nathan DM, Krolewski AS, Stampfer MJ, Willett WC, Hennekens CH. A prospective study of exercise and incidence of diabetes among U.S. male physicians. *JAMA* 268:63–67, 1992.

Manson JE, Willett WC, Stampfer MJ, Colditz GA, Hunter DJ, Hankinson SE, Hennekens CH, Speizer FE. Body weight and mortality among women. *N Engl J Med* 333:677–685, 1995.

Marckmann P, Sandstrom B, Jespersen J. Low fat, high fiber diet favorably affects several independent risk markers of ischemic heart disease: observations on blood lipids, coagulation and fibrinolysis from a trial of middle-aged Danes. *Am J Clin Nutr* 59:935–939, 1994.

Margetts BM, Armstrong BK, Beilin LJ, Vandongen R. Dietary fats and blood pressure. *Aust N Z J Med* 14:444–447, 1984.

Margetts BM, Beilin LJ, Vandongen R, Armstrong BK. Vegetarian diet in mild hypertension: a randomised controlled trial. *Br Med J* 293:1468–1471, 1986.

Margetts BM, Beilin LJ, Vandongen R, Armstrong BK. A randomized controlled trial of the effect of dietary fiber on blood pressure. *Clin Sci* 72:343–350, 1987.

Marshall JA, Hamman RF, Baxter J. High fat, low carbohydrate diet and the etiology of non-insulin-dependent diabetes mellitus: the San Luis Valley Diabetes Study. *Am J Epidemiol* 134:590–603, 1991.

Martinez ME, Giovannucci EL, Colditz GA, Stampfer MJ, Hunter DJ, Speizer FE, Wing A, Willett WC. Calcium, vitamin D, and the occurrence of colorectal cancer among women. *J Natl Cancer Inst* 88:1375–1382, 1996.

Martinez ME, Giovannucci E, Spiegelman D, Hunter DJ, Willett WC. Leisure time physical activity, body size, and colon cancer in women: the Nurses' Health Study Research Group. *J Natl Cancer Inst* 89:948–955, 1997.

Marx A, Neutra RR. Magnesium in drinking water and ischemic heart disease. *Epidemiol Rev* 19:258–272, 1997.

Maton KI. The stress-buffering role of spiritual support: cross-sectional and prospective investigations. *Je Sci Study Religion* 28(3):310–323, 1989.

Matthews DA, McCullough ME, Larson DB, Koenig HG, Swyers JP, Milano MG. Religious commitment and health status: a review of the research and implications for family medicine. *Arch Fam Med* 7(2):118–124, 1998.

Mattson FH, Grundy SM. Comparison of effects of dietary saturated, monounsaturated and polyunsaturated fatty acids on plasma lipids and lipoproteins in men. *J Lipid Res* 26:194–202, 1985.

Maughan RJ, Leiper JB. Limitations to fluid replacement during exercise. *Can J Appl Physiol* 24:173–187, 1999.

Mayer-Davis EJ, D'Agostino R, Karter AJ, Haffner SM, Rewers MJ, Saad M, Bergman RN. Intensity and amount of physical activity in relation to insulin sensitivity. *JAMA* 279:669–674, 1998.

Mayer-Davis EJ, Levin S, Bergman RN, D'Agostino RB, Karter AJ, Saad MF. Insulin secretion, obesity, and potential behavioral influences: results from the Insulin Resistance Atherosclerosis Study (IRAS). *Diabetes Metab Res Rev* 17:137–145, 2001.

McCarron DA, Reusser ME. Non-pharmacologic therapy in hypertension: from single components to overall dietary management. *Prog Cardiovasc Dis* 41:451–460, 1999.

McCranie EW, Watkins LO, Brandsma JM, Sisson BD. Hostility, coronary heart disease (CHD) incidence, and total mortality: lack of association in a 25-year follow-up study of 478 physicians. *J Behav Med* 29:119–125, 1986.

McCullough ME. Prayer and health: conceptual issues, research review, and research agenda. *J Psychol Theol* 23(1):15–29, 1995.

McCullough ME, Larson DB. Religion and depression: a review of the literature. *Twin Res* 2(2):126–136, 1999.

McCully KS. Homocysteine, folate, vitamin B6, and cardiovascular disease. *JAMA* 279:392–393, 1998.

McDougall J, Litzau K, Haver E, Sauders V, Spiller GA. Rapid reduction of serum cholesterol and blood pressure by a twelve-day, very low fat, strictly vegetarian diet. *J Am Coll Nutr* 14:491–496, 1995.

McGovern PG, Pankow JS, Shahar E, Doliszny KM, Folsom AR, Blackburn H, Luepker RV. Recent trends in acute coronary heart disease. *N Engl J Med* 334:884–890, 1996.

McKeown-Eyssen GF. Epidemiology of colorectal cancer revisited: are serum triglycerides and/or plasma glucose associated with risk? *Cancer Epidemiol Biomarkers Prev* 3:687–695, 1994.

McKeown-Eyssen GF and the Toronto Polyp Prevention Group. Insulin resistance and the risk of colorectal neoplasia (Abstract). *Cancer Epidemiol Biomarkers Prev* 5:235, 1996.

McTiernan A, Ulrich C, Slate S, Potter J. Physical activity and cancer etiology: associations and mechanisms. *Cancer Causes Control* 9:487–509, 1998.

Meade TW, Imeson J, Stirling Y. Effects of changes in smoking and other characteristics on clotting factors and the risk of ischemic heart disease. *Lancet* 2:986–988, 1987.

Melby CL, Goldflies DG, Toohey ML. Blood pressure differences in older black and white long-term vegetarians and nonvegetarians. *J Am Coll Nutr* 12:262–269, 1993.

Melby CL, Toohey ML, Cebrick J. Blood pressure and blood lipids among vegetarian, semivegetarian, and non-vegetarian African Americans. *Am J Clin Nutr* 59:103–109, 1994.

Melina V, Davis B, Harrison V. *Becoming Vegetarian*. Summertown, TN: Book Publishing Company, 1995.

Mendes de Leon CF, Krumholz HM, Seeman TS, Vaccarino V, Williams CS, Kasl SV, Berkman LF. Depression and risk of coronary heart disease in elderly men and women. *Arch Int Med* 158:2341–2348, 1998.

Menotti A, Seccareccia F. Cardiovascular risk factors predicting all causes of death in an occupational population sample. *Int J Epidemiol* 17:773–778, 1988.

Messina MJ, Persky VK, Setchell KDR, Barnes S. Soy intake and cancer risk: a review of the in vitro and in vivo data. *Nutr Cancer* 21:113–131, 1994.

Messina MJ. Legumes and soybeans: overview of their nutritional profiles and health effects. *Am J Clin Nutr* 70(Suppl.):439S–450S, 1999.

Messina MJ, Messina VK, Mangels R. *The Dietians Guide to Vegetarian Diets: Issues and Applications*, 2nd ed. Gaithersburg, MD: Aspen Publishers, 2001.

Messina VK, Burke KI. Position of the American Dietetic Association: vegetarian diets. *J Am Diet Assoc* 97:1317–1321, 1997.

Mezzano D, Munoz X, Martinez C, Cuevas A, Panes O, Aranda E, Guasch V, Strobel P, Munoz B, Rodriguez S, et al. Vegetarians and cardiovascular risk factors: hemostasis, inflammatory markers and plasma homocysteine. *Thromb Haemost* 81:913–917, 1999.

Michaud DS, Spiegelman D, Clinton SK, Rimm EB, Willett WC, Giovannucci EL. Fruit and vegetable intake and incidence of bladder cancer in a male prospective cohort. *J Natl Cancer Inst* 91:605–613, 1999.

Michaud DS, Feskanich D, Rimm EG, Colditz GA, Speizer FE, Willett WC, Giovannucci E. Intake of specific carotenoids and risk of lung cancer in two prospective cohorts. *Am J Clin Nutr* 72:990–997, 2000.

Michaud DS, Augustsson K, Rimm EB, Stampfer MJ, Willett WC, Giovannucci E. A prospective study on intake of animal products and risk of prostate cancer. *Cancer Causes Control* 12:557–567, 2001.

Mickley JR, Carson V, Soeken KL. Religion and adult mental health: state of the science in nursing. *Issues Ment Health Nurs* 16(4):345–360, 1995.

Mikhail N, Golub MS, Tuck ML. Obesity and hypertension. *Prog Cardiovasc Dis* 42:39–58, 1999.

Miller GJ. Environmental influences on hemostasis and thrombosis: diet and smoking. *Ann Epidemiol* 2:387–391, 1992.

Miller HW, Wen CJ. Experimental nutrition studies of soymilk in human nutrition. *Chin Med J* 50:450–459, 1936.

Miller TQ, Smith TW, Turner CW, Guijarro ML, Hallet AJ. Meta-analytic review of research on hostility and physical health. *Psychol Bull* 119(2):322–348, 1996.

Mills PK, Beeson WL, Abbey DE, Fraser GE, Phillips RL. Dietary habits and past medical history as related to fatal pancreas cancer risk among Adventists. *Cancer* 61:2578–2585, 1988.

Mills PK, Beeson WL, Phillips RL, Fraser GE. Cohort study of diet, lifestyle, and prostate cancer in Adventist men. *Cancer* 64:598–604, 1989a.

Mills PK, Beeson WL, Phillips RL, Fraser GE. Dietary habits and breast cancer incidence among Seventh-day Adventists. *Cancer* 64:582–590, 1989b.

Mills PK, Preston-Martin S, Annegers JF, Beeson WL, Phillips RL, Fraser GE. Risk factors for tumors of the brain and cranial meninges in Seventh-day Adventists. *Neuroepidemiology* 8:266–275, 1989c.

Mills PK, Newell GR, Beeson WL, Fraser GE, Phillips RL. History of cigarette smoking and risk of leukemia and myeloma: results from the Adventist Health Study. *J Natl Cancer Inst* 82:1832–1836, 1990.

Mills PK, Beeson WL, Phillips RL, Fraser GE. Bladder cancer in a low risk population: results from the Adventist Health Study. *Am J Epidemiol* 133:230–239, 1991.

Missmer SA, Smith-Warner SA, Spiegelman D, Yaun S-S, Adami H-O, Beeson WL, van den Brandt P, Fraser GE, Freudenheim JL, Goldbohm RA, et al. Meat and dairy food consumption and breast cancer: a pooled analysis of cohort studies. *Int J Epidemiol* 31:78–85, 2002.

Moore TJ, Vollmer WM, Appel LJ, Sacks FM, Svetkey LP, Vogt TM, Conlin PR, Simons-Morton DG, Carter-Edwards L, Harsha DW. Effect of dietary patterns on ambulatory blood pressure: results from the Dietary Approaches to Stop Hypertension (DASH) Trial. *Hypertension* 34:472–477, 1999.

Morris DL, Kritchevsky SB, Davis CE. Serum carotenoids and coronary heart disease. *JAMA* 272:1439–1441, 1994.

Morris JN, Marr JW, Clayton DG. Diet and heart: a postscript. *Br Med J* 2:1307–1314, 1977.

Morris MC, Manson JE, Rosner B, Buring JE, Willett WC, Hennekens CH. Fish consumption and cardiovascular disease in the Physicians' Health Study: a prospective study. *Am J Epidemiol* 142:166–175, 1995.

Morrison HI, Schaubel D, Desmeules M, Wigle DT. Serum folate and risk of fatal coronary heart disease. *JAMA* 275:1893–1896, 1996.

Morrow JD, Frei B, Longmire AT, Gaziano JM, Lynch SM, Shyr Y, Strauss WE, Oates JA, Roberts LJ. Increase in circulating products of lipid peroxidation (F_2-isoprostanes) in smokers. *N Engl J Med* 332:1198–1203, 1995.

Murphy E. Social origins of depression in old age. *Br J Psychiatry* 141:135–142, 1982.

Murphy FG, Blumenthal DS, Dickson-Smith J, Peay RP. The mortality profile of black Seventh-day Adventists residing in metropolitan Atlanta: a pilot study. *Am J Public Health* 80:984–985, 1990.

Murphy FG, Gwebu E, Braithwaite RL, Green-Goodman D, Brown L. Health values and practices among Seventh-day Adventists. *Am J Health Behav* 21:43–50, 1997.

Murphy TK, Calle EE, Rodriguez C, Kahn HS, Thun MJ. Body mass index and colon cancer mortality in a large prospective study. *Am J Epidemiol* 152:847–854, 2000.

Murray RP, Johnston JJ, Dolce JJ, Lee WW, O'Hara P. Social support for smoking cessation and abstinence: the Lung Health Study. *Addict Behav* 20:159–170, 1995.

Musick MA. Religion and subjective health among black and white elders. *J Health Soc Behav* 37(3):221–237, 1996.

Musselman DL, Evans DL, Nemeroff CB. The relationship of depression to cardiovascular disease: epidemiology, biology, and treatment. *Arch Gen Psychiatry* 55(7):580–592, 1998.

Musselman DL, Nemeroff CB. Depression and cardiovascular disease: increasing evidence of a connection. *Cardiovasc Rev Rep* 19:34–42, 1998.

Myers DG. The funds, friends, and faith of happy people. *Am Psychol* 55(1):56–67, 2000.

Nair GV, Gurbel PA, O'Connor CM, Gattis WA, Muruesan SP, Serebruany VL. Depression, coronary events, platelet inhibition, and serotonin reuptake inhibitors. *Am J Cardiol* 84:321–323, 1999.

National Academy of Sciences. *Diet, Nutrition and Cancer.* Washington DC: National Academy Press, 1982.

Nenonen MT. Rheumatoid arthritis, fasting, diet and bacteria: myths and enthusiasm. *Clin Rheumatol* 17:269–270, 1998.

Ness AR, Powles JW. Fruit and vegetables, and cardiovascular disease: a review. *Int J Epidemiol* 26:1–13, 1997.

Nestel PJ. Comment on trans fatty acids and coronary heart disease. *Am J Clin Nutr* 62:522–523, 1995.

Nicholson AS, Sklar M, Barnard ND, Gore S, Sullivan R, Browning S. Toward improving management of NIDDM: a randomized, controlled, pilot intervention using a low fat, vegetarian diet. *Prev Med* 29:87–91, 1999.

Nielsen GL, Faarvang KL, Thomsen BS, Teglbjaerg KL, Jensen LT, Hansen TM, Lervang HH, Schmidt EB, Dyerberg J, Ernst E. The effects of dietary supplementation with *n*-3 polyunsaturated fatty acids in patients with rheumatoid arthritis: a randomized, double-blind trial. *Eur J Clin Invest* 22:687–691, 1992.

Nilsson TK, Sundell IB, Hellsten G, Hallmans G. Reduced plasminogen activator inhibitor activity in high consumers of fruits, vegetables, and root vegetables. *J Int Med* 227:267–271, 1990.

Nomura A, Henderson BE, Lee J. Breast cancer and diet among the Japanese in Hawaii. *Am J Clin Nutr* 31:2020–2025, 1978.

Nomura A, Heilbrun CK, Stemmerman GN, Judd HL. Prediagnostic serum hormones and the risk of prostate cancer. *Cancer Res* 48:3515–3517, 1988.

Norrish A, North D, Yee RL, Jackson R. Do cardiovascular disease risk factors predict all-cause mortality? *Int J Epidemiol* 24:908–914, 1995.

Numbers RL. *Prophetess of Health*. Knoxville: University of Tennessee Press, 1992, pp. 48–76.

Nutrition Committee, American Heart Association. AHA dietary guidelines. Revision, 2000: a statement for healthcare professionals. *Circulation* 102:2284–2299, 2000.

O'Connor GT, Morton JR, Diehl MJ, Olmstead EM, Coffin LH, Levy DG, Maloney CT, Plume SK, Nugent W, Malenko DJ, et al. Differences between men and women in hospital mortality associated with coronary artery bypass graft surgery. *Circulation* 88:2104–2110, 1993.

Office of Communications, National Cancer Institute. *The Smoking Digest. Progress Report on a Nation Kicking the Habit*. Bethesda, MD: U.S. Department of Health, Education and Welfare, National Institutes of Health, 1977, pp. 61–62.

O'Laoire S. An experimental study of the effects of distant, intercessory prayer on self-esteem, anxiety, and depression. *Alternat Ther Health Med* 3(6):38–53, 1997.

Oliver MF. It is more important to increase the intake of unsaturated fats than to decrease the intake of saturated fats: evidence from clinical trials relating to ischemic heart disease. *Am J Clin Nutr* 66(Suppl.):980S–986S, 1997.

Olshansky SJ, Carnes BA, Cassel C. In search of Methusaleh: estimating the upper limits of human longevity. *Science* 250:634–640, 1990.

Olshansky SJ, Rudberg MA, Carnes BA, Cassel CK, Brody JA. Trading off longer life for worsening health: the expansion of morbidity hypothesis. *J Aging Health* 3:194–216, 1991.

Oman D, Reed D. Religion and mortality among the community-dwelling elderly. *Am J Public Health* 99(10):1469–1475, 1998.

Omenn GS, Goodman GE, Thornquist MD, Balmos J, Cullen MR, Glass A, Keogh JP, Meyskens FL, Valanis B, Williams JE, et al. Effects of a combination of beta-carotene and vitamin A on lung cancer and cardiovascular disease. *N Engl J Med* 334:1150–1155, 1996.

Oomen CM, Feskens EJM, Rasanen L, Fidanza F, Nissinen AM, Menotti A, Kok FJ, Kromhout D. Fish consumption and coronary heart disease mortality in Finland, Italy, and the Netherlands. *Am J Epidemiol* 15:999–1006, 2000.

Ophir O, Peer G, Gilad J, Blum M, Aviram A. Low blood pressure in vegetarians: the possible role of potassium. *Am J Clin Nutr* 37:755–762, 1983.

Orencia AJ, Daviglus ML, Dyer AR, Shekelle RB, Stamler J. Fish consumption and stroke in men: 30-year findings of the Chicago Western Electric Study. *Stroke* 27:204–209, 1996.

Ortberg J, Gorusch R, Kim G. Changing attitude and moral obligation: their independent effects on behavior. *J Sci Study Religion* 40(3):489–496, 2001.

Otvos J. Measurement of triglyceride-rich lipoproteins by nuclear magnetic resonance spectroscopy. *Clin Cardiol* 22(Suppl. 2): 21–27, 1999.

Oxman TE, Berkman LF, Kasl S, Freeman DH, Barrett J. Social support and depressive symptoms in the elderly. *Am J Epidemiol* 135:356–368, 1992.

Oxman TE, Freeman DHJ, Manheimer ED. Lack of social participation or religious strength and comfort as risk factors for death after cardiac surgery in the elderly. *Psychosom Med* 57(1):5–15, 1995.

Paffenbarger RS, Hyde RT, Wing AL, Hsieh C-C. Physical activity, all-cause mortality, and longevity of college alumni. *N Engl J Med* 314:605–613, 1986.

Pahor M, Elam MB, Garrison RJ, Kritchevsky SB, Applegate WB. Emerging noninvasive biochemical measures to predict cardiovascular disease. *Arch Int Med* 159:237–245, 1999.

Pais P, Pogue J, Gerstein H, Zachariah E, Savitha D, Jayprakash S, Nayak Pr, Yusuf S. Risk factors for acute myocardial infarction in Indians: a case-control study. *Lancet* 348:358–363, 1996.

Pan W-H, Chin C-J, Sheu C-T, Lee M-H. Hemostatic factors and blood lipids in young Buddhist vegetarians and omnivores. *Am J Clin Nutr* 58:354–359, 1993.

Pandey DK, Shekelle R, Selwyn BJ, Tangney C, Stamler J. Dietary vitamin C and β-carotene and risk of death in middle-aged men: the Western Electric Study. *Am J Epidemiol* 142:1269–1278, 1995.

Pargament KI, Kennell J, Hathaway W, Grevengoed N, Newman J, Jones W. Religion and the problem-solving process: three styles of coping. *J Sci Study Religion* 27(1):90–104, 1988.

Pargament KI. God help me: toward a theoretical framework of coping for the psychology of religion. In: M. L. Lynn and D. O. Moberg (eds.), *Research in the Social Scientific Study of Religion*. Greenwich, CT: JAI Press, 1990, vol. 2, pp. 195–224.

Pargament KI, Olsen H, Reilly B, Falgout K, Ensing DS, Van Haitsma K. God help me: II. The relationship of religious orientations to religious coping with negative life events. *J Sci Study Religion* 31(4):504–513, 1992.

Pargament KI, Brant CR. Religion and coping. In: H. G. Koenig (ed.), *Handbook of Religion and Mental Health*. San Diego: Academic Press, 1998, pp. 111–128.

Pargament KI, Smith BW, Koenig HG, Perez L. Patterns of positive and negative religious coping with major life stressors. *J Sci Study Religion* 37(4):710–724, 1998a.

Pargament KI, Zinnbauer BJ, Scott AB, Butter EM., Zerowin J, Stanik P. Red flags and religious coping: identifying some religious warning signs among people in crisis. *J Clin Psychol* 54(1):77–89, 1998b.

Payne IR, Bergin AE, Bielema KA, Jenkins PH. Review of religion and mental health: prevention and the enhancement of psychosocial functioning. *Prev Hum Serv* 9(2):11–40, 1991.

Pekkanen J, Marti B, Nissinen A, Tuomilehto J. Reduction of premature mortality by high physical activity: a 20-year follow-up of middle-aged Finnish men. *Lancet* 1:1473–1477, 1987.

Peltonen R, Nenoren M, Helve T, Hanninen O, Toivanen P, Eerola E. Faecal microbial flora and disease activity in rheumatoid arthritis during a vegan diet. *Br J Rheumatol* 36:64–68, 1997.

Pennebaker JW. Confession, inhibition, and disease. In: L. Berkowitz (ed.), *Advances in Experimental Social Psychology*. San Diego: Academic Press, 1989, vol. 22, pp. 211–244.

Pennebaker JW (ed.). *Emotion, Disclosure, and Health*. Washington, DC: American Psychological Association, 1995.

Penninx BWJH, Kriegsman DMW, van Eijk JTM, Boeke AJP, Deeg DJH. Differential effect of social support on the course of chronic disease: a criteria-based literature study. *Fam Syst Health* 14(2):223–244, 1996.

Penninx BWJH, Geerlings SW, Deeg DJH, van Eijk JTM, van Tilburg W, Beekman, ATF. Minor and major depression and the risk of death in older persons. *Arch Gen Psychiatry* 56(10):889–895, 1999.

Persky VW, Chatterton RT, Van Horn LV, Grant MD, Langenberg P, Marvin J. Hormone levels in vegetarian and nonvegetarian teenage girls: potential implications for breast cancer risk. *Cancer Res* 52:578–583, 1992.

Peterson C, Seligman ME, Vaillant GE. Pessimistic explanatory style is a risk factor for physical illness: a thirty-five-year longitudinal study. *J Personal Soc Psychol* 55:23–27, 1988.

Peterson C. Explanatory style and health. In: G. M. Buchanan and M. E. P. Seligman (eds.), *Explanatory Style*. Hillsdale, NJ: Lawrence Erlbaum Associates, 1995, pp. 233–246.

Peterson, C. The future of optimism. *Am Psychol* 55(1):44–55, 2000.

Phillips RL. Role of lifestyle and dietary habits in risk of cancer among Seventh-day Adventists. *Cancer Res* 35(Suppl.):3513–3522, 1975.

Phillips RL, Lemon FR, Beeson WL, Kuzma JW. Coronary heart disease mortality among Seventh-day Adventists with differing dietary habits: a preliminary report. *Am J Clin Nutr* 32(Suppl.):S191–S198, 1978.

Phillips RL, Kuzma JW, Beeson WL, Lotz T. Influence of selection versus lifestyle on risk of fatal cancer and cardiovascular disease among Seventh-day Adventists. *Am J Epidemiol* 112:296–314, 1980a.

Phillips RL, Garfinkel L, Kuzma JW, Beeson WL, Lotz T, Brin B. Mortality among California Seventh-day Adventists for selected cancer sites. *J Natl Cancer Inst* 65:1097–1107, 1980b.

Phillips RL, Snowdon DA. Dietary relationships with fatal colorectal cancer among Seventh-day Adventists. *J Natl Cancer Inst* 74:307–317, 1985.

Pietinen P, Rimm EB, Korhonen P, Hartman AM, Willett WC, Albanes D, Virtamo J. Intake of dietary fiber and risk of coronary heart disease in a cohort of Finnish men. *Circulation* 94:2720–2727, 1996.

Pietinen P, Ascherio A, Korhonen P, Hartman AM, Willett WC, Albanes D, Virtamo J. Intake of fatty acids and risk of coronary heart disease in a cohort of Finnish men. *Am J Epidemiol* 145:876–887, 1997.

Pike MC, Spicer DV, Dahmoush L, Press MF. Estrogens, progestogens, normal breast cell proliferation, and breast cancer risk. *Epidemiol Rev* 15:17–35, 1993.

Pino AM, Valladares LE, Palma MA, Mancilla AM, Yanez M, Albala C. Dietary isoflavones affect sex hormone-binding globulin levels in postmenopausal women. *J Clin Endocrinol Metab* 85:2797–2800, 2000.

Pinto RJ. Risk factors for coronary heart disease in Asian Indians: clinical implications for prevention of coronary heart disease. *Indian J Med Sci* 52:49–54, 1998.

Polkinghorne J. *One World. The Interaction of Science and Theology.* The Longdunn Press, Bristol, UK, 1993, p. 9.

Pollner M. Divine relations, social relations, and well-being. *J Health Soc Behav* 30(1):92–104, 1989.

Poloma MM, Pendleton BF. The effects of prayer and prayer experiences on measures of general well-being. Special issue: Spirituality: perspectives in theory and research. *J Psychol Theol* 19(1):71–83, 1991.

Potishman N, Swanson CA, Siiteri P, Hoover RN. Reversal of relation between body mass and endogenous estrogen concentrations with menopausal status. *J Natl Cancer Inst* 88:756–758, 1996.

Potter JD (ed.). *Food, Nutrition and the Prevention of Cancer: A Global Perspective.* Washington, DC: World Cancer Research Fund and American Institute of Cancer Research, 1997.

Powles JW, Day NE, Sanz MA, Bingham SA. Protective foods in winter and spring: a key to lower vascular mortality? (Letter). *Lancet* 348:898–899, 1996.

Pratt LA, Ford DE, Crum RM, Armenian HK, Gallo JJ, Eaton WW. Depression, psychotropic medication, and risk of myocardial infarction. *Circulation* 94:3123–3129, 1996.

Prescott SL, Jenner DA, Beilin LJ, Margotts BM, Vandongen R. A randomized controlled trial of the effect on blood pressure of dietary non-meat protein versus meat protein in normotensive omnivores. *Clin Sci* 74:665–672, 1988.

Pribis P. Association between nutrient intake and risk of coronary heart disease in California Seventh-day Adventists. Ph.D. diss., Loma Linda University, 1996. (Available from University Microfilms International, Ann Arbor, Michigan.)

Prineas RJ, Crow RS, Blackburn H. *The Minnesota Code Manual of Electrocardiographic Findings.* Littleton, MA: John Wright, 1982.

Prineas RJ, Kushi LH, Folsom AR, Bostick RM, Wu Y. Walnuts and serum lipids (Letter). *N Engl J Med* 329:359, 1993.

Probst-Hensch NM, Lin HJ, Witte JS, Longnecker MP, Sinha R, Ingles SA, Frankl HD, Lee ER, Haile RW. Meat preparation, fast acetylator trait, glutathione *S*-transferase (M1) null genotype, and colorectal adenomas. *Cancer Causes Control* 8:175–183, 1997.

Psaty BM, Koepsell TD, Manolio TA, Longstreth WT, Wagner EH, Wahl PW, Krommal RA. Risk ratios and risk differences in estimating the effect of risk factors for cardiovascular disease in the elderly. *J Clin Epidemiol* 43:961–970, 1990.

Purvis JR, Movahed A. Magnesium disorders and cardiovascular diseases. *Clin Cardiol* 15:556–568, 1992.

Puska P, Nissinen A, Vartiainen E, Dougherty R, Mutanen M, Iacono JM, Korhonen HJ, Pietinen P, Leino U, Moisio S, Huttunen J. Controlled randomised trial of the effect of dietary fat on blood pressure. *Lancet* 1:1–5, 1983.

Puska P, Iacono JM, Nissinen A, Vartiainen E, Dougherty R, Pietinen P, Leino U, Uusitalo U, Kuusi T, Kostiainen E, et al. Dietary fat and blood pressure: an intervention study on the effects of a lowfat diet with two levels of polyunsaturated fat. *Prev Med* 14:573–584, 1985.

Ragland DR, Brand RJ. Type A behavior and mortality from coronary heart disease. *N Engl J Med* 318:65–69, 1988.

Rajaram S, Burke K, Connell B, Myint T, Sabaté J. A monounsaturated fatty acid-rich pecan-enriched diet favorably alters the serum lipid profile of healthy men and women. *J Nutr* 131:2275–2279, 2001.

Rauma A-L, Torronen R, Hanninen O, Mykkanen H. Vitamin B-12 status of long-term adherents of a strict uncooked vegan diet ("Living Food Diet") is compromised. *J Nutr* 125:2511–2515, 1995a.

Rauma A-L, Torronen R, Hanninen O, Verhagen H, Mykkanen H. Antioxidant status in long-term adherents to a strict uncooked vegan diet. *Am J Clin Nutr* 62:1221–1227, 1995b.

Reddy BS, Simi B, Engle A. Effects of types of fiber on colonic DAG in women. *Gastroenterology* 105:883–889, 1994.

Reed D, McGee D, Yano K, Feinleib M. Social networks and coronary heart disease among Japanese men in Hawaii. *Am J Epidemiol* 117:384–396, 1983.

Reed DM, Foley DJ, White LR, Heimovitz H, Burchfiel CM, Masaki K. Predictors of healthy aging in men with high life expectancies. *Am J Public Health* 88:1463–1468, 1998.

Resnicoff M, Abraham D, Yutanawiboonchai W, Rotman HL, Kajstura J, Rubin R, Zoltick P, Baserga R. The insulin-like growth factor I receptor protects tumor cells from apoptosis in vivo. *Cancer Res* 55:2463–2469, 1995.

Rexrode KM, Manson JE. Antioxidants and coronary heart disease: observational studies. *J Cardiovasc Risk* 3:363–367, 1996.

Rimm EB, Stampfer MJ, Ascherio A, Giovannucci E, Colditz GA, Willett WC. Vitamin E consumption and the risk of coronary heart disease in men. *N Engl J Med* 328:1450–1456, 1993.

Rimm EB, Stampfer MJ, Giovannucci E, Ascherio A, Spiegelman D, Colditz GA, Willett WC. Body size and fat distribution as predictors of coronary heart disease among middle-aged and older U.S. males. *Am J Epidemiol* 141:1117–1127, 1995.

Rimm EB, Ascherio A, Giovannucci E, Spiegelman D, Stampfer MJ, Willett WC. Vegetable, fruit, and cereal fiber intake and risk of coronary heart disease among men. *JAMA* 275:447–451, 1996a.

Rimm EB, Katan MB, Ascherio A, Stampfer MJ, Willett WC. Relation between intake of flavonoids and risk for coronary heart disease in male health professionals. *Ann Int Med* 125:384–389, 1996b.

Rimm EB, Willett WC, Hu FB, Sampson L, Colditz GA, Manson JE, Hennekens C, Stampfer MJ. Folate and vitamin B_6 from diet and supplements in relation to risk of coronary heart disease among women. *JAMA* 279:359–364, 1998.

Rinzler SH. Primary prevention of coronary heart disease by diet. *Bull N Y Acad Med* 44:936–949, 1968.

Risch HA, Jain M, Marrett LD, Howe G. Dietary fat intake and risk of epithelial ovarian cancer. *J Natl Cancer Inst* 86:1409–1415, 1994.

Rissanen T, Voutilainen S, Nyyssonen K, Lakka TA, Salonen JT. Fish oil-derived fatty acids, docosahexaenoic acid and docosapentaenoic acid, and the risk of acute coronary events. *Circulation* 102:2677–2679, 2000.

Roberts TL, Wood DA, Riemersma RA, Gallagher PJ, Lampe FC. *Trans* isomers of oleic and linoleic acids in adipose tissue and sudden cardiac death. *Lancet* 345:278–282, 1995.

Robinson K, Arheart K, Refsum H, Brattstrom L, Boers G, Ueland P, Rubba P, Palma-Reis R, Meleady R, Daly L, et al. Low circulating folate and vitamin B$_6$ concentrations: risk factors for stroke, peripheral vascular disease, and coronary artery disease. *Circulation* 97:437–443, 1998.

Rodriguez BL, Sharp DS, Abbott RD, Burchfiel CM, Masaki K, Chyou PH, Huang B, Yano K, Curb JD. Fish intake may limit the increase in risk of coronary heart disease morbidity and mortality among heavy smokers: the Honolulu Heart Program. *Circulation* 94:952–956, 1996.

Rogers P, Hassan J, Bresnihan B, Feighery C, Whelan A. Antibodies to Proteus in rheumatoid arthritis. *Br J Rheumatol* 27(Suppl 2):90–94, 1988.

Rohan TE, Howe GR, Friedenreich CM, Jain M, Miller AB. Dietary fiber, vitamins A, C, and E, and risk of breast cancer: a cohort study. *Cancer Causes Control* 4:29–37, 1993.

Rosenman RH, Brand RJ, Jenkins CD, Friedman M, Straus R, Wurm M. Coronary heart disease in the Western Collaborative Group Study. *JAMA* 233:872–877, 1975.

Rosetti RG, Seiler CM, DeLuca P, Laposata M, Zurier RB. Oral administration of unsaturated fatty acids: effects on human peripheral blood T lymphocyte proliferation. *J Leukoc Biol* 62:438–443, 1997.

Roshanai F, Sanders TAB. Assessment of fatty acid intakes in vegans and omnivores. *Hum Nutr Appl Nutr* 38A:345–354, 1984.

Rosner B, Spiegelman D, Willett W. Correction of logistic regression relative risk estimates and confidence intervals for measurement error: the case of multiple covariates measured with error. *Am J Epidemiol* 132:734–745, 1990.

Ross R. The pathogenesis of atherosclerosis: a perspective for the 1990's. *Nature* 362:801–809, 1993.

Rouse IL, Armstrong BK, Beilin LJ. The relationship of blood pressure to diet and lifestyle in two religious populations. *J Hypertens* 1:65–71, 1983a.

Rouse IL, Beilin LJ, Armstrong BK, Vandongen R. Blood-pressure-lowering effect of a vegetarian diet: controlled trial in normotensive subjects. *Lancet* 1:5–10, 1983b.

Rouse IL, Armstrong BK, Beilin LJ, Vandongen R. Vegetarian diet, blood pressure and cardiovascular risk. *Aust N Z J Med* 14:439–443, 1984.

Rowland IR, Granli T, Bockman OC, Key PE, Massey RC. Endogenous N-nitrosation in man assessed by measurement of apparent total N-nitroso compounds in faeces. *Carcinogens* 12:1359–1401, 1991.

Rozen F, Yang XF, Huynh H, Polak M. Antiproliferative action of vitamin D–related compounds and insulin-like growth factor-binding protein 5 accumulation. *J Natl Cancer Inst* 89:652–656, 1997.

Rubenowitz E, Molin I, Axelsson G, Rylander R. Magnesium in drinking water in relation to morbidity and mortality from acute myocardial infarction. *Epidemiology* 11:416–421, 2000.

Ruoslahti E. How cancer spreads. *Sci Am*, Special Issue 275(3):72–77, 1996.

Ruys J, Hickie JB. Serum cholesterol and triglyceride levels in Australian adolescent vegetarians. *Br Med J* 2:87, 1976.

Sabaté J, Fraser GE, Burke K, Knutsen S, Bennett H, Lindsted KD. Effects of walnuts on serum lipid levels and blood pressure in normal men. *N Engl J Med* 328:603–607, 1993.

Sabate J, Haddad E, Tanzman J, Jambazian T, Rajaram S. Serum lipid response to a graded enrichment of a step I diet with almonds: a randomized feeding trial. *Am J Clin Nutrition* (in press).

Sabaté J (ed.). *Vegetarian Nutrition*. Boca Raton, FL: CRC Press, 2001.

Sacks FM, Rosner B, Kass EH. Blood pressure in vegetarians. *Am J Epidemiol* 100:390–398, 1974.

Sacks FM, Castelli WP, Donner A, Kass EH. Plasma lipids and lipoproteins in vegetarians and controls. *N Engl J Med* 292:1148–1151, 1975.

Sacks FM, Donner A, Castelli WP, Gronemeyer J, Pletka P, Margolius HS, Landsberg L, Kass EH. Effect of ingestion of meat on plasma cholesterol in vegetarians. *JAMA* 246:640–644, 1981.

Sacks FM, Marais GE, Handysides G, Salazar J, Miller L, Foster JM, Rosner B, Kass EH. Lack of effect of dietary saturated fat and cholesterol on blood pressure in normotensives. *Hypertension* 6:193–198, 1984a.

Sacks FM, Wood PG, Kass EH. Stability of blood pressure in vegetarians receiving dietary protein supplements. *Hypertension* 6:199–201, 1984b.

Sacks FM, Rouse IL, Stampfer MJ, Biship LM, Lenherr CF, Walther RJ. Effects of dietary fats and carbohydrate on blood pressure of mildly hypertensive patients. *Hypertension* 10:452–460, 1987a.

Sacks FM, Stampfer MJ, Munoz A, McManus K, Canessa M, Kass EH. Effect of linoleic and oleic acids on blood pressure, blood viscosity, and erythrocyte cation transport. *J Am Coll Nutr* 6:179–185, 1987b.

Sahyoun NR, Jacques PF, Russell RM. Carotenoids, vitamins C and E, and mortality in an elderly population. *Am J Epidemiol* 144:501–511, 1996.

Salmeron J, Ascherio A, Rimm EB, Colditz GA, Spiegelman D, Wing AL, Willett WC. Diet and risk of non-insulin-dependent diabetes mellitus in men. (Abstract). Diabetes Care 18:A22, 1995.

Salmeron J, Manson JE, Stampfer MJ, Colditz GA, Wing AL, Willett WC. Dietary fiber, glycemic load, and risk of non-insulin-dependent diabetes mellitus in women. *JAMA* 277:472–477, 1997.

Salovey P, Rothman AJ, Detweiler JB, Steward WT. Emotional states and physical health. *Am Psychologist* 55:110–121, 2000.

Sanders TAB, Ellis FR, Dickerson JWT. Studies of vegans: the fatty acid composition of plasma choline phosphoglycerides, erythrocytes, adipose tissue, and breast milk, and some indicators of susceptibility to ischemic heart disease in vegan and omnivore controls. *Am J Clin Nutr* 31:805–813, 1978.

Sanders TAB, Key TJ. Blood pressure, plasma renin activity and aldosterone concentrations in vegans and omnivore controls. *Hum Nutr Appl Nutr* 41A:204–211, 1987.

Sandler RS, Baron JA, Tosteson TD, Mandel JS, Haile RW. Rectal mucosal proliferation and risk of colorectal adenomas: results from a randomized controlled trial. *Cancer Epidemiol Biomarkers Prev* 9:653–656, 2000.

Sandvik L, Erikksen J, Thaulow E, Erikksen G, Mundal R, Rodahl K. Physical fitness as a predictor of mortality among healthy, middle-aged Norwegian men. *N Engl J Med* 328:533–537, 1993.

Schaefer EJ, Audelin MC, McNamara JR, Shah PK, Tayler T, Daly JA, Augustin JL, Seman LJ, Rubenstein JJ. Comparison of fasting and postprandial plasma lipoproteins, in subjects with and without coronary heart disease. *Am J Cardiol* 88:1129–1133, 2001.

Scheier MF, Carver CS. Effects of optimism on psychological and physical well-being: theoretical overview and empirical update. *Cogn Ther Res* 16(2):201–228, 1992.

Schmieder RE, Schobel HP. Is endothelial dysfunction reversible? *Am J Cardiol* 76:117A–121A, 1995.

Schottenfeld D, Fraumeni JF. Part 3: The causes of cancer. *Cancer Epidemiology and Prevention*. New York: Oxford University Press, 1996.

Schuck L, Bucy J. Family rituals: implications for early intervention. *Top Early Child Special Educ* 17(4):477–493, 1998.

Schuman LM, Mandel JS, Radke A, Seal U, Halberg F. Some selected features of the epidemiology of prostatic cancer: Minneapolis–St. Paul, Minnesota case-control study, 1976–1979. In: K. Magnus (ed.), *Trends in Cancer Incidence: Causes and Implications*. Washington, DC: Hemisphere Publishing, 1982, pp. 345–354.

Schuurman AG, Goldbohm RA, Dorant E, van den Brandt PA. Vegetable and fruit consumption and prostate cancer risk: a cohort study in the Netherlands. *Cancer Epidemiol Biomarkers Prev* 7:673–680, 1998.

Schuurman AG, van den Brandt PA, Dorant E, Brants HAM, Goldbohm RA. Association of energy and fat intake with prostate carcinoma risk. *Cancer* 86:1019–1027, 1999.

Schwartz GG, Wang MH, Zang M, Singh RK, Siegal GP. 1-α-25 dihydroxy vitamin D (calcitriol) inhibits the invasiveness of human prostate cancer cells. *Cancer Epidemiol Biomarkers Prev* 6:727–732, 1997.

Schwarz RW. *John Harvey Kellogg: Father of the Health Food Industry*. Berrien Springs, MI: Andrews University Press, 1970.

Schwarzer R, Renner B. Social-cognitive predictors of health behavior: action self-efficacy and coping self-efficacy. *Health Psychol* 19:487–495, 2000.

Sciarrone SE, Strahan MT, Beilin LJ, Burke V, Rogers P, Rouse JL. Biochemical and neurohormonal responses to the introduction of a lacto-ovo-vegetarian diet. *J Hypertens* 11:849–860, 1993.

Scott LW, Dunn JK, Pownall HJ, Brauchi DJ, McMann MC, Herd JA, Harris KB, Savell JW, Cross HR, Gotto AM. Effects of beef and chicken consumption on plasma lipid levels in hypercholesterolemic men. *Arch Int Med* 154:1261–1267, 1994.

Seidell JC. Dietary fat and obesity: an epidemiologic perspective. *Am J Clin Nutr* 67(Suppl.):545S–550S, 1998.

Sellers TA, Bazyk AE, Bostick RM, Kushi LH, Olson JE, Anderson KE, Lazovich D, Folsom AR. Diet and risk of colon cancer in a large prospective study of older women: an analysis stratified on family history (Iowa, United States). *Cancer Causes Control* 9:357–367, 1998.

Sesso HD, Paffenbarger RS, Lee I-M. Physical activity and breast cancer risk in the College Alumni Health Study (United States). *Cancer Causes Control* 9:433–439, 1998.

Severson RK, Nomura AMY, Grove JS, Stemmermann GN. A prospective study of demographics, diet, and prostate cancer among men of Japanese ancestry in Hawaii. *Cancer Res* 49:1857–1860, 1989.

Shapiro JA, Koepsell TD, Voigt LF, Dugowson CE, Kestin M, Nelson JL. Diet and rheumatoid arthritis in women: a possible protective effect of fish consumption. *Epidemiology* 7:256–263, 1996.

Shekelle RB, Shryock AM, Paul O, Lepper M, Stamler J, Liu S, Rayner WJ. Diet, serum cholesterol and death from coronary heart disease: the Western Electric Study. *N Engl J Med* 304:65–70, 1981.

Shekelle RB, Gale M, Ostfeld AM, Paul O. Hostility, risk of coronary heart disease, and mortality. *Psychosom Med* 45:109–114, 1983.

Shekelle RB, Hulley SB, Neaton JD, Billings JH, Borhani NO, Gerace TA, Jacobs DR, Lasser NL, Mittlemark MB, Stamler J. The MRFIT behavior pattern study: II. Type A behavior and incidence of coronary heart disease. *Am J Epidemiol* 122:559–570, 1985.

Shepherd J, Packard CJ, Patsch JF, Gotto AM, Taunton OD. Effects of dietary polyunsaturated and saturated fat on the properties of high density lipoproteins and the metabolism of apolipoprotein A-1. *J Clin Invest* 61:1582–1592, 1978.

Shepherd JT, Weiss SM. *Conference on Behavioral Medicine and Cardiovascular Disease.* Circulation Monograph, No. 6. Dallas: American Heart Association, 1987.

Shi X, Summers RW, Schedl HP, Flanagan SW, Chang R, Gisolfi GV. Effects of carbohydrate type and concentration and solution osmolality on water absorption. *Med Sci Sports Exerc* 27:1607–1615, 1995.

Shibata A, Paganini-Hill A, Ross RK Henderson BE. Intake of vegetables, fruits, beta-carotene, vitamin C and vitamin supplements and cancer incidence among the elderly: a prospective study. *Br J Cancer* 66:673–679, 1992.

Shimomura Y, Tamura T, Suzuki M. Less body fat accumulation in rats fed safflower oil diet than in rats fed a beef tallow diet. *J Nutr* 120:1291–1296, 1990.

Shu XO, Jin F, Dai Q, Wen W, Potter JD, Kushi LH, Ruan Z, Gao Y-T, Zheng W. Soy food intake during adolescence and subsequent risk of breast cancer among Chinese women. *Cancer Epidemiol Biomarkers Prev* 10:483–8, 2001.

Shultz TD, Leklem JE. Nutrient intake and hormonal status of premenopausal vegetarian Seventh-day Adventists and premenopausal vegetarians. *Nutr Cancer* 4:247–259, 1983.

Shurtleff W. Dr. Harry Miller: taking soy foods around the world. *Soy Foods* 1(4):28–36, 1981.

Signorello LB, Tzonou A, Mantzaros CS, Lipworth L, Lagion P, Hsieh C-C, Stampfer M, Trichopoulos D. Serum steroids in relation to prostate cancer risk in a case-control study (Greece). *Cancer Causes Control* 8:632–636, 1997.

Siiteri PK. Adipose tissue as a source of hormones. *Am J Clin Nutr* 45:277–282, 1987.

Silverman DT, Hartge P, Morrison AS, Devesa SS. Epidemiology of bladder cancer. *Hematol Oncol Clin North Am* 6:1–30, 1992.

Simons LA, Gibson JC, Paino C, Hosking M, Bullock J, Trim J. The influence of a wide range of absorbed cholesterol on plasma cholesterol levels in man. *Am J Clin Nutr* 31:1334–1339, 1978.

Singh PN, Fraser GE. Dietary risk factors for colon cancer in a low risk population. *Am J Epidemiol* 148:761–774, 1998.

Singh PN. Body weight and mortality among adults who never smoked. Ph.D. diss., Loma Linda University, 1999.

Sirtori CR, Tremoli E, Gatti E, Montanari G, Sirtori M, Colli S, Gianfranceschi G, Maderna P, Dentone CZ, Testolin G, Galli C. Controlled evaluation of fat intake in the Mediterranean diet: comparative activities of olive oil and corn oil on plasma lipids and platelets in high-risk patients. *Am J Clin Nutr* 44:635–642, 1986.

Slattery ML, Edwardo SL, Ma KN, Friedman GD, Potter JD. Physical activity and colon cancer: a public health perspective. *Ann Epidemiol* 7:137–145, 1997.

Slattery ML, Potter JD, Samovitz W, Schaffer D, Leppert M. Methylene *tetra* hydrofolate reductase, diet and risk of cancer. *Cancer Epidemiol Biomarkers Prev* 8:513–518, 1999.

Slavin J, Jacobs DR, Marquart L. Whole grain consumption and chronic disease: protective mechanisms. *Nutr Cancer* 27:14–21, 1997.

Sloan RP, Bagiella E, Powell T. Religion, spirituality, and medicine. *Lancet* 353:664–667, 1999.

Snowdon DA, Phillips RL, Fraser GE. Meat consumption and fatal ischemic heart disease. *Prev Med* 13:490–500, 1984.

Snowdon DA, Phillips RL. Does a vegetarian diet reduce the occurrence of diabetes? *Am J Public Health* 75:507–512, 1985.

Sowers MF, Sigler C. Complex relation between increasing fat mass and decreasing high density lipoprotein cholesterol levels: evidence from a population-based study of premenopausal women. *Am J Epidemiol* 149:47–54, 1999.

Spady DK, Kearney DM, Hobbs HH. Polyunsaturated fatty acids up-regulate hepatic scavenger receptor B1 (SR-BI) expression in the hamster. *J Lipid Res* 40:1384–1394, 1999.

Spiller GA, Gates JE, Jenkins DAJ, Bosello O, Nichols SF, Cragen L. Effect of two foods high in monounsaturated fat on plasma cholesterol and lipoproteins in adult humans (Abstract). *Am J Clin Nutr* 51:524, 1990.

Spiller GA, Jenkins DJA, Cragen LN, Gates JE, Bosello O, Berra K, Rudd C, Stevenson M, Superko R. Effects of a diet high in monounsaturated fat from almonds on plasma cholesterol and lipoproteins. *J Am Coll Nutr* 11:126–130, 1992.

Spiller GA, Jenkins DAJ, Bosello O, Gates JE, Cragen LN, Bruce B. Nuts and plasma lipids: an almond-based diet lowers LDL-C while preserving HDL-C. *J Am Coll Nutr* 17:285–290, 1998.

Spitz MR, Duphorne CM, Detry MA, Pillow PC, Amos CI, Lei L, de Andrade M, Gu X, Hong WK, Wu X. Dietary intake of isothiocyanates: evidence of a joint effect with glutathione *S*-transferase polymorphisms in lung cancer risk. *Cancer Epidemiol Biomarkers Prev.* 9:1017–1020, 2000.

Stamler J. Epidemiologic findings on body mass and blood pressure in adults. *Ann Epidemiol* 1:347–362, 1991.

Stamler J, Caggiula A, Grandits GA, Kjelsberg M, Cutler JA. Relationship of blood pressure to combinations of dietary macronutrients: findings of the Multiple Risk Factor Intervention Trial (MRFIT). *Circulation* 94:2417–2423, 1996.

Stamler J. The INTERSALT study: background, methods, findings and implications. *Am J Clin Nutr* 65(Suppl.):626S–642S, 1997.

Stamler J, Stamler R, Neaton JD, Wentworth D, Daviglus ML, Garside D, Dyer AR, Liu K, Greenland P. Low risk-factor profile and long-term cardiovascular and non cardiovascular mortality and life expectancy: findings for five large cohorts of young adult and middle-aged men and women. *JAMA* 282:2012–2018, 1999.

Stampfer MJ, Malinow MR, Willett WC, Newcomer LM, Upson B, Ullmann D,

Tishler PV, Hennekens CH. A prospective study of plasma homocyst(e)ine and risk of myocardial infarction in U.S. physicians. *JAMA* 268:877–881, 1992.

Stampfer MJ, Hennekens CH, Manson JE, Colditz GA, Rosner B, Willett WC. Vitamin E consumption and the risk of coronary disease in women. *N Engl J Med* 328:1444–1449, 1993.

Stampfer MJ, Hu FB, Manson JE, Rimm EB, Willett WC. Primary prevention of coronary heart disease in women through diet and lifestyle. *N Engl J Med* 343:16–22, 2000.

Stasse-Wolthuis M, Albers HFF, van Jeveren JGC, de Jong JW, Hautvast JGAJ, Hermus RJJ, Katan MB, Brydon WG, Eastwood MA. Influence of dietary fiber from vegetables and fruits, bran or citrus pectin on serum lipids, fecal lipids, and colonic function. *Am J Clin Nutr* 33:1745–1756, 1980.

Stein JH, Keevil JG, Wiebe DA, Aeschlimann S, Folts JD. Purple grape juice improves endothelial function and reduces the susceptiblility of LDL cholesterol to oxidation in patients with coronary artery disease. *Circulation* 100:1050–1055, 1999.

Steineck G, Norell SE, Feychting M. Diet, tobacco and urothelial cancer. *Acta Oncol* 27:323–327, 1988.

Steinmetz KA, Kushi LH, Bostick RM, Folsom AR, Potter JD. Vegetables, fruit and colon cancer in the Iowa Women's Health Study. *Am J Epidemiol* 139:1–15, 1994.

Stephens NG, Parsons A, Schofield PM, Kelly F, Cheeseman K, Mitchinson MJ, Brown MJ. Randomized controlled trial of vitamin E in patients with coronary disease: Cambridge Heart Antioxidant Study (CHAOS). *Lancet* 347:781–786, 1996.

Stevens J, Keil JE, Rust PF, Tyroler HA, Davis CE, Gazes PC. Body mass index and body girths as predictors of mortality in black and white women. *Arch Int Med* 152:1257–1262, 1992.

Stevens J, Cai J, Pamuk ER, Williamson DF, Thun MJ, Wood JL. The effect of age on the association between body mass index and mortality. *N Engl J Med* 338:1–7, 1998.

Stone NJ. Diet, lipids, and coronary heart disease. *Endocrinol Metab Clin North Am* 19:321–344, 1990.

Strawbridge WJ, Cohen RD, Shema SJ., Kaplan GA. Frequent attendance at religious services and mortality over 28 years. *Am J Public Health* 87(6):957–961, 1997.

Strawbridge WJ, Shema SJ, Cohen RD, Roberts RE, Kaplan GA. Religiosity buffers effects of some stressors on depression but exacerbates others. *J Gerontol B Psychol Sci Soc Sci* 53(3):S118–S126, 1998.

Sturmer T, Sun Y, Sauerland S, Zeissig I, Gunther K-P, Puhl W, Brenner H. Serum cholesterol and arthritis. the baseline examination of the Ulm Osteoarthritis Study. *J Rheumatol* 25:1827–1832, 1998.

Suomi SJ. Early determinants of behavior: evidence from primate studies. *Br Med Bull* 53:170–184, 1997.

Surveillance, Epidemiology and End Results (SEER). CD ROM. Bethesda, MD: U.S. Department of Health and Human Services, National Cancer Institute, 1998.

Suzman RM, Willis DP, Manton KG. *The Oldest Old*. Oxford University Press, New York, 1992.

Sweet M. Eating meat more than 10 times a week almost doubles chances of bowel cancer (News Extra). *Br Med J* 324:1544, 2002

Targ, E. Evaluating distant healing: a research review. *Alternat Ther Health Med* 3(6):74–78, 1997.

Tavani A, LaVecchia C, Gallus S, Lagiou P, Trichopoulos D, Levi F, Negri E. Red meat intake and cancer risk: a study in Italy. *Int J Cancer* 86:425–428, 2000.

Taylor SE, Kemeny ME, Reed GM, Bower JE, Gruenewald TL. Psychological resources, positive illusions, and health. *Am Psychol* 55(1):99–109, 2000.

Thefeld W, Rottka H, Melchert H-U. Verhaltensweisen und Gesundheitszustand von Vegetariern. *Akt Ernähr* 11:127–135, 1986.

Thomas D, Stram D, Dwyer J. Exposure measurement error: influence on exposure–disease relationships and methods of correction. *Annu Rev Public Health* 14:69–93, 1993.

Thomas HV, Reeves GK, Key TJ. Endogenous estrogen and postmenopausal breast cancer: a quantitative review. *Cancer Causes Control* 8:922–928, 1997.

Thomas HV, Davey GK, Key TJ. Oestradiol and sex hormone-binding globulin in premenopausal and post-menopausal meat-eaters, vegetarians, and vegans. *Br J Cancer* 80:1470–1475, 1999.

Thomas PD, Goodwin JM, Goodwin JS. Effect of social support on stress-related changes in cholesterol level, uric acid level, and immune function in an elderly sample. *Am J Psychiatry* 142:735–737, 1985.

Thompson LU, Robb P, Serraino M, Cheung F. Mammalian lignan production from various foods. *Nutr Cancer* 16:43–52, 1991.

Thomsen KK, Larsen S, Schroll M. Do CHD risk factors still count in the aged? A follow-up survey of the 1914 population in Glostrup. *Am J Geriatr Cardiol* 4:20–35, 1995.

Thorogood M, Carter R, Benfield L, McPherson K, Mann JI. Plasma lipids and lipoprotein cholesterol concentrations in people with different diets in Britain. *Br Med J* 295:351–353, 1987.

Thorogood M, Mann J, Appleby P, McPherson K. Risk of death from cancer and ischemic heart disease in meat and non-meat eaters. *Br Med J* 308:1667–1670, 1994.

Thorogood M. The epidemiology of vegetarianism and health. *Nutr Res Rev* 8:179–92, 1995.

Thune I, Brenn T, Lund E, Gaard M. Physical activity and risk of breast cancer. *N Engl J Med* 336:1269–75, 1997.

Tiemersma EW, Kampman E, Bas Bueno de Mesquita H, Bunschoten A, Van Schothorst EM, Kok FJ, Kromhout D. Meat consumption, cigarette smoking, and genetic susceptibility in the etiology of colorectal cancer: results from a Dutch prospective study. *Cancer Causes Control* 13:383–393, 2002.

Tomlinson, G. *Treasury of Religious Quotations*. Englewood Cliffs, NJ: Prentice Hall, 1991.

Tomaino RM, Decker EA. High-fat meals and endothelial function. *Nutrition Rev* 56:182–185, 1998.

Toniolo P, Riboli E, Shore RE, Pasternack BS. Consumption of meat, animal products, protein, and fat and risk of breast cancer: a prospective cohort study in New York. *Epidemiology* 5:391–397, 1994.

Toniolo P, Van Kappel AL, Akhmedkanov A, Ferrari P, Kato I, Shore RE, Riboli

E. Serum carotenoids and breast cancer. *Am J Epidemiol* 153:1142–1147, 2001.

Toohey ML, Harris MA, Williams DeW, Foster G, Schmidt WD, Melby CL. Cardiovascular disease risk factors are lower in African-American vegans compared to lacto-ovo-vegetarians. *J Am Coll Nutr* 17:425–434, 1998.

Toretsky A, Helman LJ. Involvement of IGF-II in human cancer. *J Endocrinol* 149:367–372, 1996.

Triandis HC. Self and social behavior in differing social contexts. *Psychol Rev* 96:269–289, 1989.

Trichopoulos D, Li FP, Hunter DJ. What causes cancer? *Sci Am*, Special Issue 275(3):80–87, 1996.

Trichopoulou A, Kouris-Blazos A, Wahlqvist ML, Gnardellis C, Lagiou P, Polychronopoulos E, Vassilakou T, Lipworth L, Trichopoulos D. Diet and overall survival in elderly people. *Br Med J* 311:1457–1460, 1995.

Trichopoulou A, Vasilopoulou E, Lagiou A. Mediterranean diet and coronary heart disease: are antioxidants critical? *Nutr Rev* 57:253–255, 1999.

Trieber FA, Batanowski T, Broden DS, Strong WB, Levy M, Knox W. Social support for exercise: relationship to physical activity in young adults. *Prev Med* 20:737–750, 1991

Troyer H. Review of cancer among four religious sects: evidence that life-styles are distinctive sets of risk factors. *Soc Sci Med* 26(10):1007–1017, 1988.

Tsai SP, Hardy RJ, Wen CP. The standardized mortality ratio and life expectancy. *Am J Epidemiol* 135:824–831, 1992.

Tsevat J, Weinstein MC, Williams LW, Tosteson ANA, Goldman L. Expected gains in life expectancy from various coronary heart disease risk factor modifications. *Circulation* 83:1194–1201, 1991.

Turpeinen O, Karvonen MJ, Pekkarinen M, Miettinen M, Elosuo R, Paavilainen E. Dietary prevention of coronary heart disease: the Finnish Mental Hospital Study. *Int J Epidemiol* 8:99–118, 1979.

Tzonou A, Hsieh C-C, Polychronopoulou A, Kaprinis G, Toupadaki N, Trichopoulou A, Karakatsoni A, Trichopoulos D. Diet and ovarian cancer: a case-control study in Greece. *Int J Cancer* 55:411–414, 1993.

Uchino BN, Cacioppo JT, Kiecolt-Glaser JK. The relationship between social support and physiological processes: a review with emphasis on underlying mechanisms and implications for health. *Psychol Bull* 119(3):488–531, 1996.

Uchino BN, Uno D, Holt-Lunstad J. Social support, physiological processes, and health. *Curr Dir Psychol Sci* 8(5):145–148, 1999.

Ursini F, Tubaro F, Rong J, Sevanian A. Optimization of nutrition: Polyphenols and vascular protection. *Nutrition Reviews* 57:241–249, 1999.

U.S. Department of Agriculture, Agricultural Research Service. *USDA Nutrient Database for Standard Reference, Release 15*. Nutrient Data Laboratory Home Page; available at http://www.nal.usda.gov/fnic/foodcomp, accessed 1-13-2003.

U.S. Department of Health and Human Services. *Report of the Secretary's Task Force on Black and Minority Health*, Vol. 1. Washington, DC: U.S. Department of Health and Human Services, 1985.

Van Dam RM, Willett WC, Rimm EB, Stampfer MJ, Hu FB. Dietary fat and meat intake in relation to risk of type 2 diabetes in men. *Diabetes Care* 25:417–424, 2002.

van den Brandt PA, Van't Veer P, Goldbohm RA, Dorant E, Volovics A, Hermus RJ, Sturmans F. A prospective cohort study on dietary fat and the risk of postmenopausal breast cancer. *Cancer Res* 53:75–82, 1993.

Vanharanta M, Voutilainen S, Lakka TA, van der Lee M, Adlercreutz H, Salonen J. Risk of acute coronary events according to serum concentrations of enterolactone: a prospective population-based case-control study. *Lancet* 354:2112–2115, 1999.

Van Horn L. Fiber, lipids, and coronary heart disease. *Circulation* 95:2701–2704, 1997.

Van Weel C, Michels J. Dying, not old age, to blame for costs of health care. *Lancet* 350:1159–1160, 1997.

Vardan S, Mookherjee S, Vardan S, Sinha AK. Special features of coronary heart disease in people of the Indian sub-continent. *Indian Heart J* 47:399–407, 1995.

Vaupel JW. How change in age-specific mortality affects life expectancy. *Popul Stud* 40:147–157, 1986.

Vaux K. Religion and health. *Prev Med* 5:522–536, 1976.

Veierod MB, Laake P, Thelle DS. Dietary fat intake and risk of prostate cancer: a prospective study of energy and fat intake with prostate carcinoma risk. *Int J Cancer* 73:634–638, 1997.

Verhoeven DT, Goldbohm RA, van Poppel G, Verhagen H, van den Brandt PA. Epidemiologic studies on brassica vegetables and cancer risk. *Cancer Epidemiol Biomarkers Prev* 5:733–748, 1996.

Virtamo J, Rapola JM, Ripatti S, Heinonen OP, Taylor PR, Albanes D, Huttunen JK. Effect of vitamin E and beta-carotene on the incidence of primary nonfatal myocardial infarction and fatal coronary heart disease. *Arch Int Med* 158:668–675, 1998.

Vita AJ, Terry RB, Hubert HB, Fries JF. Aging, health risks, and cumulative disability. *N Engl J Med* 338:1035–1041, 1998.

Vollset, Heuch I, Bjelke E. Fish consumption and mortality from coronary heart disease. *N Engl J Med* 313:820–821, 1985.

Voorrips LE, Goldbohm RA, Brants HA, van Poppel GA, Sturmans F, Hermus RJ, van den Brandt PA. A prospective cohort study on antioxidant and folate intake and male lung cancer risk. *Cancer Epidemiol Biomarkers Prev* 9:357–365, 2000.

Voutilainen S, Lakka TA, Porkkala-Sarataho E, Rissanen T. Low serum folate concentrations are associated with an excess incidence of acute coronary events. *Eur J Clin Nutr* 54:424–428, 2000.

Voutilainen S, Rissanen TH, Virtanen J, Lakka TA, Salonen JT. Low dietary folate intake is associated with an excess incidence of acute coronary events. *Circulation* 103:2674–2680, 2001.

Waaler H, Hjort PF. Hoyere leavealder hos norske adventister 1960–1977: et budskap om livsstil og helse? *Tidsskr Nor Laegeforen* 101:623–627, 1981. (Translated to English: Low mortality among Norwegian Seventh-day Adventists 1960–1977: A message on lifestyle and health?)

Walker SR, Tonigan S, Miller WR, Corner S, Kahlich L. Intercessory prayer in the treatment of alcohol abuse and dependence: a pilot investigation. *Alternat Ther Health Med* 3(6):79–86, 1997.

Wallace Jr, JM, Forman TA. Religion's role in promoting health and reducing risk among American youth. *Health Educ Behav* 25(6):721–742, 1998.

Wang H, Griffiths S, Williamson G. Effect of glucosinolate breakdown products on B-naphthoflavone-induced expression of human cytochrome $P_{450}1A1$ via the Ah receptor in HepG2 cells. *Cancer Lett* 114:121–125, 1997.

Watson PJ, Morris RJ, Hood RW. Sin and self-functioning: II. Grace, guilt, and psychological adjustment. *J Psychol Theol* 16(3):270–281, 1988.

Watson S, Shively CA, Kaplan JR, Line SW. Effects of chronic social separation on cardiovascular risk factors in female cynomolgus monkeys. *Atherosclerosis* 137:259–266, 1998.

Weaver AJ, Flannelly LT, Flannelly KJ, Koenig HG, Larson DB. An analysis of research on religious and spiritual variables in three major mental health nursing journals, 1991–1995. *Issues Ment Health Nurs* 19(3):263–276, 1998.

Weaver AJ, Samford JA, Morgan VJ, Lichton AI, Larson DB, Garbarino J. Research on religious variables in five major adolescent research journals: 1992 to 1996. *J Nerv Ment Dis* 188(1):36–44, 2000.

Weaver CM, Plawecki KL. Dietary calcium: adequacy of a vegetarian diet. *Am J Clin Nutr* 59(Suppl.):1238S–1241S, 1994.

Weaver CM, Proulx WR, Heaney R. Choices for achieving adequate dietary calcium with a vegetarian diet. *Am J Clin Nutr* 70(Suppl.):543S–548S, 1999

Wei H, Bowen R, Cai Q, Barnes S, Wang Y. Antioxidant and antipromotional effects of the soybean isoflavone genistein. *Proc Soc Exp Biol Med* 208:124–130, 1995.

Weinberg RA. How cancer arises. *Sci Am*, Special Issue 275(3):62–70, 1996.

West RO, Hayes OB. Diet and serum cholesterol levels: a comparison between vegetarians and non-vegetarians in a Seventh-day Adventist group. *Am J Clin Nutr* 21:853–862, 1968.

Westlake CA, St. Leger AS, Burr ML. Appendicectomy and dietary fibre. *J Hum Nutr* 34:267–272, 1980.

Whelton PK, Jiang H, Cutler JA, Brancati FL, Appel LJ, Follman D, Klag MJ. Effects of oral potassium on blood pressure: meta-analysis of randomized controlled clinical trials. *JAMA* 277:1624–1632, 1997.

White E, Kushi LH, Pepe MS. The effect of exposure variance and exposure measurement error on study sample size: implications for the design of epidemiologic studies. *J Clin Epidemiol* 47:873–880, 1994.

White EG. *The Story of Patriarchs and Prophets*. Pacific Press Publishing Association, Mountain View, CA. 1890, p. 600. Reprinted 1958.

White EG. A cause of mortality. Letter 72, 1896. Reprinted in E. G. White, *Medical Ministry*. Mountain View, CA: Pacific Press, 1963, p. 278.

White EG. *The Ministry of Healing*. Pacific Press Publishing Assoc., Mountain View, CA, 1905. Reprinted 1942.

White EG. *Counsels on Diet and Foods*. Washington DC: Review and Herald, 1938, p. 81.

White EG. Flesh meats and stimulants. (Testimony 15, 1868). Reprinted in E. G. White, *Testimonies for the Church*. Mountain View, CA: Pacific Press, 1948, vol. 2, p. 63.

White EG. *Counsels on Health*. Mountain View, CA: Pacific Press, 1951.

Whittemore AS, Kolonel LN, Wu AH, John EM, Gallagher RP, Howe GR, Burch JD, Hankin J, Dreon DM, West DW, et al. Prostate cancer in relation to diet, physical activity, and body size in blacks, whites, and Asians in the United States and Canada. *J Natl Cancer Inst* 87:652–661, 1995.

Whorton JC. Historical development of vegetarianism. *Am J Clin Nutr* 59(Suppl.):1103S–1109S, 1994.

Willett WC, Stampfer MJ, Colditz GA, Rosner BA, Speizer FE. Relation of meat, fat, and fiber intake to the risk of colon cancer in a prospective study among women. *N Engl J Med* 323:1664–1672, 1990.

Willett WC, Hunter DJ, Stampfer MJ, Colditz G, Manson JE, Spiegelman D, Rosner B, Hennekens CH, Speizer FE. Dietary fat and fiber in relation to risk of breast cancer: an eight year follow-up. *JAMA* 268:2037–2044, 1992.

Willett WC, Stampfer MJ, Manson JE, Colditz GA, Speizer FA, Rosner BA, Sampson LA, Hennekens CH. Intake of *trans* fatty acids and risk of coronary heart disease among women. *Lancet* 341:581–585, 1993.

Willett WC. *Nutritional Epidemiology*. Oxford University Press, New York, 1998a. chapter 12; pp. 288–291.

Willett WC. Is dietary fat a major determinant of body fat? *Am J Clin Nutr* 67(Suppl.):556S–562S, 1998b.

Williams JK, Vita JA, Manuck SB, Selwyn AP, Kaplan JR. Psychosocial factors impair vascular responses of coronary arteries. *Circulation* 84:2146–2153, 1991.

Williams PT. Interactive effects of exercise, alcohol, and vegetarian diet on coronary artery disease risk factors in 9242 runners: the National Runners' Health Study. *Am J Clin Nutr* 66:1197–1206, 1997.

Williams RB. Refining the type A hypothesis: emergence of the hostility complex. *Am J Cardiol* 60(Suppl.):27J–32J, 1987a.

Williams RB. Psychological factors in coronary artery disease: epidemiologic evidence. *Circulation* 76(Suppl. 1):117–123, 1987b

Williams RB, Barefoot JC, Haney TL, Harrell FE, Blumenthal JA, Pryor DB, Peterson B. Type A behavior and angiographically documented coronary atherosclerosis in a sample of 2289 patients. *Psychosom Med* 50:136–152, 1988.

Wing RR. Physical activity in the treatment of the adult overweight and obesity: current evidence and research issues: *Med Sci Sports Exerc* 31(Suppl.):S547–S552, 1999.

Witt S. Parental influence on children's socialization to gender roles. *Adolescence* 32(126):253–259, 1997.

Witztum JL. The oxidation hypothesis of atherosclerosis. *Lancet* 344:793–795, 1994.

Wolk A, Manson JE, Stampfer MJ, Colditz GA, Hu FB, Speizer FE, Hennekens CH, Willett WC. Long-term intake of dietary fiber and decreased risk of coronary heart disease. *JAMA* 281:1998–2004, 1999.

Wolk A, Gridley G, Svensson M, Nyren O, McLaughlin JK, Fraumeni JF, Adami H-O. A prospective study of obesity and cancer risk (Sweden). *Cancer Causes Control* 12:13–21, 2001.

Woods TE, Antoni MH, Ironson GH, Kling DW. Religiosity is associated with affective and immune status in symptomatic HIV-infected gay men. *J Psychosom Res* 46(2):165–176, 1999.

Wu AH, Ziegler RG, Horn-Ross PL, Nomura AMY, West DW, Kolonel LN, Rosenthal JF, Hoover RN, Pike MC. Tofu and risk of breast cancer in Asian-Americans. *Cancer Epidemiol Biomarkers Prev* 5:901–906, 1996.

Wu AH, Pike MC, Stram DO. Meta-analysis: dietary fat intake, serum estrogen levels, and risk of breast cancer. *J Natl Cancer Inst* 91:529–534, 1999.

Wu AH, Stanczyk FZ, Hendrich S, Murphy PA, Zhang C, Wan P, Pike MC. Effects of soy foods on ovarian function in premenopausal women. *Br J Cancer* 82:1879–1886, 2000.

Wulsin LR, Vaillant GE, Wells VE. A systematic review of the mortality of depression. *Psychosom Med* 61(1):6–17, 1999.

Yang SK, Silverman BD. *Polycyclic Aromatic Hydrocarbon Carcinogenesis: Structure-Activity Relationships*. Vol. 1. Boca Raton, FL: CRC Press, 1998.

Yavelow J, Finlay TH, Kennedy AR, Troll W. Bowman–Birk soybean protease inhibitor as an anticarcinogen. *Cancer Res* 43(Suppl.):2454S–2459S, 1983.

Young VR, Pellett PL. Plant proteins in relation to human protein and amino acid nutrition. *Am J Clin Nutr* 59(Suppl.):1203S–1212S, 1994.

Zambon D, Sabaté J, Munoz S, Campero B, Casals E, Mérlos M, Laguna JC, Ros É. Substituting walnuts for monounsaturated fat improves the lipid profile of hypercholesterolemic men and women. *Ann Int Med* 132:538–546, 2000.

Zhang SM, Hunter DJ, Rosner BA, Giovannucci EL, Colditz GA, Speizer FE, Willett WC. Intake of fruits, vegetables, and related nutrients and the risk of non-Hodgkins lymphoma among women. *Cancer Epidemiol Biomarkers Prev* 9:477–485, 2000.

Zhao B, Seow A, Lee EJD, Poh W-T, Teh M, Eng P, Wang Y-T, Tan W-C, Yu MC, Lee H-P. Dietary isothiocyanates glutathione *S*-transferase: M1-T1 polymorphisms and lung cancer risk among chinese women in Singapore. *Cancer Epidemiol Biomarkers Prev.* 10:1063–1067, 2001.

Zheng W, McLaughlin JK, Gridley G, Bjelke E, Schuman LM, Silverman DT, Wacholder S, Co-Chien HT, Blot WJ, Fraumeni JF. A cohort study of smoking, alcohol and dietary factors for pancreatic cancer (United States). *Cancer Causes Control* 4:477–482, 1993.

Zheng W, Xie D, Corhan JR, Sellers TA, Wen W, Folsom AR. Sulfotransferase 1A1 polymorphism, endogenous estrogen exposure, well-done meat intake, and breast cancer risk. *Cancer Epidemiol Biomarkers Prev* 10:89–94, 2001.

Zurier RB, Rossetti RG, Jacobson EW, DeMarco DM, Liu NY, Temming JE, White BM, LaPosata M. Gamma-linolenic acid treatment of rheumatoid arthritis. *Arth Rheum* 39:1808–1817, 1996.

Index

Page references followed by *f* or *t* indicate figures or tables, respectively.